THE NETTER COLLECTION OF MEDICAL ILLUSTRATIONS

VOLUME 3

A Compilation of Paintings on the
Normal and Pathologic Anatomy of the

DIGESTIVE SYSTEM

PART I

UPPER DIGESTIVE TRACT

Prepared by

FRANK H. NETTER, M.D.

Edited by

ERNST OPPENHEIMER, M.D.

Commissioned and published by

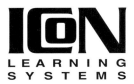

LEARNING
SYSTEMS

OTHER PUBLISHED VOLUMES OF
THE NETTER COLLECTION OF MEDICAL ILLUSTRATIONS
(Formerly THE CIBA COLLECTION OF MEDICAL ILLUSTRATIONS)
By
FRANK H. NETTER, M.D.

NERVOUS SYSTEM, PART I:
ANATOMY AND PHYSIOLOGY

NERVOUS SYSTEM, PART II:
NEUROLOGIC AND NEUROMUSCULAR DISORDERS

REPRODUCTIVE SYSTEM

DIGESTIVE SYSTEM, PART II:
LOWER DIGESTIVE TRACT

DIGESTIVE SYSTEM, PART III:
LIVER, BILIARY TRACT AND PANCREAS

ENDOCRINE SYSTEM AND
SELECTED METABOLIC DISEASES

HEART

KIDNEYS, URETERS, AND URINARY BLADDER

RESPIRATORY SYSTEM

MUSCULOSKELETAL SYSTEM, PART I:
ANATOMY, PHYSIOLOGY, AND METABOLIC DISORDERS

MUSCULOSKELETAL SYSTEM, PART II:
DEVELOPMENTAL DISORDERS, TUMORS, RHEUMATIC DISEASES, AND
JOINT REPLACEMENT

MUSCULOSKELETAL SYSTEM, PART III:
TRAUMA, EVALUATION, AND MANAGEMENT

Copies of all NETTER COLLECTION books, ATLAS OF HUMAN ANATOMY, CLINICAL SYMPOSIA reprints, and color slides of all illustrations contained in them are available from Icon Learning Systems, 295 North Street, Teterboro, NJ 07608, call 1-800-631-1181 or visit us at www.netterart.com

First Printing, 1959
Second Printing, 1966
Third Printing, 1971
Fourth Printing, 1975
Fifth Printing, 1978
Sixth Printing, 1983
Seventh Printing, 1989
Eighth Printing, 1997
Ninth Printing, 2000

ISBN 0-914168-76-2
Library of Congress Catalog No: 97-76569

Printed in U.S.A.

Original Printing by Colorpress, New York, N.Y.
Color Engravings by Embassy Photo Engraving Co., Inc., New York, N.Y.
Offset Conversion by R. R. Donnelley & Sons Company, Crawfordsville, IN
Ninth Printing by Hoechstetter Printing Company, Inc.

3M • 12/2000 • HPC

CONTRIBUTORS AND CONSULTANTS

The artist, editor and publishers express their appreciation
to the following authorities for their generous collaboration:

WILLIAM H. BACHRACH, M.D., PH.D.
Associate Clinical Professor of Medicine, University of Southern California School of
Medicine; Associate Chief, Gastroenterology Section, Wadsworth General Medical and
Surgical Hospital, Veterans Administration Center, Los Angeles, Calif.

JOHN FRANKLIN HUBER, M.D., PH.D.
Professor and Head of the Department of Anatomy, Temple University School of
Medicine, Philadelphia, Pa.

NICHOLAS A. MICHELS, M.A., D.Sc.
Professor of Anatomy, Daniel Baugh Institute of Anatomy, Jefferson Medical College,
Philadelphia, Pa.

G. A. G. MITCHELL, O.B.E., T.D., M.B., CH.M., D.Sc.
Professor of Anatomy and Director of the Anatomical Laboratories, Dean of the Medical
School, University of Manchester, England.

RUDOLF NISSEN, M.D.
Professor of Surgery, Head of the Department of Surgery, University of Basle,
Switzerland.

MAX L. SOM, M.D., F.A.C.S.
Assistant Clinical Professor of Otolaryngology, New York University Post-Graduate
Medical School, New York, N. Y.; Associate Otolaryngologist, The Mount Sinai Hospital, New York, N. Y.; Attending Endoscopist and Chairman of Head and Neck Group
of the Surgical Service, Montefiore Hospital, New York, N. Y.

LEO STERN, JR., D.D.S.
Associate Attending Dental and Oral Surgeon, The Mount Sinai Hospital, New York,
N. Y.

BERNARD S. WOLF, M.D.
Director, Department of Radiology, The Mount Sinai Hospital, New York, N. Y.;
Associate Clinical Professor of Radiology, Columbia University College of Physicians
and Surgeons, New York, N. Y.

GERHARD WOLF-HEIDEGGER, M.D., PH.D.
Professor and Director of the Anatomical Institute, Faculty of Medicine, University of
Basle, Switzerland.

INTRODUCTION

The making of pictures is a stern discipline. One may "write around" a subject where one is not quite sure of the details, but, with brush in hand before the drawing board, one must be precise and realistic. The white paper before the artist demands the truth, and it will not tolerate blank areas or gaps in continuity. Often in the production of the pictures contained in this volume, I would find myself confronted with problems to which I did not have the answers, problems which I had not anticipated when making the preliminary studies and research and which were brought to light only when I began to put the subject on paper. Then I had to stop and seek out the additional facts or information I needed, and, on occasion, when I had found it, a complete revision and redesigning of the picture took place. In the course of such research, I would sometimes be frustrated by a maze of conflicting data in the literature. Then came the problem of finding someone who could give me the correct answers.

It was on one such quest related to the nerve supply of the gastro-intestinal tract that I first made the acquaintance of Dr. G. A. G. Mitchell, Professor of Anatomy and Dean of the Medical School at the University of Manchester, England. From having studied his published volumes and articles, I felt sure that here was a man who could give me the solution to many of the problems which were troubling me. I was, therefore, most delighted when, in response to my inquiry, he so cordially agreed to act as a consultant for the plates on the innervation of the esophagus, stomach and duodenum and also for the general intrinsic nervous organization of the alimentary tract, a field in which he has made so many valuable contributions and in which his publications are classics. My joys were not unfounded, for, when I visited him in England in connection with this work, I discovered him to be even more helpful than I had anticipated and in addition a most gracious and friendly host. Dr. Mitchell's subsequent visit to this country gave me the opportunity also to avail myself of his advice and criticism not only for those plates which we had planned together but also those in Section IV on the nervous regulation of the upper digestive tract (mastication, salivation, deglutition, gastric activity, vomiting). Dealing in these latter plates with rather complex problems, a great deal of which has come to light in only relatively recent neurophysiologic investigations, I also received most willing counsel from Dr. W. R. Ingram, Iowa State University, with whom I had previously collaborated on the series of 18 pictures on the hypothalamus which have been published as a supplement in Volume 1 of THE CIBA COLLECTION OF MEDICAL ILLUSTRATIONS.

Another consultant with whom scientific collaboration has developed into a warm and lasting friendship was Dr. John Franklin Huber, Professor of Anatomy at Temple University, Philadelphia. His practical point of view, coupled with his profound knowledge of the subject, was of tremendous aid to me in portraying the complex and difficult anatomy of the mouth and pharynx. It was, indeed, a pleasure to visit him repeatedly, to see him among his students, and then in his "sanctum-sanctorum" to work out with him the program for this section as well as the innumerable details involved.

For the illustrations depicting the vascular anatomy of the esophagus, stomach and duodenum, it became necessary for me to seek out the man who has contributed as no other to the knowledge in this particular field of medical science. This was Dr. Nicholas A. Michels who, with his co-workers, especially Dr. P. C. Schroy, has spent many years in elucidating with special techniques the complex and varied course of the vessels of the upper intestinal tract. At Dr. Michels's suggestion four of the illustrations already published in

Part III of this volume have been reprinted here, so that the entire story of the multifarious arrangement of the arteries and anastomoses is presented as completely as possible and compatible with the limited aims of the CIBA COLLECTION, and at the same time the reader will be spared the necessity of referring to another book of this volume.

It has been only in the last decade or so that our knowledge and understanding of the anatomy, function and diseases of the esophagus have begun to crystallize. For this reason I was most fortunate in having the advice and collaboration of Dr. Max L. Som of New York City, who has contributed so much to our knowledge of these subjects. He was consultant for the sections on the anatomy and diseases of the esophagus, as well as for the plates on diseases of the pharynx. His brilliance and his incredible store of information in these fields were to me an unending source of amazement. In addition, his wit and his delightful manner in explaining a point made it sheer pleasure to work with him.

Medicine is, by its very nature, international. This fact is recognized in this volume by the inclusion, for the first time in this series, of consultants from countries other than the United States. This innovation is exemplified not only by Dr. Mitchell, whom I have mentioned above, but also by Dr. Rudolf Nissen, Professor of Surgery at the University of Basle, Switzerland, and also Dr. med. et phil. G. Wolf-Heidegger, Professor of Anatomy at the University of Basle, Switzerland. Professor Nissen and his associates, Dr. Mario Rosetti and Dr. W. Hess, collaborated with me on the section for diseases of the stomach and duodenum, and Professor Wolf-Heidegger on the anatomy of the same structures. The days that I spent with these men in Basle were an unforgettable experience, not only because of their splendid hospitality but even more because of the stimulus of their interest, their knowledge and their discernment. Their devotion to the task made it possible to overcome the difficulties which would ordinarily have arisen because of our geographic separation.

Oral pathology, though a specialty in itself, has many phases of vital interest to the internist, the gastro-enterologist, the surgeon, the radiologist, the dentist, the pathologist and other specialists. The field is so vast that I was delighted to see how much thought and study Dr. Leo Stern, Jr., who was consultant for this section, devoted to the selection of topics. Because of his experience in having supplied, for CLINICAL SYMPOSIA in 1953, an article on the pathology of the mouth and because of his constant reference to the literature, I feel that we were able to present with judicious restraint a fair survey of oral pathology. For the histopathologic material on pages 121, 122-129 and its description, I sincerely thank Dr. Lester R. Cahn, Associate Professor of Oral Pathology, Faculty of Medicine, Columbia University, and Oral Pathologist at The Mount Sinai Hospital.

In Section IV on the physiology of the upper digestive tract, I was confronted with what seemed to me a challenge of the first magnitude. Physiology or function, after all, implies motion, and to present this in static pictures was a task which I approached with some trepidation. I needed a pilot competent in the field of experimental physiology as well as in clinical gastro-enterology. It was a rare stroke of destiny that brought me to Dr. William H. Bachrach as the principal consultant for this section. His unflagging, always cheerful, guidance through the voluminous literature and through the many intricacies that stood in the way of a clear, simplified, yet correct visual demonstration caused my misgivings to fade away and the pictures to take form in my mind.

Dr. Bachrach was most desirous that his "irreversible

indebtedness" to his teacher and master, Dr. A. C. Ivy, "from whose unpublished *Physiology of the Gastro-intestinal Tract* much of the material discussed has been drawn, often verbatim", should be given full recognition. I take the opportunity here of doing this. Dr. Bachrach and I, furthermore, received most effective help from several members of the Gastroenterology Department at the Veterans Administration General Hospital in Los Angeles. Dr. M. I. Grossman documented his genuine concern with significant suggestions during the preparatory phase and with his constructive criticism of the final paintings. Drs. S. Tuttle and F. Goetz displayed their interest with a series of elaborate demonstrations.

The two double plates in the same section on the physiologic aspects (pages 74-77), describing graphically the process of deglutition, were developed under the personal direction of an investigator, Dr. Bernard Wolf, who himself was instrumental in the clarification of the motor phenomena

in the esophagus. With his assistance, the plate and text on inferior esophageal ring formation (Section V, page 144) was developed also.

I must express here my sincere gratitude for the very valuable advice and actual information so graciously supplied to me by Dr. Hans Popper, Director of Pathology at The Mt. Sinai Hospital, New York City. Throughout the preparation of this volume, I often called on him for information or suggestions. Despite his busy schedule he always found time to give of his tremendous store of medical knowledge in his characteristic dynamic fashion. My thanks go also to Dr. H. M. Spiro of Yale University, School of Medicine, for his personal communication on the subject of indirect (tubeless) gastric analysis.

Throughout the trials and tribulations of this project, the optimism and faith of the editor have been to me a source of satisfaction.

FRANK H. NETTER, M.D.

This Part I of Volume 3 of THE CIBA COLLECTION OF MEDICAL ILLUSTRATIONS contains altogether 172 full-color plates illustrating the anatomy, the diseases and some functional and diagnostic aspects of the upper intestinal tract. Together with Part II [issued in 1962] and Part III [issued in 1957], the present book presents our attempt to cover pictorially those topics and features of the digestive system that are of interest for the practicing physician and the student of medicine alike.

The principles guiding the consultants, artist and editor have been repeatedly set forth in the introductions to preceding volumes and need not be restated here. It may be worth emphasizing again, however, that completeness in presenting each and every detail in the anatomic and pathologic aspects of normal and diseased organs and tissues has never been our aim. In this book, as in the previous ones, we have tried to supplement graphically the standard reference works rather than to replace them. From the number of copies of the previous volumes and of Part III of *Digestive System* ordered continuously month after month and year after year, and from the thousands of requests for projection slides of the illustrations, it seems permissible to conclude that the selection of topics and the type of presentation strike a happy medium and definitely fill a demand. We hope our endeavors with this present compilation will have a similarly gratifying success.

Though his relations to the consultants are quite different from those of the artist, the editor likewise feels a deep gratitude to all those who have contributed to the generation, growth and maturation of this book. I am aware of the fact that the editor's functions cannot have left the pleasant memories which the creative co-operation of artist and consultant awake and leave behind. The obligations of the editor connect him with the rôle of an exhorter, monitor or

admonisher, who endeavors to get the texts and the bibliographic references and who may have caused annoyance in his efforts to produce a book fairly uniform in style, appearance and nomenclature. I have not received any sign of misgiving, and it is, therefore, more than thankfulness — it is esteem mounting to admiration that I hold for the understanding of our contributors, their patience and willingness to bear with my interference.

It remains for me to express our indebtedness to those who have placed at our disposal some didactically most valuable material in the form of slides or microphotographs. To Dr. J. R. Rintoul and Mr. P. Howarth, both of the Department of Anatomy in the University of Manchester, England, we owe the pictures demonstrating the nerve cells of the alimentary tract. Dr. Leo Kaplan, Director of the Clinical and Anatomic Laboratories of Mount Sinai Hospital in Los Angeles, was kind enough to supply the photomicrographs on page 102. Dr. Sadeo Otani provided the slide reproduced on page 154.

Our thanks go, furthermore, as in previous volumes, to Paul W. Roder, Mrs. L. A. Oppenheim, Felton Davis, Jr., Wallace and Anne Clark, to Harold B. Davison of Embassy Photo Engraving Co., Inc., and to Colorpress for their tremendous efforts in solving the innumerable problems of such highly diversified character. We wish also to express our appreciation for the valuable assistance and encouragement which Mrs. Vera Netter gave in many ways not only to her artist husband but to all concerned in this project.

It gives us, finally, great pleasure to introduce to our readership Dr. Hans H. Zinsser, Assistant Clinical Professor of Surgery at the College of Physicians and Surgeons, Columbia University, who joined us as Associate Editor in May, 1958, just in time to support us in the most critical phase of getting this book ready for press.

E. OPPENHEIMER, M.D.

CONTENTS

Information on THE NETTER COLLECTION Volumes

CONTENTS OF COMPLETE VOLUME 3
DIGESTIVE SYSTEM

Section I

ANATOMY OF THE MOUTH AND PHARYNX

by

FRANK H. NETTER, M.D.

in collaboration with

JOHN FRANKLIN HUBER, M.D., Ph.D.

ORAL CAVITY

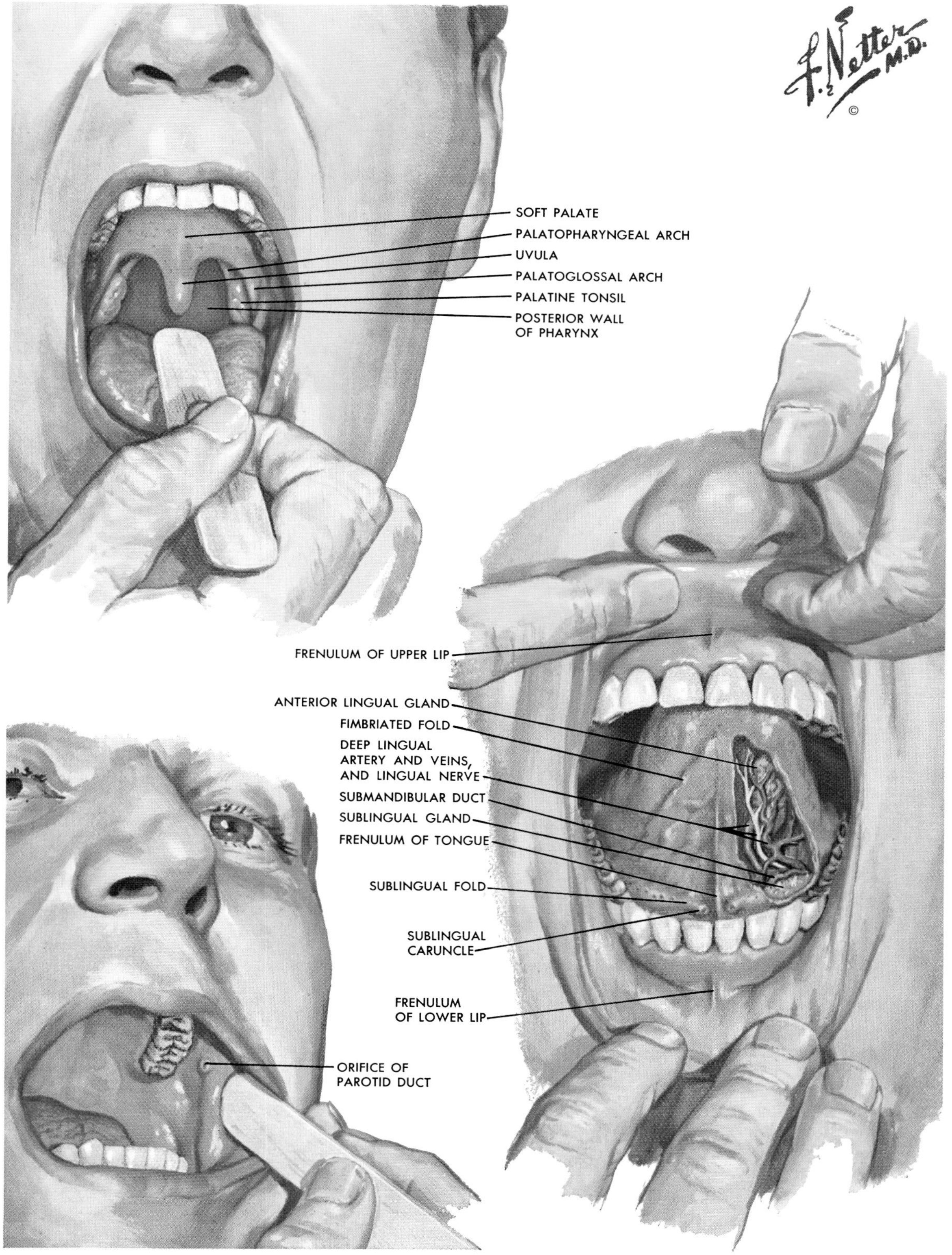

SOFT PALATE
PALATOPHARYNGEAL ARCH
UVULA
PALATOGLOSSAL ARCH
PALATINE TONSIL
POSTERIOR WALL OF PHARYNX

FRENULUM OF UPPER LIP

ANTERIOR LINGUAL GLAND
FIMBRIATED FOLD
DEEP LINGUAL ARTERY AND VEINS, AND LINGUAL NERVE
SUBMANDIBULAR DUCT
SUBLINGUAL GLAND
FRENULUM OF TONGUE

SUBLINGUAL FOLD

SUBLINGUAL CARUNCLE

FRENULUM OF LOWER LIP

ORIFICE OF PAROTID DUCT

The mouth, or oral cavity, is the beginning of the alimentary canal. Its roof is formed by the palate, the tongue rises up out of its floor, and the cheeks and lips bound it laterally and anteriorly. Communicating anteriorly with the exterior by the rima oris, or oral orifice, and posteriorly with the pharynx through the isthmus faucium, it is divided into the vestibule and oral cavity proper by the teeth and alveolar processes of the mandible and maxilla. When the mouth is closed, these two parts are connected only by the small spaces between the teeth and a variable gap between the last molar tooth and the ramus of the mandible, through which a catheter can be passed for feeding when the jaws are closed tightly by muscle spasm.

When the lips are everted, a midline fold of mucous membrane, known as the *frenulum*, can be seen extending from each lip to the adjacent gum. These frenula may cause some problem in the fitting of artificial dentures. Also in the vestibule, opposite the crown of the second maxillary molar tooth, is a small eminence through which the *duct of the parotid gland* opens. Many small glands are located in the mucous membrane of the lips (labial glands) and of the cheeks (buccal glands), which empty their secretions directly into the vestibule. The above structures in the vestibule usually can all be readily felt by the tongue.

The lips (upper and lower) are extremely mobile folds, which form the margins of the rima oris and meet laterally at the angle of the mouth, where they are continuous with the cheeks. The framework of the lip is formed by the orbicularis oris muscle (see page 8), external to which lies skin with its subcutaneous tissue and internal to which is the mucous membrane (see page 11). At the red area of the lip the covering has an intermediate structure between the skin and the mucous membrane.

The general structure of the cheek is similar to that of the lip. The framework is formed by the buccinator muscle, strengthened by a firm fascial layer (see pages 8 and 9), with skin and subcutaneous tissue external to it and mucous membrane internal to it (see page 15). On the outer surface of the buccinator muscle at the anterior border of the masseter muscle lies a pad of fat, which is especially prominent in the infant and may be referred to as the suctorial pad.

When the tip of the tongue is turned up and back, several structures come into view. In the midline is the *frenulum of the tongue*, and just to each side of its lower end is a *sublingual caruncle*, at the apex of which is the opening of the duct of the submandibular gland. Running posterolaterally from the sublingual caruncle is the sublingual fold caused by the *sublingual gland*, with openings of several small ducts of this gland scattered along it. At each side of the under surface of the tongue is the *fimbriated fold* and, medial to that, the *deep lingual vessels* are visible through the mucous membrane.

By direct examination of the open mouth, in addition to the structures described above, one can see the palate (see page 7), the palatopharyngeal fold and the palatoglossal fold, with the palatine tonsil between them (see page 16), the teeth (see pages 12 and 13) and the tongue (see pages 10 and 11).

In an at-rest state the upper and lower teeth are apt to be slightly separated from each other, the tongue is at least partially in contact with the palate, and the vestibule is obliterated by the lips and cheeks lying against the teeth and gums.

MANDIBLE

The *mandible,* or lower jawbone, forms the bony framework for the lower part of the oral cavity and the skeleton of the lower part of the face. It has a U-shaped body, with a broad flat ramus running superiorly from each end of the body.

The area of fusion of the right and left halves of the body of the mandible at the midline anteriorly is known as the symphysis. At the lower part of the outer surface of the symphysis is a triangular elevation called the *mental protuberance,* the lower outer angles of which are the *mental tubercles.* At the lower part of the inner surface of the symphysis is a variable elevation, the *mental spine* or spines, which may be present as a single eminence or as two eminences, one above the other, or as two pairs of tubercles, also called the genial tubercles. These give origin to the geniohyoid and genioglossus muscles (see pages 6 and 11).

Each half of the body of the mandible has an upper and a lower part and an outer and an inner surface. The lower part has an arch wider than that of the upper part. The upper part is the alveolar process, so called because it contains the sockets for the teeth. The lower part, known as the base, or *body,* has a much greater proportion of compact bone which greatly strengthens it. Just lateral to the symphysis on the lower border is an oval depression or roughened area for the attachment of the digastric muscle (see page 6), the *digastric fossa.* On the outer surface of the body below the second premolar tooth or on the internal surface between the two premolars is the *mental foramen,* by which the mental branches of the inferior alveolar nerve and vessels leave the mandibular canal. Also on the outer surface a rather ill-defined *oblique line* runs from the mental tubercle to the anterior border of the ramus. Sometimes it seems to start from the lower border of the mandible below the molar teeth, or there may appear to be lines from each of these places, which meet as they run posterosuperiorly. On the inner surface of the body, a ridge of bone runs obliquely from the digastric fossa to the level of the socket of the last molar tooth. This ridge gives attachment to the mylohyoid muscle (see page 6) and is therefore known as the *mylohyoid line.* Superior to the mylohyoid line is a shallow sublingual fossa, in relation to which lies the sublingual gland, and inferior to the mylohyoid line is the *fossa for the submandibular gland.*

The *ramus* presents a medial and a lateral surface and an anterior, a superior and a posterior border. The remaining border of the ramus depends on an arbitrary decision as to the dividing line between the ramus and the body. This

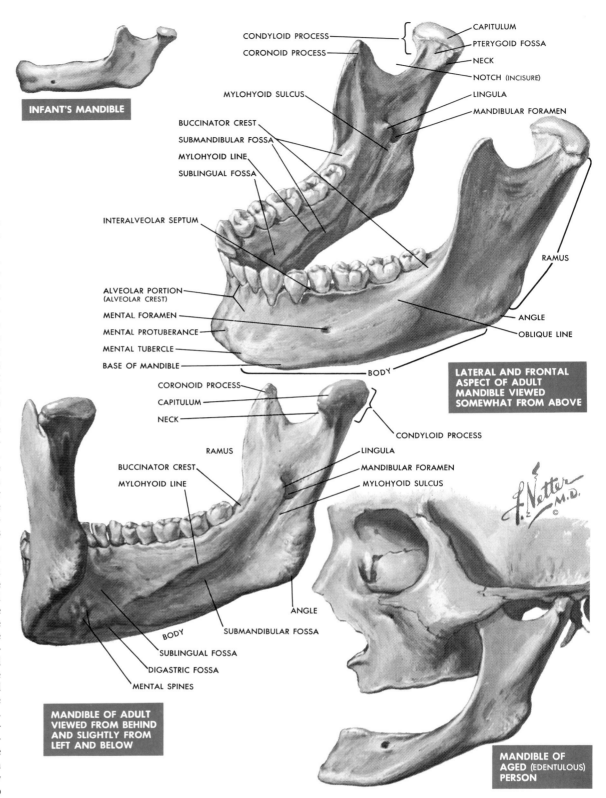

INFANT'S MANDIBLE

CONDYLOID PROCESS
CORONOID PROCESS
CAPITULUM
PTERYGOID FOSSA
NECK
NOTCH (INCISURE)
LINGULA
MANDIBULAR FORAMEN
MYLOHYOID SULCUS
BUCCINATOR CREST
SUBMANDIBULAR FOSSA
MYLOHYOID LINE
SUBLINGUAL FOSSA
INTERALVEOLAR SEPTUM
RAMUS
ALVEOLAR PORTION (ALVEOLAR CREST)
MENTAL FORAMEN
MENTAL PROTUBERANCE
MENTAL TUBERCLE
BASE OF MANDIBLE
ANGLE
OBLIQUE LINE
BODY

LATERAL AND FRONTAL ASPECT OF ADULT MANDIBLE VIEWED SOMEWHAT FROM ABOVE

CORONOID PROCESS
CAPITULUM
NECK
CONDYLOID PROCESS
RAMUS
BUCCINATOR CREST
MYLOHYOID LINE
LINGULA
MANDIBULAR FORAMEN
MYLOHYOID SULCUS
ANGLE
SUBMANDIBULAR FOSSA
BODY
SUBLINGUAL FOSSA
DIGASTRIC FOSSA
MENTAL SPINES

MANDIBLE OF ADULT VIEWED FROM BEHIND AND SLIGHTLY FROM LEFT AND BELOW

MANDIBLE OF AGED (EDENTULOUS) PERSON

line is not agreed upon by various authors, some of whom consider the ramus as forming the posterior part of the inferior border of the mandible and some of whom consider the region of junction of the body and ramus as at the angle of the mandible. About the center of the medial surface of the ramus is the *mandibular foramen* — the beginning of the mandibular canal which transmits the inferior alveolar nerve, artery and vein. The *lingula* projects partly over the foramen from in front of it, and the mylohyoid groove, or sulcus, runs antero-inferiorly from it for a short distance. Projecting upward from the superior border of the ramus are the triangular *coronoid process* anteriorly and the *condyloid process* posteriorly, with the *mandibular notch* between the two. The condyloid process is made up of the head and neck. The muscle attachments which the ramus provides are pictured and described on pages 8 and 11.

The *angle of the mandible* is the area of junction of the posterior and inferior borders of the mandible. It is usually slightly obtuse in the young adult and flares slightly laterally.

The mandible changes with age. The two halves usually have fused by the second year. The position of the mental foramen indicates changes in the body. At birth it is near the lower border, since the alveolar process comprises most of the body. After full development it is about halfway between the upper and the lower borders. When the *individual* becomes *edentulous,* much of the alveolar process is resorbed, and the mental foramen is located near or on the upper border. The angle of the mandible is more obtuse in the infant than after it has become fully developed. Again, in the edentulous state, it appears more obtuse, although this may be at least in part due to a backward tilt of the condyloid process.

TEMPOROMANDIBULAR JOINT

The bony structures which enter into the formation of this joint are the head of the mandible below and the articular, or mandibular, fossa and *articular tubercle* of the temporal bone above. The head of the mandible is ellipsoidal, with the long axis directed medially and slightly backward. This articular surface is markedly convex from before backward and slightly convex from side to side. The articular surface on the temporal bone is concavoconvex from behind forward. An *articular disk* is interposed between the two surfaces just described. Each surface of the disk more or less conforms to the articular surface to which it is related, but the shape of the disk is quite variable. The disk is usually described as being made up of fibrocartilage, but the tissue apparently has very few or no cartilage cells present. The cartilages covering the bony articular surfaces differ from those of most joints in that they are fibrocartilage or even fibrous tissue rather than hyaline cartilage, although they have a gross appearance similar to the articular cartilages of other joints.

The temporomandibular joint is a true or synovial joint, with two separate synovial cavities — one above the articular disk and one below it. This joint can be further classified as a ginglymo-arthrodial joint, with the *hinge motion* in the lower joint and the *sliding motion* in the upper joint.

The capsular ligament is rather loosely arranged, being attached superiorly to the margins of the articular surface on the temporal bone and affixed inferiorly around the neck of the mandible. The capsular ligament is firmly attached to the entire circumference of the articular disk, which some authors list as a ligament of the joint. Forming a pronounced thickening of the lateral aspect of the capsule is the *temporomandibular ligament,* which runs downward and backward from the lower border of the zygomatic process of the temporal bone to the side and back of the neck of the mandible. Two accessory ligaments are not blended with the capsule. The rather thin *sphenomandibular ligament* runs

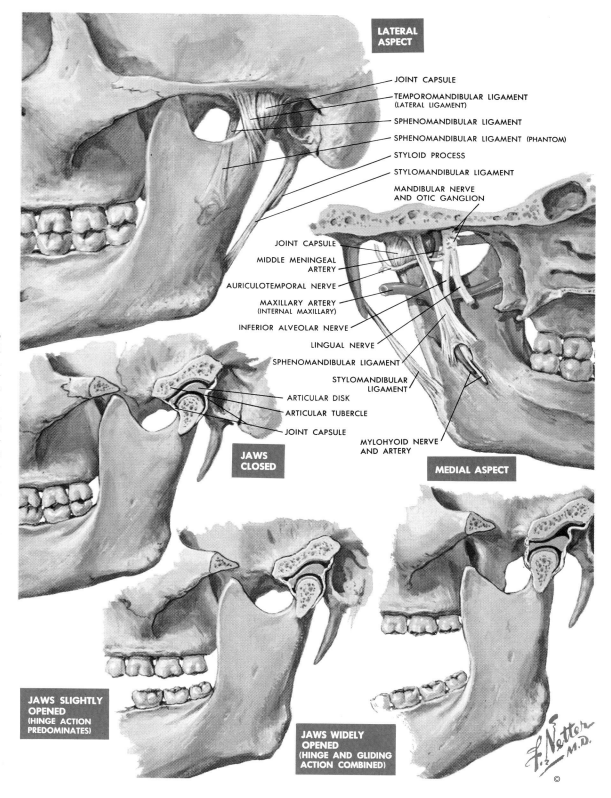

LATERAL ASPECT

JOINT CAPSULE
TEMPOROMANDIBULAR LIGAMENT (LATERAL LIGAMENT)
SPHENOMANDIBULAR LIGAMENT
SPHENOMANDIBULAR LIGAMENT (PHANTOM)
STYLOID PROCESS
STYLOMANDIBULAR LIGAMENT
MANDIBULAR NERVE AND OTIC GANGLION
JOINT CAPSULE
MIDDLE MENINGEAL ARTERY
AURICULOTEMPORAL NERVE
MAXILLARY ARTERY (INTERNAL MAXILLARY)
INFERIOR ALVEOLAR NERVE
LINGUAL NERVE
SPHENOMANDIBULAR LIGAMENT
STYLOMANDIBULAR LIGAMENT
ARTICULAR DISK
ARTICULAR TUBERCLE
JOINT CAPSULE
MYLOHYOID NERVE AND ARTERY

JAWS CLOSED

MEDIAL ASPECT

JAWS SLIGHTLY OPENED (HINGE ACTION PREDOMINATES)

JAWS WIDELY OPENED (HINGE AND GLIDING ACTION COMBINED)

from the spine of the sphenoid bone to the lingula of the mandible, and the *stylomandibular ligament,* a thickened band of deep cervical fascia, runs from the styloid process to the lower part of the posterior border of the ramus of the mandible.

The temporomandibular joint receives its nerve supply by twigs from the *auriculotemporal* and *masseteric branches* of the *mandibular* division of the *trigeminal nerve* (see page 29), and its arterial supply via branches of the internal maxillary and superficial temporal arteries from the external carotid artery (see also page 24).

The basic movements which are allowed in the temporomandibular joint are: (1) the gliding forward and backward on the temporal bone articular surface by the articular disk, accompanied by the head of the mandible, which moves with the disk because the disk is attached to the capsule near the

attachment of the capsule to the neck of the mandible, and the external pterygoid muscle attaches to both, and (2) the hinge movement which takes place between the head of the mandible and the articular disk. In the opening of the mouth, both movements are involved, with the hinge movement predominating in slight opening and the gliding movement predominating in wide opening. In the chewing motion, one condyle remains more or less in position, while the other moves backward and forward. This is combined with slight elevation and depression of the mandible. If the mouth is opened just enough so that the upper and lower incisor teeth can clear each other, the jaw can be protracted and retracted, with the movement occurring in the upper joint.

The muscles which produce the movements occurring at the temporomandibular joint are described on pages 8 and 9.

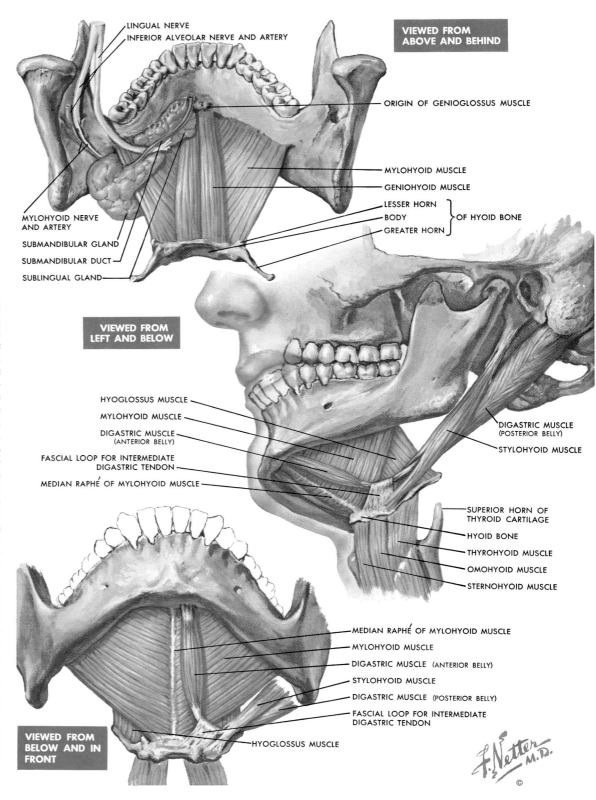

VIEWED FROM ABOVE AND BEHIND

LINGUAL NERVE
INFERIOR ALVEOLAR NERVE AND ARTERY
ORIGIN OF GENIOGLOSSUS MUSCLE
MYLOHYOID MUSCLE
GENIOHYOID MUSCLE
LESSER HORN
BODY } OF HYOID BONE
GREATER HORN
MYLOHYOID NERVE AND ARTERY
SUBMANDIBULAR GLAND
SUBMANDIBULAR DUCT
SUBLINGUAL GLAND

VIEWED FROM LEFT AND BELOW

HYOGLOSSUS MUSCLE
MYLOHYOID MUSCLE
DIGASTRIC MUSCLE (ANTERIOR BELLY)
FASCIAL LOOP FOR INTERMEDIATE DIGASTRIC TENDON
MEDIAN RAPHÉ OF MYLOHYOID MUSCLE
DIGASTRIC MUSCLE (POSTERIOR BELLY)
STYLOHYOID MUSCLE
SUPERIOR HORN OF THYROID CARTILAGE
HYOID BONE
THYROHYOID MUSCLE
OMOHYOID MUSCLE
STERNOHYOID MUSCLE

MEDIAN RAPHÉ OF MYLOHYOID MUSCLE
MYLOHYOID MUSCLE
DIGASTRIC MUSCLE (ANTERIOR BELLY)
STYLOHYOID MUSCLE
DIGASTRIC MUSCLE (POSTERIOR BELLY)
FASCIAL LOOP FOR INTERMEDIATE DIGASTRIC TENDON

VIEWED FROM BELOW AND IN FRONT
HYOGLOSSUS MUSCLE

FLOOR OF MOUTH

The term "floor of the mouth" is used differently by different authors, but in all cases it is applied to the floor of the "oral cavity proper" and does not include the "vestibule". It is sometimes used to mean the structures which actually bound the cavity inferiorly. In this sense the structures which comprise it would be the upper and lateral surfaces of the anterior part of the tongue (see pages 10 and 11) and the mucous membrane which is reflected from the side of the tongue to the inner aspect of the mandible. Other authors have used the term to mean the muscular and other structures which fill the interval bounded by the mandible and the hyoid bone. This would mean primarily the mylohyoid muscle, which is then thought of as the boundary between the mouth above the muscle and the submandibular triangle of the neck below the muscle.

The right and left *mylohyoid muscles* form a diaphragm which is stretched between the two halves of the mandible and the body of the *hyoid bone*. The mandibular attachment of each muscle is the respective mylohyoid line (see page 4) of the mandible. The posterior fibers of each muscle insert on the body of the hyoid bone, and from here forward to the symphysis of the mandible the right and left muscles meet each other in a midline raphé. The mylohyoid muscle is supplied by the mylohyoid branch of the *inferior alveolar nerve,* a branch of the mandibular division (see also page 29) of the trigeminal nerve.

A little to each side of the midline, the *anterior belly of the digastric muscle* lies against the inferior surface of the mylohyoid muscle. Anteriorly it attaches to the digastric fossa of the mandible, and posteriorly it ends in the *intermediate tendon,* by means of which it is continuous with the *posterior belly,* which attaches to the mastoid notch of the temporal bone. The intermediate tendon is anchored to the hyoid bone by a *fascial loop.* The anterior belly is supplied by the mylohyoid nerve (see page 29) and the posterior belly by a branch from the facial nerve.

Closely related to the posterior belly of the digastricus, the *stylohyoid muscle* extends from near the root of the styloid process to the greater cornu (horn) of

the hyoid bone near the body. It usually attaches to the hyoid by two slips, between which the posterior belly of the digastricus passes. The stylohyoid is supplied by a branch of the facial nerve.

The right and left *geniohyoid muscles,* one on each side of the midline, rest on the superior surface of the mylohyoid muscle (see page 11). They are attached anteriorly to the mental spine (inferior genial tubercles) (see page 18) and posteriorly to the body of the hyoid bone. The geniohyoid muscle is supplied by fibers from the first and second cervical nerves which accompany the hypoglossal nerve (see page 29).

With the foregoing description of the related muscles in mind, the hyoid bone can be thought of as held in a muscular sling hung between the mandible and the stylomastoid area of the temporal bone, thus making the floor of the mouth quite mobile. All of these muscles can help in the elevation of the hyoid

bone and, thus, the floor of the mouth. The geniohyoid and stylohyoid muscles determine the anterior-posterior position of the hyoid bone, lengthening and shortening the floor of the mouth. The strap muscles (*omohyoid, sternohyoid, sternothyroid* [just inferior to the thyrohyoid muscle as visible in the middle picture] and *thyrohyoid*) pull the hyoid bone and floor of the mouth downward.

A usage of the term "floor of the mouth", which is less technical than the two previously given, is to think of it as the mucous membrane which is reflected from the side of the tongue to the mandible. This area has been pictured and described on page 3. The attachment of the mucous membrane of this area to the mandible, where it is continuous with the gum, is along a line drawn from the posterior end of the mylohyoid line (see page 4) to a point just above the mental spine.

ROOF OF MOUTH

The roof of the mouth, or palate, forms the superior and posterosuperior boundary of the "oral cavity proper", which it thus separates from the nasal cavity and the nasopharynx (see pages 16 and 18). Approximately the anterior two thirds of the palate has a bony framework and is, therefore, the "hard palate"; the posterior third is the "soft palate". The palate is variably arched both anteroposteriorly and transversely, the transverse curve being more pronounced in the hard palate.

The bony framework of the hard palate is formed by the palatine processes of the two maxillae and the horizontal processes of the two palatine bones (see page 12), which meet in the midline. These bony structures also form the framework of the floor of the nasal cavity, and this common bony wall is traversed near the midline anteriorly by the *incisive canals*, which transmit blood vessels and nerves from the mucous membrane of the nose to the mucous membrane of the palate. Usually one canal begins at each side of the midline on the nasal side, and each of these canals divides into two before reaching the oral side, where all four resulting canals open into a single midline fossa. In a posterolateral position at each side of the bony palate are located the *greater and lesser palatine foramina* for the transmission of the *greater and lesser palatine vessels and nerves*. The oral surface of the bony palate is covered by mucoperiosteum (mucous membrane and periosteum fused together) which exhibits a faint midline ridge, the *palatine raphé*, at the anterior end of which is a slight elevation called the *incisive papilla*. Running laterally from the anterior part of the raphé are about six transverse ridges, the *transverse plicae (rugae)*.

The soft palate is continuous anteriorly with the hard palate and ends posteroinferiorly in a free margin, which forms an arch with the palatoglossal and the palatopharyngeal folds on each side as its pillars (see page 3). The uvula, greatly variable as to length and shape, is a projection which hangs inferiorly from the free margin of the soft palate. The framework of the soft palate is formed by a strong, thin fibrous sheet, known as the *palatine aponeurosis,* which is, at least in part, formed by the spreading out *tendons of the tensor veli palatini muscles*. In addition to the aponeurosis, the thickness of the soft palate is made up of the *palatine* muscles, many mucous *glands* on the oral side and mucous membrane on both the oral and pharyngeal surfaces. The mass of glands extends forward onto the hard palate as far anteriorly as a line between the canine teeth.

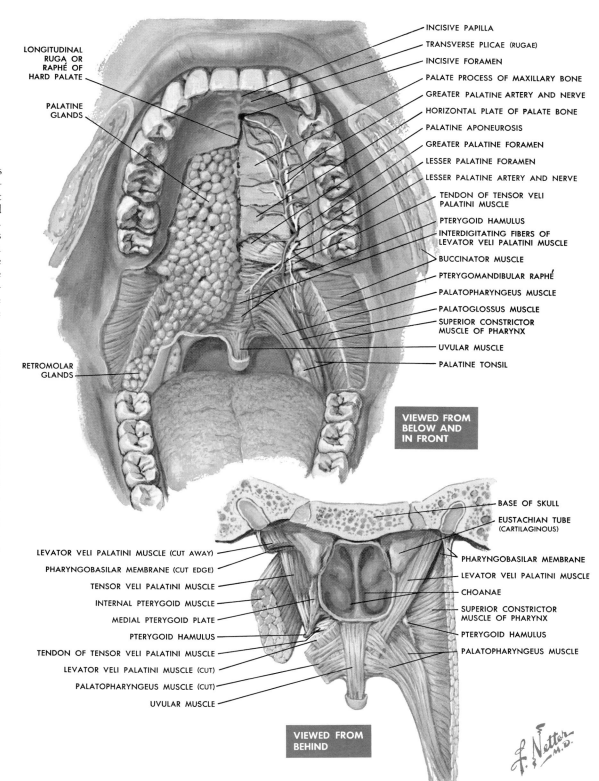

LONGITUDINAL RUGA OR RAPHÉ OF HARD PALATE
PALATINE GLANDS
RETROMOLAR GLANDS

INCISIVE PAPILLA
TRANSVERSE PLICAE (RUGAE)
INCISIVE FORAMEN
PALATE PROCESS OF MAXILLARY BONE
GREATER PALATINE ARTERY AND NERVE
HORIZONTAL PLATE OF PALATE BONE
PALATINE APONEUROSIS
GREATER PALATINE FORAMEN
LESSER PALATINE FORAMEN
LESSER PALATINE ARTERY AND NERVE
TENDON OF TENSOR VELI PALATINI MUSCLE
PTERYGOID HAMULUS
INTERDIGITATING FIBERS OF LEVATOR VELI PALATINI MUSCLE
BUCCINATOR MUSCLE
PTERYGOMANDIBULAR RAPHÉ
PALATOPHARYNGEUS MUSCLE
PALATOGLOSSUS MUSCLE
SUPERIOR CONSTRICTOR MUSCLE OF PHARYNX
UVULAR MUSCLE
PALATINE TONSIL

VIEWED FROM BELOW AND IN FRONT

LEVATOR VELI PALATINI MUSCLE (CUT AWAY)
PHARYNGOBASILAR MEMBRANE (CUT EDGE)
TENSOR VELI PALATINI MUSCLE
INTERNAL PTERYGOID MUSCLE
MEDIAL PTERYGOID PLATE
PTERYGOID HAMULUS
TENDON OF TENSOR VELI PALATINI MUSCLE
LEVATOR VELI PALATINI MUSCLE (CUT)
PALATOPHARYNGEUS MUSCLE (CUT)
UVULAR MUSCLE

BASE OF SKULL
EUSTACHIAN TUBE (CARTILAGINOUS)
PHARYNGOBASILAR MEMBRANE
LEVATOR VELI PALATINI MUSCLE
CHOANAE
SUPERIOR CONSTRICTOR MUSCLE OF PHARYNX
PTERYGOID HAMULUS
PALATOPHARYNGEUS MUSCLE

VIEWED FROM BEHIND

F. Netter, M.D.

The muscles of the soft palate can be briefly described as follows: (1) The *levator veli palatini* arises from the posteromedial side of the cartilaginous portion of the auditory tube and the adjacent lower surface of the petrous portion of the temporal bone, and its anterior fibers insert in the palatine aponeurosis, while the posterior ones are continuous with those of the opposite side; (2) the *tensor veli palatini* arises from the anterolateral side of the cartilaginous portion of the auditory tube and the adjacent angular spine and the scaphoid fossa of the sphenoid bone, and it inserts by a tendon which passes around the pterygoid hamulus and then spreads out into the palatine aponeurosis; (3) the *uvular muscle* arises from the posterior nasal spine and palatine aponeurosis, and it unites with the one of the other side to end in the mucous membrane of the uvula; (4) the *palatoglossus* runs from the soft palate to the side of the tongue (see page 11); (5) the *palatopharyngeus* runs from the soft palate inferiorly into the pharyngeal wall. These muscles are supplied by the vagus nerve by fibers, probably from the cranial part of the spinal accessory nerve, except for the tensor veli palatini, which is supplied by the trigeminal nerve.

By means of the rather easily visualized actions of the described muscles, the soft palate can be positioned as necessary for swallowing, breathing and phonation. It can be brought into contact with the dorsum of the tongue, and it can be brought up against the wall of the pharynx, which is important in closing off the nasopharynx from the oropharynx during swallowing.

The arterial supply of the palate and the nerve supply of its mucous membrane are shown in the accompanying figure. The sources of the arteries and nerves are considered on pages 24, 25 and 29.

MUSCLES INVOLVED IN MASTICATION

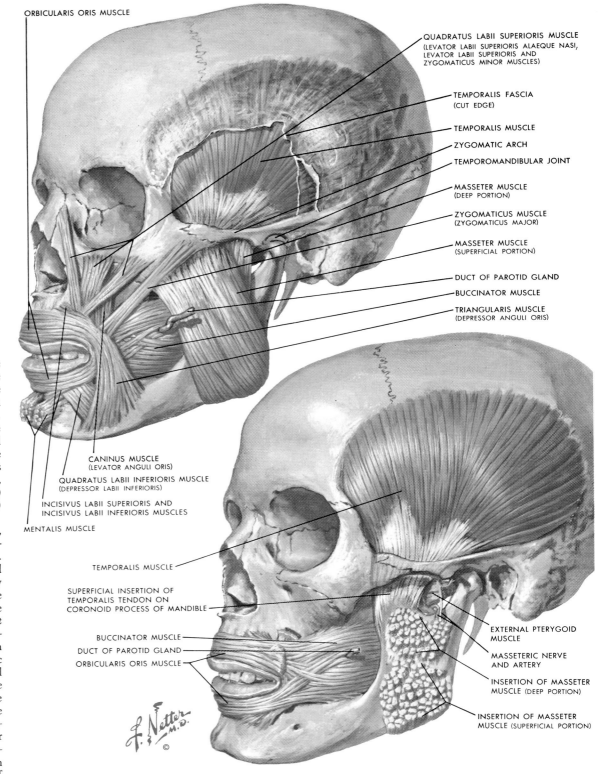

Chewing, or mastication, is one of the important functions carried on in the mouth, and a number of muscles are involved either directly or indirectly in this activity (see also pages 72 and 73). However, the four muscles which are primarily responsible for the forceful chewing movements of the mandible are classified by most authors as the "muscles of mastication". These are the masseter, the temporalis, the external (lateral) pterygoid and the internal (medial) pterygoid.

The *masseter muscle* is a flat, thick, quadrangular muscle, which is superficially placed and thus readily palpable. It is described as having a superficial and a deep part, which can be rather easily separated in the posterior portion of the muscle but are blended together in the anterior portion. The *superficial part* arises from the lower border of the anterior two thirds of the zygomatic arch (zygomatic process of maxilla, zygomatic bone and zygomatic process of temporal bone) and runs inferiorly and a little posteriorly to insert on the lateral surface of the lower part of the ramus of the mandible. The area of insertion continues all the way down to the inferior border of the mandible. The *deep portion* of the masseter muscle arises from the inner surface of the whole length of the zygomatic arch and runs almost vertically downward to insert on the lateral surface of the coronoid process and upper part of the ramus of the mandible. The deepest fibers frequently blend with the adjacent portion of the temporalis muscle. The masseter muscle is supplied by a branch from the mandibular division of the trigeminal nerve (see page 29), which reaches the deep surface of the muscle by passing through the mandibular notch.

The *temporalis muscle*, spread out broadly on the side of the skull, is a thin sheet, except where its fibers converge toward the tendon of insertion. It arises from the whole temporal fossa (the extensive area between the inferior temporal line and the infratemporal crest)

and from the inner surface of the *temporal fascia* which covers the muscle. The temporalis muscle inserts by means of a thick tendon which passes medial to the zygomatic arch (see page 20) and attaches to the apex and deep surface of the coronoid process of the mandible and the anterior border of the ramus almost as far as the last molar tooth, some of the fibers frequently becoming continuous with the buccinator muscle. Two or three deep temporal branches of the mandibular nerve enter the deep surface of the temporalis muscle.

The *external pterygoid muscle* is somewhat conical in shape and runs horizontally deep in the infratemporal fossa. It arises by an upper and a lower head. The upper head attaches to the infratemporal surface of the greater wing of the sphenoid bone, and the lower head attaches to the lateral surface of the lateral pterygoid plate (see page 20). The two heads join

and form a tendon of insertion, which ends on the front of the neck of the condyle of the mandible and on the anterior aspect of the capsule and articular disk of the mandibular joint. An external pterygoid nerve (see page 29) from the mandibular branch of the trigeminal enters the deep surface of this muscle.

The *internal pterygoid muscle,* located medial to the ramus of the mandible, is thick and quadrangular. Its main origin is from the medial surface of the lateral pterygoid plate and from the portion of the pyramidal process of the palatine bone between the two pterygoid plates. A small slip of origin lateral to the lateral pterygoid plate comes from the tuberosity of the maxilla and the adjacent surface of the pyramidal process of the palatine bone. The internal pterygoid muscle inserts on the medial surface of the ramus of the mandible between the mylohyoid groove and

(Continued on page 9)

ARTICULAR DISK

ARTICULAR TUBERCLE

EXTERNAL PTERYGOID MUSCLE

SPHENOMANDIBULAR LIGAMENT

INTERNAL PTERYGOID MUSCLE

PTERYGOMANDIBULAR RAPHÉ

BUCCINATOR MUSCLE

DUCT OF PAROTID GLAND

BUCCINATOR CREST

F. Netter M.D. ©

LATERAL VIEW

MUSCLES INVOLVED IN MASTICATION

(Continued from page 8)

AURICULOTEMPORAL NERVE

MAXILLARY ARTERY (INTERNAL MAXILLARY)

INFERIOR ALVEOLAR NERVE

MIDDLE MENINGEAL ARTERY

SPHENOMANDIBULAR LIGAMENT

LINGUAL NERVE

OTIC GANGLION

CHOANAE

EUSTACHIAN TUBE (CARTILAGINOUS)

LATERAL PTERYGOID PLATE

TEMPOROMANDIBULAR JOINT

ARTICULAR DISK

EXTERNAL PTERYGOID MUSCLE

MEDIAL PTERYGOID PLATE

INTERNAL PTERYGOID MUSCLE

HAMULAR PROCESS

MYLOHYOID NERVE

POSTERIOR VIEW

the angle. The internal pterygoid nerve from the mandibular runs down along the medial side of the muscle to enter it (see page 29).

The muscles of mastication all pass across the temporomandibular joint. They are the major muscles producing the movements allowed at this joint (see page 5). Elevation of the mandible is brought about by the masseter, the temporalis and the internal pterygoid. They are able to bring the lower teeth powerfully up against the upper teeth. They also are acting against gravity in most positions of the head in keeping the mouth closed. If they are relaxed, the weight of the jaw can open the mouth. The muscle of mastication, which actively opens the mouth, is the external pterygoid. It does this by pulling the articular disk and condyle of the mandible forward. Other muscles which may help in opening the mouth against resistance are the suprahyoid and infrahyoid muscles and the platysma. Protrusion of the jaw is brought about primarily by the external pterygoid, since in this movement, also, the articular disk and condyle of the mandible are brought forward. The superficial portion of the masseter and the internal pterygoid can give some aid in protrusion. Retraction of the mandible is accomplished mostly by the posterior part of the temporalis muscle, some of the fibers of which run almost horizontally. Other muscles which can contribute to retraction are the digastricus and the geniohyoid when the hyoid bone is anchored.

All of the muscles of mastication are employed in the act of chewing, because it involves the four movements of the mandible described above (see also pages 5 and 72), *i.e.,* elevation, depression, protrusion and retraction, and one or more of the muscles of mastication is involved in each of these movements. For the most part, chewing is done either on one side or the other, and the condyle of the side on which the chewing is being done remains more or less in position while the

condyle of the other side moves back and forth, as in protrusion and retraction. This is combined in proper sequence with slight elevation and depression to bring about the grinding action on the food.

In order that the grinding can be carried on efficiently, the food must be kept between the teeth by the tongue (see pages 10 and 11) on one side of the teeth, and the cheek and lips on the other side of the teeth. The muscular framework of the cheek and lips is, of course, of importance in accomplishing this. The framework of the cheek is formed by the *buccinator muscle,* which takes its origin from the outer surfaces of the maxilla and mandible in the region of the molar teeth and between the posterior ends of these lines of attachment from the pterygomandibular raphé (see page 22), by means of which it is continuous with the superior constrictor of the pharynx. From this U-shaped origin the fibers of the muscle

run horizontally forward, apparently to continue into the *orbicularis oris muscle,* with the uppermost and lowermost fibers going into the upper and lower lips, respectively, and the intermediate fibers crossing near the corner of the mouth, so that the upper fibers of this intermediate group go into the lower lip and the lower fibers of the intermediate group go into the upper lip. The buccinator muscle is supplied by a branch from the facial nerve. The framework of the lips is formed by the orbicularis oris muscle. In addition to the fibers which appear to be the forward prolongations of the buccinator muscle, fibers come into the orbicularis oris from all of the muscles which are inserted in the vicinity. These are illustrated in the upper figure on the opposite page. The orbicularis oris muscle is also supplied by the facial nerve.

The act of mastication is illustrated and described on pages 72 and 73.

TONGUE

The tongue is an extremely mobile mass of striated muscle, covered by mucous membrane. Arising from the floor of the mouth, the tongue practically fills the oral cavity when all its parts are at rest and the individual is in an upright position. The shape of the tongue may change extensively and rapidly during the various activities it has to perform.

The areas of the tongue covered by the mucous membrane are the *apex* or tip (directed against the lower incisor teeth), the *dorsum,* the right and left margins and the inferior surface. These are obvious topographic designations, except for the dorsum, which needs further description. The dorsum linguae extends from the apex to the reflection of the mucous membrane to the anterior surface of the *epiglottis* at the *vallecula,* forming an arch which, in its anterior or palatine two thirds, is directed superiorly, whereas its posterior or pharyngeal one third is directed posteriorly. Several divisions of the tongue have been proposed. Sometimes the *sulcus terminalis* has been said to separate the *body* and the *root* of the tongue, while in other instances the portion called the root has been limited to the posterior and inferior attachment of the tongue or has even been restricted to mean the general region of attachment through which muscles and other structures enter and leave the tongue. From the practical point of view, it is rather irrelevant where one permits the root to start and the body to end, or vice versa, but it is important to realize that the posterior third of the tongue is not visible by simple inspection even if the tongue is protruded and that one must make it visible either by using a mirror or by pressing the tongue down with the aid of a spatula.

At the posterior end of the body, or of the anterior two thirds, a small blind pit is seen, known as the *foramen cecum,* the remnant of the thyroglossal duct, from which the fetal development of the thyroid gland started. Angling anterolaterally toward each side from the cecal foramen is the sulcus terminalis, which is usually referred to as the dividing line between the anterior and posterior parts of the tongue. This groove, or sulcus, represents the junction of the two anlagen of the tongue and is of practical significance as far as the nerve supply is concerned (see page 30). (The real dividing line may run just in front of the circumvallate papillae.) A *median sulcus,* not always very distinct, is related to the median septum of the tongue.

The mucous membrane over the apex and body is normally moist and pink. Owing to its being thickly studded with papillae, it is rough, to provide friction for the handling of food. The majority of the *papillae* are of the *filiform* type, in which the epithelium ends in tapered points. Scattered about the field of filiform papillae are the larger, rounded

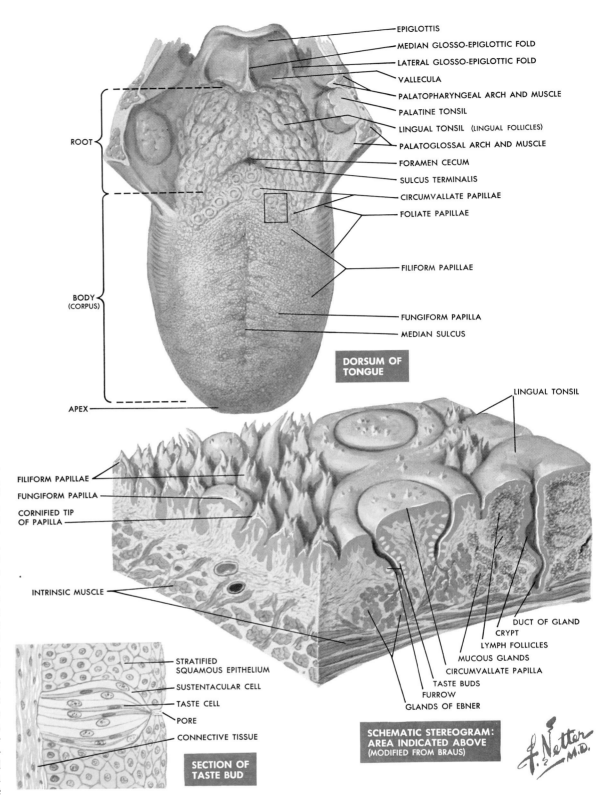

ROOT
BODY (CORPUS)
APEX

EPIGLOTTIS
MEDIAN GLOSSO-EPIGLOTTIC FOLD
LATERAL GLOSSO-EPIGLOTTIC FOLD
VALLECULA
PALATOPHARYNGEAL ARCH AND MUSCLE
PALATINE TONSIL
LINGUAL TONSIL (LINGUAL FOLLICLES)
PALATOGLOSSAL ARCH AND MUSCLE
FORAMEN CECUM
SULCUS TERMINALIS
CIRCUMVALLATE PAPILLAE
FOLIATE PAPILLAE
FILIFORM PAPILLAE
FUNGIFORM PAPILLA
MEDIAN SULCUS

DORSUM OF TONGUE

LINGUAL TONSIL

FILIFORM PAPILLAE
FUNGIFORM PAPILLA
CORNIFIED TIP OF PAPILLA
INTRINSIC MUSCLE

STRATIFIED SQUAMOUS EPITHELIUM
SUSTENTACULAR CELL
TASTE CELL
PORE
CONNECTIVE TISSUE

SECTION OF TASTE BUD

DUCT OF GLAND
CRYPT
LYMPH FOLLICLES
MUCOUS GLANDS
CIRCUMVALLATE PAPILLA
TASTE BUDS
FURROW
GLANDS OF EBNER

SCHEMATIC STEREOGRAM: AREA INDICATED ABOVE (MODIFIED FROM BRAUS)

fungiform papillae. In front of the sulcus terminalis runs a V-shaped row of eight to twelve circumvallate papillae, which are still larger, but which rise far more sparsely over the basic surface of the mucous membrane than do the two other types of papillae. The circumvallate, or vallate, papillae are surrounded by a *furrow,* or moat, in the bottom of which the ducts of the glands of Ebner open (see below). The whole mucosa of the anterior two thirds of the tongue is firmly adherent to the underlying tissue.

The mucous membrane of the posterior one third or pharyngeal part of the tongue, though smooth and glistening, has an uneven or nodular surface, which owes its existence to the presence of a varying number (35 to 100) of rounded elevations with a crypt in the center. These elevations, or "nodules", consist of lymphoid tissue lying under the epithelium. The lymphoid nodules, or lymph follicles, are grouped

around the epithelium-lined crypt or pit and, taken collectively, are called the *lingual tonsil.*

On both margins of the tongue, the mucous membrane is thinner and, for the most part, devoid of papillae, though a variable number of vertical folds may be found on the posterior part of each margin. They are called "folia", or *foliate papillae,* and represent rudimentary structures of the well-developed foliate papillae seen in rodents.

The mucous membrane of the inferior surface is thin, smooth, devoid of papillae and more loosely attached to the underlying tissue. It exhibits the midline frenulum and some rather rudimentary fimbriated folds, which run posterolaterally from the tip of the tongue. The frenulum is a duplication of the mucous membrane and connects the inferior lingual surface with the floor of the mouth (see also pages

(*Continued on page 11*)

TONGUE

(Continued from page 10)

3 and 14). The deep lingual veins usually shine through the mucosa between the frenulum and the fimbriated folds on each side.

Many small glands are scattered in and beneath the mucous membrane and are also partly embedded in the muscle. *Mucous glands* are located in the posterior third of the dorsum, with their ducts opening on the dorsum and into the pits of the lingual tonsil. In the region of the circumvallate papillae, the purely serous *glands of Ebner* send numerous ducts (from four to thirty-eight) into the furrows surrounding each of these papillae. Glands of a mixed type, the lingual glands of Blandin and Nuhn, are found to each side of the midline under the apex of the tongue and a little behind it.

The receptor organs for the sense of taste, the *taste buds,* are pale oval bodies (about 70μ in their long axis), seen microscopically in the epithelium of the tongue and to a much lesser extent in the epithelium of the soft palate, pharynx and epiglottis. The greatest number of taste buds is situated in the epithelial lining of the furrows surrounding the circumvallate papillae. A few taste buds are present on the fungiform papillae and also, though occasionally only in a rather scattered fashion, on the foliate papillae. A taste bud reaches from the basement membrane to the epithelial surface, where a *pore* is situated, into which the taste hairs of the neuro-epithelial *taste cells* extend. From four to twenty taste cells are intermingled with the more numerous supporting (*sustentacular*) cells of the taste buds. A general chemical gustatory sensibility probably exists in regions where no taste buds occur.

The greater mass of the tongue is made up of voluntary striated muscles, which are, as seen microscopically, composed of bundles of fasciculi, interlaced in many directions. An incomplete median septum (see page 15) divides the tongue into symmetrical halves. One group of muscles, the extrinsic ones, originates outside of the tongue, whereas the intrinsic group of lingual muscles originates and inserts entirely within the tongue. The *genioglossus muscle* arises from the superior mental spine of the mandible and fans out to the entire length of the dorsum, with the lowest fibers having some attachment to the hyoid bone. Lateral to this muscle is the *hyoglossus muscle,* which arises from the body of the hyoid bone and from the entire length of the greater and lesser cornua, whence it runs vertically upward. (The part coming from the lesser cornu may be somewhat distinct and is sometimes called the chondroglossus.) The *styloglossus muscle* arises from near the tip of the styloid process and an adjacent part of the stylomandibular ligament. It runs as a band downward and forward onto the side of the tongue. The *palatoglossus muscle* descends from the soft palate,

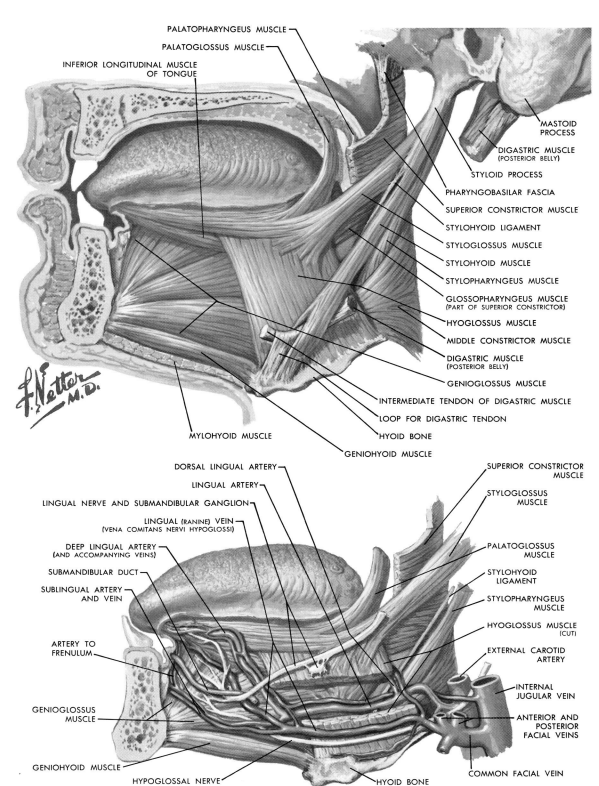

PALATOPHARYNGEUS MUSCLE
PALATOGLOSSUS MUSCLE
INFERIOR LONGITUDINAL MUSCLE OF TONGUE
MASTOID PROCESS
DIGASTRIC MUSCLE (POSTERIOR BELLY)
STYLOID PROCESS
PHARYNGOBASILAR FASCIA
SUPERIOR CONSTRICTOR MUSCLE
STYLOHYOID LIGAMENT
STYLOGLOSSUS MUSCLE
STYLOHYOID MUSCLE
STYLOPHARYNGEUS MUSCLE
GLOSSOPHARYNGEUS MUSCLE (PART OF SUPERIOR CONSTRICTOR)
HYOGLOSSUS MUSCLE
MIDDLE CONSTRICTOR MUSCLE
DIGASTRIC MUSCLE (POSTERIOR BELLY)
GENIOGLOSSUS MUSCLE
INTERMEDIATE TENDON OF DIGASTRIC MUSCLE
LOOP FOR DIGASTRIC TENDON
MYLOHYOID MUSCLE
HYOID BONE
GENIOHYOID MUSCLE

DORSAL LINGUAL ARTERY
LINGUAL ARTERY
LINGUAL NERVE AND SUBMANDIBULAR GANGLION
LINGUAL (RANINE) VEIN (VENA COMITANS NERVI HYPOGLOSSI)
DEEP LINGUAL ARTERY (AND ACCOMPANYING VEINS)
SUBMANDIBULAR DUCT
SUBLINGUAL ARTERY AND VEIN
ARTERY TO FRENULUM
GENIOGLOSSUS MUSCLE
GENIOHYOID MUSCLE
HYPOGLOSSAL NERVE
HYOID BONE
SUPERIOR CONSTRICTOR MUSCLE
STYLOGLOSSUS MUSCLE
PALATOGLOSSUS MUSCLE
STYLOHYOID LIGAMENT
STYLOPHARYNGEUS MUSCLE
HYOGLOSSUS MUSCLE (CUT)
EXTERNAL CAROTID ARTERY
INTERNAL JUGULAR VEIN
ANTERIOR AND POSTERIOR FACIAL VEINS
COMMON FACIAL VEIN

forming the framework of the palatoglossal fold (see also pages 15 and 16).

The intrinsic lingual muscles (see page 15) are named according to the three spatial dimensions in which their fascicles run. Of the two longitudinal muscles, the superior stretches along just under the mucous membrane of the dorsum. The inferior longitudinal muscle spreads between the genioglossus and hyoglossus muscles on the undersurface of the tongue.

The contraction of both longitudinal muscles shortens the tongue. The transverse lingual muscle, which is covered by the superior longitudinal muscle, furnishes nearly all of the transversely running fibers and is intermingled with fascicles of the extrinsic muscle group. The vertical lingual muscle is made up of all the vertical fibers, except those supplied by extrinsic muscles, with which it forms a closely woven network.

By the combined actions of all these muscles, the shape of the tongue can be extensively altered, *i.e.,* lengthened, shortened, broadened, narrowed, curved in various directions, protruded and drawn back into the mouth.

The innervation of the tongue (see also pages 29 and 30) involves the following nerves: (1) the hypoglossal nerve, (2) the lingual nerve, which is accompanied by the chorda tympani, and (3) the glossopharyngeal nerve. The hypoglossal nerve supplies all the muscles except the palatoglossus, which receives its innervation from the cranial part of the spinal accessory nerve through the pharyngeal plexus. The functions of the two other nerves are described on page 30.

(Concerning the blood supply and venous or lymphatic drainage see pages 24, 26 and 27, respectively.)

Teeth

The teeth are the structures which are differentiated for the purpose of biting or tearing off the pieces of solid food which enter the oral cavity and for chopping and grinding this food as it is being mixed with saliva in preparation for swallowing. In this process the muscles of mastication are responsible for the movements of the lower teeth in relation to the upper teeth, and the tongue and cheeks are responsible for placing and keeping the food between the teeth as necessary (see pages 72 and 73).

Man develops two sets of teeth, a deciduous set (milk teeth), which begin to come in at about the age of 6 months, and a so-called permanent set, which gradually begin to replace the deciduous set at about the age of 6 years.

The *deciduous teeth* number twenty in all, five on each side of the jaw. Starting at the midline of each jaw and progressing laterally and posteriorly to each side, the deciduous teeth are named in order: *central* (medial) *incisor, lateral incisor, canine* (cuspid), *first molar* and *second molar.* The four teeth of the same name are differentiated by designating which jaw and which side of the jaw, as right or left upper (maxillary) or lower (mandibular) central incisor. The deciduous teeth are smaller than the permanent teeth.

The *permanent teeth,* once all have come in, number thirty-two, eight on each side of the jaw. Starting at the midline of each jaw and progressing laterally and posteriorly to each side, the permanent teeth are named in order: *central* (medial) *incisor, lateral incisor, canine* (cuspid), *first premolar* (bicuspid), *second premolar* (bicuspid), *first molar, second molar* and *third molar* (wisdom tooth). The incisors, and to some extent the canines, are adapted for biting the food, whereas the molars, and to some extent the premolars, are adapted for grinding and pounding the food.

Normally, the upper dental arch is wider than the lower dental arch, and the upper incisors and canines overlap the lower incisors and canines. When the jaws are closed (in occlusion), the teeth of the two jaws come into contact in such a way that their chewing surfaces fit each other, which means that the teeth of one jaw are not exactly opposite the corresponding teeth of the other jaw. In spite of this, since the lower molars, especially the third molars, are longer anteroposteriorly, the dental arches end at approximately the same place posteriorly. The labial or buccal surface, the lingual surface and the contact, masticating or occlusal, surface of a tooth

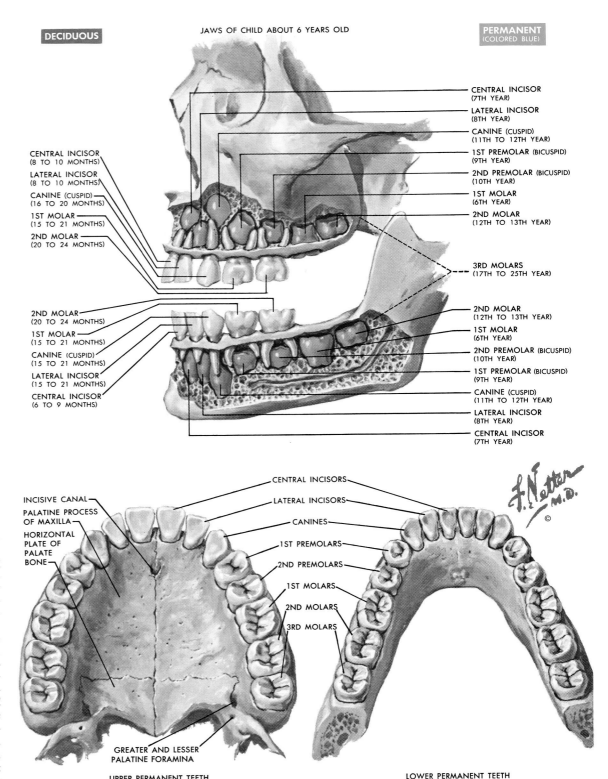

are descriptive terms which are self-explanatory.

Ordinarily, none of the teeth have erupted before birth, but all of the deciduous teeth usually come in between the sixth month and the end of the second year. The time of eruption of the individual teeth varies considerably as does any timetable of development. The possible range of the time at which each deciduous tooth may erupt is indicated in the parentheses below the name of each tooth in the accompanying illustration.

From the end of the second year until the sixth year, as a rule, no visible change in the teeth takes place. At about the sixth year, the first permanent molar comes in behind the second deciduous molar, and it is important that this be recognized as a permanent tooth and given the care which a permanent tooth merits. Starting with the seventh year, a gradual replacement of the deciduous teeth by the perma-

nent teeth takes place, which is usually completed by the twelfth year. The second molar, as a rule, emerges about this time, and the third molar, if it erupts at all, several years later. The approximate time at which each permanent tooth may erupt is specified in the picture below the name of the tooth. The developing permanent teeth are in the jaw long before the time of their eruption. Obviously, during the eruption of the teeth, growth changes must occur in the jaws.

The *crown* of a tooth is the portion of the tooth projecting beyond the gum. It differs in shape in different types of teeth, the difference being related to the functional adaptation of the tooth. The crown of an incisor is chisel-shaped, that of a canine is large and more conical, and the crowns of the premolars and molars are flattened and broad, with tubercles.

(*Continued on page 13*)

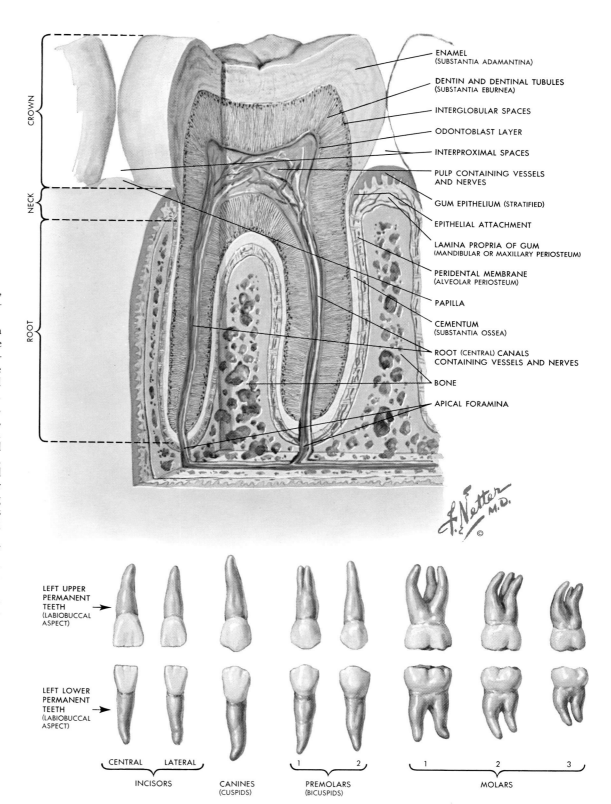

ENAMEL
(SUBSTANTIA ADAMANTINA)

DENTIN AND DENTINAL TUBULES
(SUBSTANTIA EBURNEA)

INTERGLOBULAR SPACES

ODONTOBLAST LAYER

INTERPROXIMAL SPACES

PULP CONTAINING VESSELS
AND NERVES

GUM EPITHELIUM (STRATIFIED)

EPITHELIAL ATTACHMENT

LAMINA PROPRIA OF GUM
(MANDIBULAR OR MAXILLARY PERIOSTEUM)

PERIDENTAL MEMBRANE
(ALVEOLAR PERIOSTEUM)

PAPILLA

CEMENTUM
(SUBSTANTIA OSSEA)

ROOT (CENTRAL) CANALS
CONTAINING VESSELS AND NERVES

BONE

APICAL FORAMINA

CROWN

NECK

ROOT

LEFT UPPER
PERMANENT
TEETH
(LABIOBUCCAL
ASPECT)

LEFT LOWER
PERMANENT
TEETH
(LABIOBUCCAL
ASPECT)

CENTRAL   LATERAL

INCISORS

CANINES
(CUSPIDS)

1   2

PREMOLARS
(BICUSPIDS)

1   2   3

MOLARS

TEETH

(Continued from page 12)

The *neck* of a tooth is the short, faintly constricted portion which connects the crown and the root.

The *root* of a tooth is the portion embedded in the alveolar process of the jaw. It is long, tapering, conical or flattened and is well fitted to its socket. The root of an incisor is usually single and conical, the canine has a single long root, and that of a premolar is usually single, flattened anteroposteriorly and grooved, with some tendency to division. Each molar has two roots, an anterior root and a posterior root, which is apt to be wide, flattened anteroposteriorly, grooved and perhaps partially divided. At the tip or tips of each root is a minute opening called the *apical foramen,* which allows passage into a related root canal for blood vessels and nerves.

In the interior of a tooth is a space of some size called the cavity of the tooth (pulp cavity), which is filled in the natural state by loose connective tissue, *capillaries, nerves* and *lymphatics,* collectively called the *pulp,* on the outer surface of which is a layer of cells called *odontoblasts.* The cavity is prolonged into each root as the slender tapering *root canal,* which ends at the apical foramen.

Surrounding the cavity is the *dentin* (ivory), which constitutes the mass of the tooth and is a hard, highly calcified (only 28 per cent organic matter), homogeneous material. It is traversed by *dentinal tubules* (dental canaliculi) extending from the cavity to the outer margin of the dentin. The dentinal tubules are occupied by processes of the odontoblasts.

Forming a cap over the dentin of the crown is the *enamel,* which is the hardest (containing only about 3 per cent organic material) and most resistant material in the body. It is dense, white and glistening and is made up of solid, hexagonal prisms (enamel prisms) which are oriented essentially perpendicular to the related surface of the crown.

Cementum, a modified bone having lamellae, canaliculi and lacunae, covers the dentin of the roots of the teeth. It is very thin at its beginning at the neck and increases in thickness toward the apex of the root.

The root of the tooth is united to the wall of the socket by an important layer of vascular fibrous connective tissue, the alveolar periosteum or *peridental* (perio-

dontal) *membrane.* This layer is continuous with the lamina propria of the gum at the margin of the alveolar process (region of the neck of the tooth).

The covering of the internal and external surfaces of the alveolar processes of the maxilla and mandible, the *gums* or *gingivae,* is made up of stratified *squamous epithelium,* resting on a thick, strong *lamina propria,* which is firmly attached to the underlying bone. This, being a fusion of mucous membrane and periosteum, could be called mucoperiosteum. The gum forms a free fold, which surrounds the base of the crown of the tooth for a short distance like a collar.

The blood vessels and nerves of the teeth go partly to the pulp cavity and partly to the surrounding peridental membrane. The branches to the pulp cavity reach it by way of the apical foramen and root canal. The vessels form a rich capillary plexus under the odontoblast layer. It is not known whether the nerves

send branches into the dentinal tubules. The arteries and nerves are branches of the superior and inferior alveolar arteries (see page 25) and nerves (see page 29).

The enamel of the tooth comes from the oral ectoderm, and the rest of the tooth comes from the mesenchymal tissue of the maxillary and mandibular arches. An invagination of oral ectoderm in relation to each jaw forms a dental lamina internal to the labial groove and twenty cup-shaped expansions from the lamina form the enamel organs of the twenty deciduous teeth. Each enamel organ caps over condensed mesenchyme, called a dental papilla. Enamel organs for the permanent incisor, canine and premolar teeth arise from the stalks of the enamel organs of the corresponding deciduous teeth, and the enamel organs for the three molars of each jaw come from a process from the posterior end of the dental lamina.

SALIVARY GLANDS

Numerous glands pour the watery, more or less viscous fluid, known as saliva, into the oral cavity. Small salivary glands are widely scattered under the lining of the oral cavity and are named, according to their location, labial, buccal, palatine (see pages 7 and 16) and lingual (see page 10) glands. The three chief, large, paired salivary glands are the parotid, the submandibular and the sublingual.

The *parotid gland,* the largest of the salivary glands, is roughly a three-sided wedge, which is fitted in below and in front of the external ear. The triangular superficial surface of the wedge is practically subcutaneous, with one side of the triangle almost as high as the zygomatic arch and the opposing angle at the level of the angle of the mandible. The anteromedial side of the wedge abuts against and overlaps the ramus of the mandible and the related masseter and internal pterygoid muscles. The posteromedial side of the wedge turns toward the external auditory canal, the mastoid process and the sternocleidomastoid and digastric (posterior belly) muscles (see page 15). The *parotid* (Stensen's) *duct* leaves the anterior border of the gland and passes forward superficial to the *masseter muscle,* at the anterior border of which it turns medially to pierce the *buccinator muscle* and then the mucous membrane of the cheek near the second maxillary molar tooth (see page 3).

The *submandibular* (submaxillary) *gland* lies in the submandibular triangle but overlaps all three sides of the triangle, extending superficial to the anterior and posterior bellies of the *digastric muscle* and deep to the mandible, where it lies in the submandibular fossa (see page 4). The bulk of the gland is superficial to the *mylohyoid muscle,* but a deep process extends deep to this muscle (compare page 15, lower figure). The submandibular (Wharton's) duct (visible on pages 3 and 6) runs forward at first with the deep process of the gland, then in relation to the sublingual gland (first inferior and then medial to it) to reach the *sublingual caruncle* at the summit of which it opens.

The *sublingual gland,* the smallest of the three paired large salivary glands, is

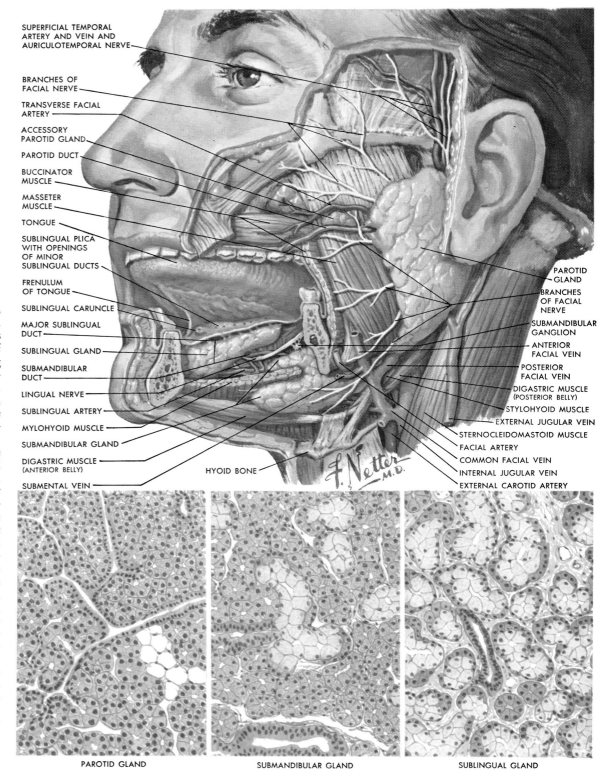

SUPERFICIAL TEMPORAL ARTERY AND VEIN AND AURICULOTEMPORAL NERVE

BRANCHES OF FACIAL NERVE

TRANSVERSE FACIAL ARTERY

ACCESSORY PAROTID GLAND

PAROTID DUCT

BUCCINATOR MUSCLE

MASSETER MUSCLE

TONGUE

SUBLINGUAL PLICA WITH OPENINGS OF MINOR SUBLINGUAL DUCTS

FRENULUM OF TONGUE

SUBLINGUAL CARUNCLE

MAJOR SUBLINGUAL DUCT

SUBLINGUAL GLAND

SUBMANDIBULAR DUCT

LINGUAL NERVE

SUBLINGUAL ARTERY

MYLOHYOID MUSCLE

SUBMANDIBULAR GLAND

DIGASTRIC MUSCLE (ANTERIOR BELLY)

SUBMENTAL VEIN

HYOID BONE

PAROTID GLAND

BRANCHES OF FACIAL NERVE

SUBMANDIBULAR GANGLION

ANTERIOR FACIAL VEIN

POSTERIOR FACIAL VEIN

DIGASTRIC MUSCLE (POSTERIOR BELLY)

STYLOHYOID MUSCLE

EXTERNAL JUGULAR VEIN

STERNOCLEIDOMASTOID MUSCLE

FACIAL ARTERY

COMMON FACIAL VEIN

INTERNAL JUGULAR VEIN

EXTERNAL CAROTID ARTERY

PAROTID GLAND   SUBMANDIBULAR GLAND   SUBLINGUAL GLAND

located beneath the mucous membrane of the floor of the mouth, where it produces the sublingual fold (see page 3). It lies superior to the mylohyoid muscle in relation with the sublingual fossa on the mandible (see page 4). In contrast to the parotid and submandibular glands, which have quite definite fibrous capsules, the lobules of the sublingual gland are loosely held together by connective tissue. About twelve *sublingual ducts* leave the superior aspect of the gland and, for the most part, open individually through the mucous membrane of the sublingual fold. Some of the ducts from the anterior part of the gland may combine and empty into the submandibular duct. This is apparently quite an individually variable situation.

The nerve supply of the large salivary glands is discussed on page 31.

Microscopically, the large salivary glands appear as compound tubulo-alveolar glands. The tubulo-alveolar portions of the glands are serous and mucous and mucous with serous demilunes (see also page 71), with different proportions of these in different glands. As can be seen, the parotid gland is entirely serous in nature, the submandibular gland is predominantly serous but with some mucous alveoli with serous demilunes, and the sublingual gland varies to quite an extent in composition in different parts of the gland but, for the most part, is predominantly mucous with serous demilunes. In the parotid and submandibular glands, the alveoli are joined by intercalated ducts with low epithelium to portions of the duct system, which are thought to contribute water and salts to the secretion and, hence, are called secretory ducts. The epithelium of the ducts is at first columnar, then pseudostratified and finally stratified near the opening of the duct.

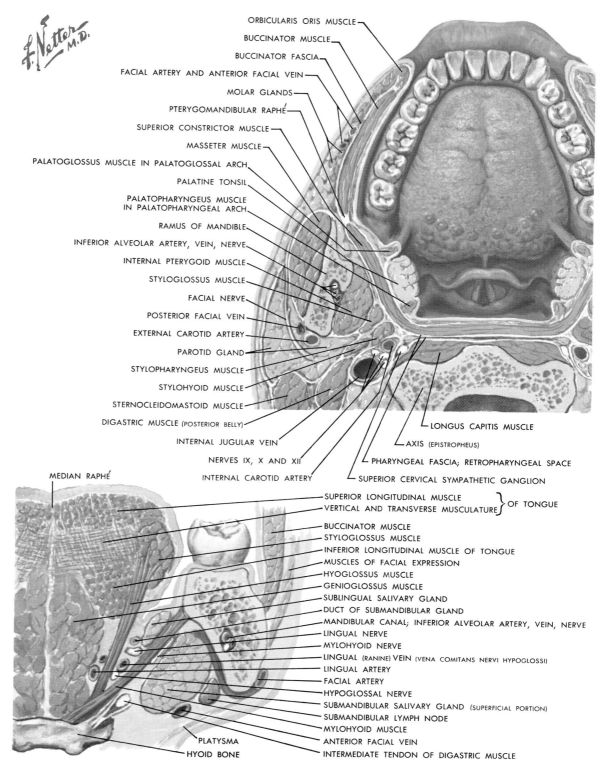

F. Netter M.D.

ORBICULARIS ORIS MUSCLE
BUCCINATOR MUSCLE
BUCCINATOR FASCIA
FACIAL ARTERY AND ANTERIOR FACIAL VEIN
MOLAR GLANDS
PTERYGOMANDIBULAR RAPHÉ
SUPERIOR CONSTRICTOR MUSCLE
MASSETER MUSCLE
PALATOGLOSSUS MUSCLE IN PALATOGLOSSAL ARCH
PALATINE TONSIL
PALATOPHARYNGEUS MUSCLE IN PALATOPHARYNGEAL ARCH
RAMUS OF MANDIBLE
INFERIOR ALVEOLAR ARTERY, VEIN, NERVE
INTERNAL PTERYGOID MUSCLE
STYLOGLOSSUS MUSCLE
FACIAL NERVE
POSTERIOR FACIAL VEIN
EXTERNAL CAROTID ARTERY
PAROTID GLAND
STYLOPHARYNGEUS MUSCLE
STYLOHYOID MUSCLE
STERNOCLEIDOMASTOID MUSCLE
DIGASTRIC MUSCLE (POSTERIOR BELLY)
INTERNAL JUGULAR VEIN
NERVES IX, X AND XII
INTERNAL CAROTID ARTERY

LONGUS CAPITIS MUSCLE
AXIS (EPISTROPHEUS)
PHARYNGEAL FASCIA; RETROPHARYNGEAL SPACE
SUPERIOR CERVICAL SYMPATHETIC GANGLION

MEDIAN RAPHÉ

SUPERIOR LONGITUDINAL MUSCLE } OF TONGUE
VERTICAL AND TRANSVERSE MUSCULATURE }
BUCCINATOR MUSCLE
STYLOGLOSSUS MUSCLE
INFERIOR LONGITUDINAL MUSCLE OF TONGUE
MUSCLES OF FACIAL EXPRESSION
HYOGLOSSUS MUSCLE
GENIOGLOSSUS MUSCLE
SUBLINGUAL SALIVARY GLAND
DUCT OF SUBMANDIBULAR GLAND
MANDIBULAR CANAL; INFERIOR ALVEOLAR ARTERY, VEIN, NERVE
LINGUAL NERVE
MYLOHYOID NERVE
LINGUAL (RANINE) VEIN (VENA COMITANS NERVI HYPOGLOSSI)
LINGUAL ARTERY
FACIAL ARTERY
HYPOGLOSSAL NERVE
SUBMANDIBULAR SALIVARY GLAND (SUPERFICIAL PORTION)
SUBMANDIBULAR LYMPH NODE
MYLOHYOID MUSCLE
ANTERIOR FACIAL VEIN
INTERMEDIATE TENDON OF DIGASTRIC MUSCLE

PLATYSMA
HYOID BONE

FRONTAL SECTION BEHIND 1ST MOLAR TOOTH

SECTIONS THROUGH MOUTH AND JAW

At Atlas Level and Behind First Molar

The structures illustrated and discussed individually in the preceding pages are shown in these sections — one vertical, the other frontal — in their mutual topographic relationships. The cheek is formed essentially by the *buccinator muscle* and its fascia, with the skin and its appendages, including fat, glands and connective tissue, covering it on the outside and the oral mucosa on the inside.

The continuity of oral and oropharyngeal wall, as it becomes visible in this cross section, may attain some practical significance in abscess formation and other pathologic processes. One should realize that the buccinator muscle is separated only by the small fascial structure, the pterygomandibular raphé, from the superior constrictor muscle of the pharynx, which constitutes the most substantial component of the oropharyngeal wall. The thin *pharyngeal fascia*, creating by the looseness of its structure a retropharyngeal space, separates the posterior wall of the pharynx from the vertebral column and prevertebral muscles.

The tonsillar bed (see page 16), as it lies between the anterior (*palatoglossal*) and the posterior (*palatopharyngeal*) arch, is easier to comprehend in a cross section.

Supplementing the picture of the external aspect of the *parotid gland* (see page 14), the cross section demonstrates the thin medial margin of the gland and its relation to the muscles arising from the styloid process (*stylohyoid, stylopharyngeus* and *styloglossus muscles*), the *internal jugular vein* and the *internal carotid artery*. Noteworthy, furthermore, is the closeness of the most medial part of the parotid gland to the lateral wall of the pharynx and the location within the glandular substance of the *posterior facial vein* (beginning above the level of the cross section by the confluence of the superficial temporal and maxillary veins, see page 26), the facial nerve and the external carotid artery, which latter

divides higher up, but still within the gland, into the superficial temporal and internal maxillary arteries (see page 25).

The frontal or coronal section of the tongue brings into view the mutual relationships of its muscular components (discussed on pages 10 and 11) and, particularly, the median septum dividing the tongue into symmetrical halves. The *lingual artery* takes its course medial to the genioglossus muscle, whereas the main *lingual vein,* the *hypoglossal* and *lingual nerves* and the *duct of the submandibular gland* lie lateral to the genioglossus and medial to the mylohyoid muscle. Located inferior and lateral to the latter muscle is the main body of the submandibular gland. Its lateral margin touches the mandible, only separated from it at the level of the section by the *facial artery.* On the deep surface of the mylohyoid muscle appears also the posterior end of the third (sublin-

gual) salivary gland in a location which would be occupied by the deep process of the submandibular gland in a section made only slightly more posteriorly. As the result of the crossings of lingual nerve and submandibular duct, the apparent situation of these two structures in the cross section would be reversed if one were to obtain a more anterior section (cf. page 14).

The *mandibular canal* harbors the *inferior alveolar artery, vein* and *nerve.* The *intermediate tendon of the digastric muscle* passes through the fascial loop which anchors it to the *hyoid bone.*

With the two reflections — one from the inferior surface of the tongue across the floor of the mouth to the gum on the inner aspect of the alveolar process of the mandible, the other from the outer surface of this process to the cheek — the lining of the oral cavity by the mucous membrane becomes continuous.

FAUCES

SPHENOIDAL SINUS
PHARYNGEAL TONSIL
TORUS TUBARIUS

PHARYNGEAL TUBERCLE (OCCIPITAL BONE)
PHARYNGOBASILAR FASCIA
OPENING OF EUSTACHIAN TUBE

HARD PALATE
PHARYNGEAL RECESS
SALPINGOPHARYNGEAL FOLD
PALATINE GLANDS
SOFT PALATE

UVULA

SUPRATONSILLAR FOSSA
PALATINE TONSIL

PHARYNGOPALATINE FOLD
GLOSSOPALATINE FOLD
ORAL PHARYNX
TRIANGULAR FOLD
TONGUE (DRAWN FORWARD)
LINGUAL TONSIL
PHARYNGO-EPIGLOTTIC FOLD
EPIGLOTTIS
PIRIFORM FOSSA
VALLECULA OF EPIGLOTTIS

EUSTACHIAN TUBE (CARTILAGE)
MEDIAL PTERYGOID PLATE
TENSOR VELI PALATINI MUSCLE AND TENDON
LEVATOR VELI PALATINI MUSCLE
ASCENDING PALATINE ARTERY
ASCENDING PHARYNGEAL ARTERY (PHARYNGEAL BRANCH)
LESSER PALATINE ARTERY
SALPINGOPHARYNGEUS MUSCLE
PTERYGOID HAMULUS
PTERYGOMANDIBULAR RAPHÉ
TONSILLAR BRANCH OF LESSER PALATINE ARTERY
SUPERIOR CONSTRICTOR MUSCLE
TONSILLAR BRANCH OF ASCENDING PHARYNGEAL ARTERY
PALATOGLOSSUS MUSCLE
PALATOPHARYNGEUS MUSCLE

STYLOPHARYNGEUS MUSCLE
MIDDLE CONSTRICTOR MUSCLE
STYLOHYOID LIGAMENT
HYOGLOSSUS MUSCLE
GLOSSOPHARYNGEAL NERVE AND TONSILLAR BRANCH
TONSILLAR BRANCH OF ASCENDING PALATINE ARTERY
TONSILLAR ARTERY (BRANCH OF FACIAL ARTERY)
TONSILLAR BRANCH OF DORSAL LINGUAL ARTERY

PALATINE TONSIL (HEMATOXYLIN–EOSIN, X 39/2)

The connotation given to the term "fauces" varies. Though complete agreement exists as to the general region to which the term refers, the agreement of various authors is less complete or less definite as to exactly what is included in this area, which covers, in general, the passage from the oral cavity into the pharynx. By most authors, the designation "isthmus faucium", or oropharyngeal isthmus, is taken to mean the aperture by which the mouth communicates with the pharynx, i.e., the dividing line between the oral cavity and the oral pharynx. The boundaries of this isthmus are the soft palate superiorly, the dorsum of the tongue in the region of the sulcus terminalis inferiorly, and the left and right palatoglossal folds, which rise arch-like (anterior pillars of the fauces) on each side in the posterior limit of the oral cavity (see page 3).

Farther back, a second arch is formed by the *pharyngopalatine* (or palatopharyngeal) *folds*, also called the posterior pillars of the fauces. As a result of the projecting prominence of the anterior and posterior folds on each side, a fossa (tonsillar fossa or tonsillar sinus) comes into existence, which houses the faucial or *palatine tonsil*. On the free surface of this oval mass, which may bulge forward into the cavity of the pharynx for varying distances, twelve to fifteen orifices (fossulae tonsillares) can be recognized. These are the openings of the tonsillar crypts. The latter, also considered as recesses or pits, branch and extend deeply into the substances of the tonsils. Several quite variable folds may overlap the medial surface of the tonsils in different degrees. Most frequently found is a *triangular fold* located anteriorly and inferiorly to the tonsils. Also, between the superior portions of the palatoglossal and palatopharyngeal folds, one may encounter frequently a supratonsillar fold which contains tonsillar tissue, a fact which has prompted some authors to call the recess below this fold the intratonsillar recess (or fossa), while others designate it as "supratonsillar". The lateral surface of the tonsil has a fibrous capsule, which is separated by some loose connective tissue from the *superior constrictor muscle* of the pharynx and, to a lesser and variable degree, from the *palatopharyngeus muscle*.

The chief blood supply of the tonsil is the *tonsillar branch of the facial* (external maxillary) *artery*, but the tonsillar branches of the lesser palatine, *ascending palatine, ascending pharyngeal* and *dorsal lingual arteries* also participate in the arterial blood supply. Efferent lymphatics from the tonsil go mostly to the jugulodigastric node of the superior deep cervical group (see pages 27 and 28). The tonsil is innervated primarily by the *glossopharyngeal nerve,* though a few branches of the lesser palatine nerves enter the tonsils also.

A stratified, squamous epithelium covers the tonsil and also lines the crypts, where it may be obscured by lymphocytic infiltration. The mass of the tonsils consists of lymphatic (lymphoid) tissue, which presents itself mostly in the form of lymph nodules or follicles, which, particularly in younger individuals, contain many germinal centers. Expansions from the above-mentioned fibrous capsule on the lateral tonsillar surface enter the lymphoid tissue, forming septa between the follicles surrounding the adjacent crypts.

Present at birth and increasing in size rapidly during the first few years of life, the tonsils usually decrease in size about puberty and may become atrophic in old age.

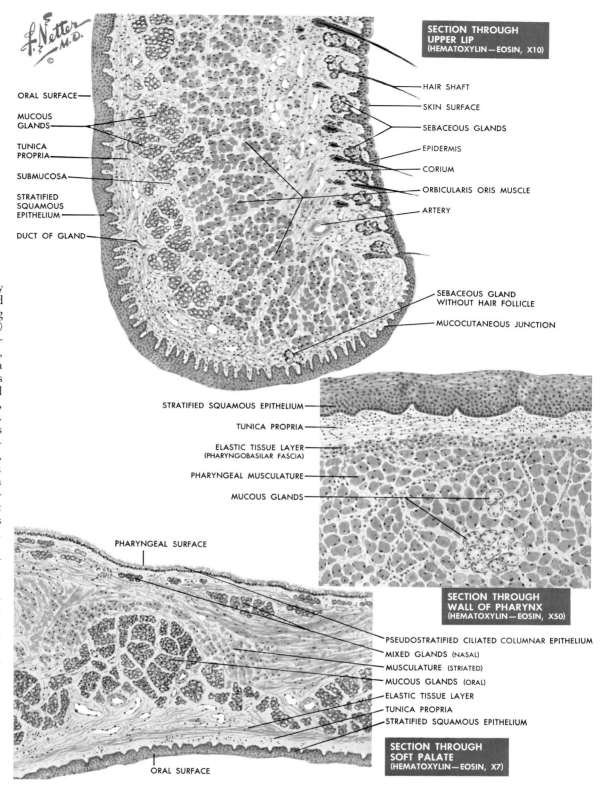

ORAL SURFACE

MUCOUS GLANDS

TUNICA PROPRIA

SUBMUCOSA

STRATIFIED SQUAMOUS EPITHELIUM

DUCT OF GLAND

SECTION THROUGH UPPER LIP (HEMATOXYLIN—EOSIN, X10)

HAIR SHAFT

SKIN SURFACE

SEBACEOUS GLANDS

EPIDERMIS

CORIUM

ORBICULARIS ORIS MUSCLE

ARTERY

SEBACEOUS GLAND WITHOUT HAIR FOLLICLE

MUCOCUTANEOUS JUNCTION

STRATIFIED SQUAMOUS EPITHELIUM

TUNICA PROPRIA

ELASTIC TISSUE LAYER (PHARYNGOBASILAR FASCIA)

PHARYNGEAL MUSCULATURE

MUCOUS GLANDS

SECTION THROUGH WALL OF PHARYNX (HEMATOXYLIN—EOSIN, X50)

PHARYNGEAL SURFACE

PSEUDOSTRATIFIED CILIATED COLUMNAR EPITHELIUM

MIXED GLANDS (NASAL)

MUSCULATURE (STRIATED)

MUCOUS GLANDS (ORAL)

ELASTIC TISSUE LAYER

TUNICA PROPRIA

STRATIFIED SQUAMOUS EPITHELIUM

SECTION THROUGH SOFT PALATE (HEMATOXYLIN—EOSIN, X7)

ORAL SURFACE

HISTOLOGY OF MOUTH AND PHARYNX

The mouth and pharynx are lined by a mucous membrane which is attached in much of the area to the supporting wall (bone, cartilage or skeletal muscle) by a fibro-elastic, gland-containing sub-mucosa which varies greatly in amount, looseness and the distinctness with which it can be delimited from the mucous membrane. The submucosa is interpreted as absent on most of the hard palate, the gums and the dorsum of the tongue. The mucosa (mucous membrane) is composed of the epithelium, which is predominantly nonkeratinizing, stratified, squamous in type; a basement membrane; and the fibro-elastic lamina propria, which has vascular papillae indenting the epithelium to varying degrees in different areas. The muscularis mucosae, which is present in the digestive tube in general, is missing in the mouth and pharynx. Its place is occupied by an elastic network in the pharynx.

The *lip* has a framework of skeletal muscle, chiefly the *orbicularis oris muscle* (see page 8). External to this are typical subcutaneous tissue and skin with hair follicles, sebaceous glands and sweat glands. On the inner side of the muscular framework is the submucosa containing rounded groups of mixed, predominantly *mucous glands* (labial glands). The *submucosa* is not definitely delimited from the covering mucous membrane, which is composed, as described above, of *tunica propria* and noncornified, *stratified, squamous epithelium*. The free margin of the lip has its characteristic red color because the epithelial cells contain much translucent eleidin, and the vascular papillae of the tunica propria indent the epithelium more deeply here. The blood in the capillaries thus shows through to a greater extent. The deeper cells of the epithelium on the free margin of the lip appear swollen and somewhat vacuolated.

The general structure of the cheek (see page 15) is very similar to that of the lip, the muscular framework being formed by the buccinator muscle. Here some glands are external to the muscular framework. In most of the area of both the lip and the cheek, the mucous membrane is quite closely bound to the muscular framework, which prevents large folds of mucous membrane from being formed, which might be easily bitten.

Near the continuity of the mucous membrane with the gums, the attachment is much looser to allow for freedom of movement.

The *soft palate* (see page 7) has a fibromuscular framework, with the fibrous constituents being more prominent near the hard palate (the expansion of the tendons of the tensor veli palatini muscles). On each side of the framework is a mucous membrane. That on the oral side has an elastic layer separating the lamina propria from a much thicker submucosa containing many glands. The *epithelium* is the typical nonkeratinizing, *stratified, squamous* variety, which rounds the free margin of the soft palate and extends for a variable distance onto the pharyngeal surface. The rest of the pharyngeal surface has *pseudostratified, ciliated, columnar epithelium*. The *tunica propria* and submucosa on this surface are much thinner and contain fewer glands.

The *wall of the pharynx* is for the most part composed of a mucous membrane, a muscular layer and a variable thin fibrous sheath outside of the muscle which attaches the pharynx to adjacent structures. The *epithelium* in the nasopharynx (except for its lower portion) is pseudostratified, ciliated, columnar, while that of the rest of the pharynx is nonkeratinizing, *stratified, squamous*. The *tunica propria* is fibro-elastic, with scattered small papillae indenting the epithelium. The deepest part of this lamina is a definite *elastic tissue layer*, many fibers of which are oriented longitudinally. A well-developed submucosa is present only in the lateral extent of the nasopharynx and near the continuity of the pharynx with the esophagus. Scattered *seromucous glands* are present, mostly where there is pseudostratified epithelium. The muscular layer, made up of skeletal muscle, is present as somewhat irregularly arranged layers.

FRONTAL SINUS

SELLA TURCICA SPHENOID SINUS

PHARYNGEAL OSTIUM OF EUSTACHIAN TUBE
PHARYNGEAL TONSIL
SPHENO-OCCIPITAL SUTURE
PHARYNGEAL TUBERCLE (OF OCCIPITAL BONE)
PHARYNGOBASILAR FASCIA
ANTERIOR LONGITUDINAL LIGAMENT
ANTERIOR ATLANTO-OCCIPITAL LIGAMENT
APICAL LIGAMENT OF DENS

NASAL SEPTUM
NASOPHARYNX
SOFT PALATE
PALATINE GLANDS
HARD PALATE
ORAL CAVITY
INCISIVE CANAL
BODY OF TONGUE
ORAL PHARYNX
PALATINE TONSIL
ORBICULARIS ORIS MUSCLE
FORAMEN CECUM
GENIOGLOSSUS MUSCLE
LINGUAL TONSIL
ROOT OF TONGUE
MANDIBLE
GENIOHYOID MUSCLE
MYLOHYOID MUSCLE
HYOID BONE
HYO-EPIGLOTTIC LIGAMENT

C1
C2
C5
C7
T1
C1
C2

EPIGLOTTIS
THYROHYOID MEMBRANE
LARYNGEAL PHARYNX (HYPOPHARYNX)
LARYNGEAL ADITUS
THYROID CARTILAGE
VOCAL CORD
TRANSVERSE ARYTENOID MUSCLE
CRICOID CARTILAGE
TRACHEA
ESOPHAGUS
CERVICAL FASCIA (ENVELOPING LAYER)
THYROID GLAND (ISTHMUS)
VERTEBRAL BODIES
PREVERTEBRAL FASCIA AND ANTERIOR LONGITUDINAL LIG.
ESOPHAGEAL MUSCULATURE
SUPRASTERNAL SPACE
STERNUM

SURFACE PROJECTION

PHARYNX

The pharynx is a musculomembranous tube, with much of its anterior wall absent, owing to the fact that the right and left nasal cavities as well as the oral and laryngeal cavities open into it from in front. It extends from the base of the skull, above, to the lower border of the cricoid cartilage at the level of the lower margin of the sixth cervical vertebra, where it is continuous with the esophagus. In addition to the cavities already listed, the pharynx also communicates by means of the auditory (*Eustachian*) *tube* with the right and left tympanic cavities (a fact worthy of mention because infection may spread from the pharynx to the middle ear), making a total of seven cavities with which it has communication. The transverse diameter exceeds the anteroposterior diameter, which is greatest superiorly and is diminished to nothing inferiorly where the anterior and posterior walls are in contact, except when separated by contents, *e.g.*, during the act of swallowing (see pages 74 and 75). The transverse diameter does not differ greatly throughout the length of the pharynx, except where it narrows rapidly at the lower end.

The posterior wall of the pharynx is attached superiorly to the *pharyngeal tubercle* on the antero-inferior surface of the basilar part of the occipital bone, its adjacent area and the undersurface of the petrous portion of the temporal bone medial to the external aperture of the carotid canal. The lateral wall is attached superiorly to the cartilaginous portion of the auditory tube, which pierces the wall in this area, and anteriorly, from above downward, to the lower part of the posterior border of the medial pterygoid plate and its hamulus, the pterygomandibular raphé, the inner surface of the mandible

near the posterior end of the mylohyoid line, the side of the root of the tongue, the hyoid bone and the thyroid and cricoid cartilages. Inferiorly, the walls of the pharynx continue into the walls of the esophagus.

The pharyngeal lining is a mucous membrane (see page 17), which is continuous with the lining of the cavities communicating with the pharynx (see above). External to the mucous membrane of the posterior and lateral walls is a sheet of fibrous tissue, more definite superiorly than inferiorly, known as the pharyngeal aponeurosis (*pharyngobasilar fascia* or *lamina*), and external to this is the muscular layer (see pages 21, 22 and 23). On the outer surface of the muscular layer is an indefinite fascial covering, the buccopharyngeal fascia. The posterior pharyngeal wall is separated from the prevertebral fascia overlying the anterior arch of atlas and the bodies of the second to the sixth cervical vertebrae (partially cov-

ered by the longus colli and longus capitis muscles) by a minimal amount of loose fibrous connective tissue which allows freedom of movement and forms a "retropharyngeal space". Under anesthesia it is possible to palpate these bony structures as far caudally as the fourth or fifth cervical vertebra.

On the basis of the openings in its anterior wall, the pharynx is divided into the *nasal pharynx* (sometimes called epipharynx), the *oral pharynx* and the *laryngeal pharynx* (also called hypopharynx).

The nasal pharynx which normally has a purely respiratory function (acting as a passageway only for air and not for food), remains patent because of the bony framework to which its walls are related. The anterior wall is entirely occupied by the *choanae* (posterior nares), with the posterior border of the *nasal septum* between them. The posterior wall and

(*Continued on page 19*)

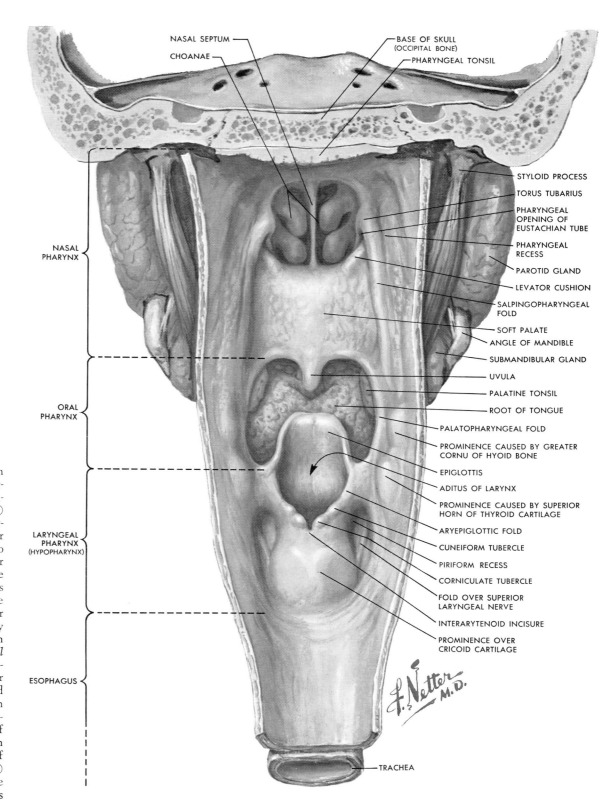

NASAL SEPTUM
CHOANAE
BASE OF SKULL (OCCIPITAL BONE)
PHARYNGEAL TONSIL

NASAL PHARYNX

STYLOID PROCESS
TORUS TUBARIUS
PHARYNGEAL OPENING OF EUSTACHIAN TUBE
PHARYNGEAL RECESS
PAROTID GLAND
LEVATOR CUSHION
SALPINGOPHARYNGEAL FOLD
SOFT PALATE
ANGLE OF MANDIBLE

ORAL PHARYNX

SUBMANDIBULAR GLAND
UVULA
PALATINE TONSIL
ROOT OF TONGUE
PALATOPHARYNGEAL FOLD
PROMINENCE CAUSED BY GREATER CORNU OF HYOID BONE
EPIGLOTTIS
ADITUS OF LARYNX
PROMINENCE CAUSED BY SUPERIOR HORN OF THYROID CARTILAGE

LARYNGEAL PHARYNX (HYPOPHARYNX)

ARYEPIGLOTTIC FOLD
CUNEIFORM TUBERCLE
PIRIFORM RECESS
CORNICULATE TUBERCLE
FOLD OVER SUPERIOR LARYNGEAL NERVE
INTERARYTENOID INCISURE
PROMINENCE OVER CRICOID CARTILAGE

ESOPHAGUS

TRACHEA

PHARYNX

(*Continued from page 18*)

roof form a continuous arched wall, with the roof extending from the superior margin of the choanae (where it is continuous with the roof of the nasal cavities) to about the midpoint of the basilar portion of the occipital bone; the posterior wall extends from this point caudally to about the lower border of the anterior arch of atlas. In the region where the roof and posterior wall meet, the mucous membrane is thrown into many variable folds, with an accumulation of nodular and diffuse lymphoid tissue (extensively developed in children, atrophied in adults) forming the *pharyngeal tonsil* (adenoids). In the midline near the anterior margin of the pharyngeal tonsil, or surrounded by it, is a minute flask-shaped depression of mucous membrane, known as the pharyngeal bursa. Also in the midline, near the anterior limit of the roof and submerged in the mucosa or lying in the periosteum, a microscopic remnant of Rathke's pouch (pharyngeal hypophysis) can be found, which is grossly visible only when it has become cystic or has formed a tumor.

The incomplete floor of the nasal pharynx is formed by the posterosuperior surface of the *soft palate* with an opening from the nasal to the oral pharynx ("pharyngeal isthmus") between the soft palate and the posterior wall of the pharynx. This opening is closed by bringing these two structures in contact.

On the lateral wall of the nasal pharynx (see also page 16) at the level of the inferior concha is the *pharyngeal ostium* of the auditory tube, with the *pharyngeal recess* (fossa of Rosenmüller) posterior to it. The prominence of the posterior lip of the opening facilitates the introduction of a catheter. The levator cushion (produced by the levator veli palatini muscle) bulges into the inferior margin of the triangular opening, and, coursing inferiorly from the posterior lip, is the *salpingopharyngeal fold* produced by the muscle of the same name. In childhood a considerable mass of lymphoid tissue (tubal tonsil) may be present in relation to the opening of the auditory tube and may cause deafness.

The *oral pharynx* extends from the "pharyngeal isthmus" to the level of the pharyngo-epiglottic folds, with the *epiglottis* protruding into it. In this part of the pharynx, the air and food pathways cross. The posterior wall is in relation to the bodies of the second to fourth cervical vertebrae, while the anterior wall is deficient superiorly where the oral pharynx and oral cavity communicate by means of the faucial isthmus. Below this isthmus the anterior wall is formed by the posterior third of the tongue. Between the tongue and epiglottis are the valleculae (see page 10), where foreign bodies may lodge. (For the structures of the lateral wall, see pages 15 and 16.)

The *laryngeal pharynx* (hypopharynx) lies posterior to the larynx and anterior to the fifth and sixth cervical vertebrae. In the cranial part of the anterior wall is the roughly triangular *laryngeal aditus*, the borders of which are formed by the margins of the epiglottis, the *aryepiglottic folds* and the *interarytenoid incisure*. Caudal to this opening the laryngeal pharynx is purely alimentary in function. The mucous membrane of the anterior wall overlies the posterior surfaces of the arytenoid cartilages and the lamina of the *cricoid cartilage* (mostly covered by laryngeal muscles). Caudal to the laryngo-epiglottic fold on each side is the *piriform sinus* (recess or fossa), located between the cricoid and arytenoid cartilages medially and the lamina of the thyroid cartilage laterally. This is one of the locations in which foreign bodies may lodge.

BONY FRAMEWORK OF MOUTH AND PHARYNX

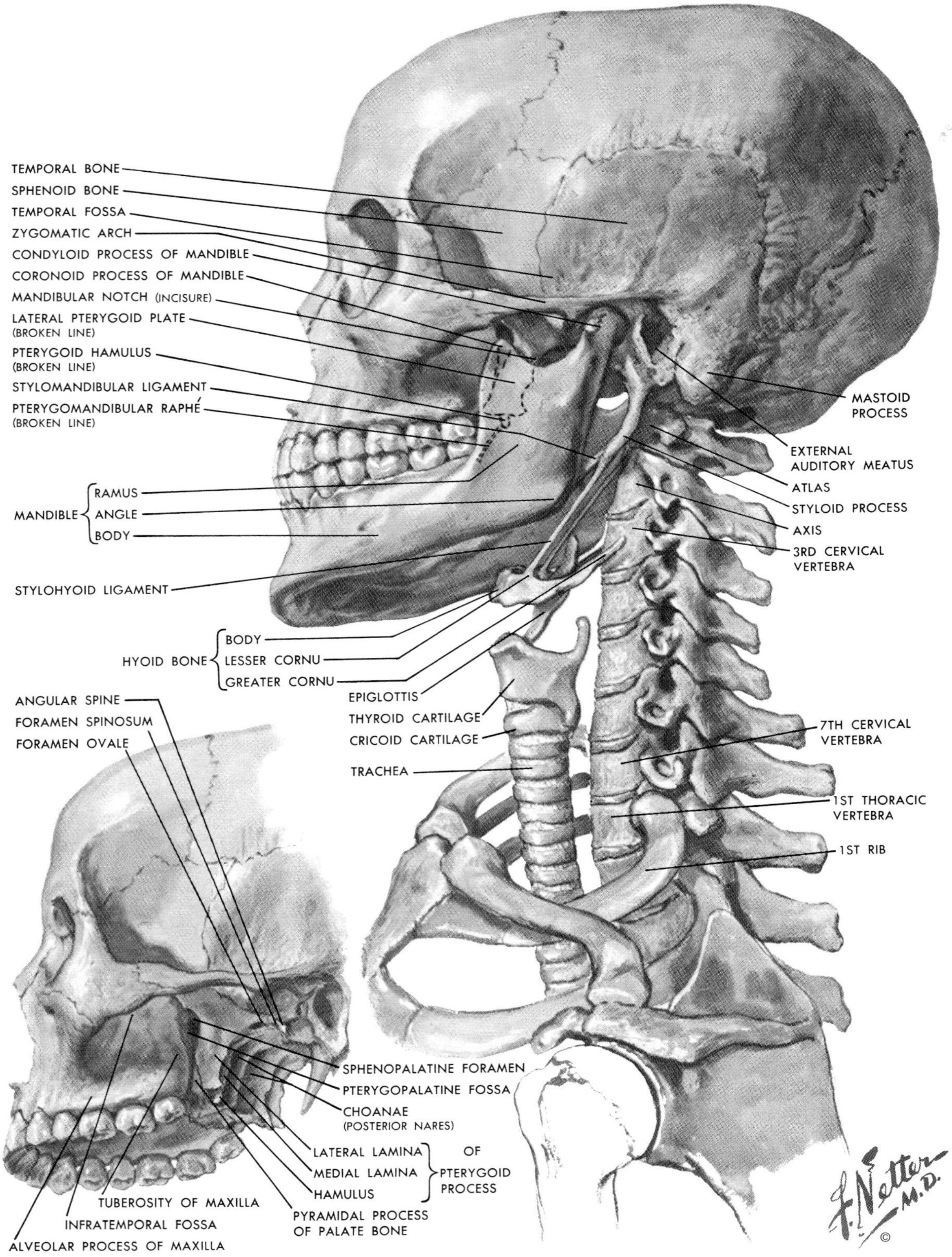

The bony framework of the mouth is composed largely of the two *maxillae,* immovably attached to other bones of the skull, and the freely movable *mandible.* The portions of the maxillae contributing to the formation of the bony palate have been previously described (see page 7, also pages 12 and 18), and the alveolar processes of the maxilla have been referred to as providing the sockets for the upper teeth (see page 13). For a description of the mandible, see page 4.

Other bony structures contributing to the framework of the mouth and pharynx or serving as attachments for muscles of the mouth and pharynx are parts of the palatine bone, parts of the *sphenoid bone,* parts of the *temporal bone,* the *zygomatic arch,* parts of the *occipital bone* and the *hyoid bone.*

The palatine bone is interposed between the maxilla and the *pterygoid process* of the sphenoid bone, and its horizontal portion forms the framework of the posterior part of the hard palate (see page 7). Its pyramidal process is articulated with the lower portions of the medial and lateral pterygoid laminae and helps to complete the pterygoid fossa.

The sphenoid bone, located in the base of the skull with the ethmoid, frontal, palatine and maxillary bones anterior to it and the occipital and temporal bones posterior to it, has the right and left *pterygoid processes* extending inferiorly, each with its lateral and its medial lamina and a hamulus (to which the *pterygomandibular raphé* attaches and around which the tendon of the tensor veli palatini muscle passes) projecting inferiorly from the medial lamina. The greater wing of the sphenoid forms the anterior parts of the *temporal* and infratemporal *fossae.* The (angular) spine of the sphenoid, to which the sphenomandibular ligament (see page 5) attaches, is just medial to the mandibular fossa of the temporal bone.

The *external acoustic (auditory) meatus* is an obvious landmark in the temporal bone to which the portions of this bone pertinent to the present discussion can be related. Posterior to the meatus is the *mastoid process,* on the medial side of which is the mastoid notch, where the posterior belly of the digastric muscle attaches. Antero-inferior to the meatus is the mandibular fossa for the articulation with the condyle of the mandible (see page 5). Inferior to the meatus and posterior to the mandibular fossa is the base of the *styloid process* (see also page 11), which projects for a variable distance inferiorly and slightly anteriorly. The squama of the temporal bone is the

Labels (upper figure):
TEMPORAL BONE
SPHENOID BONE
TEMPORAL FOSSA
ZYGOMATIC ARCH
CONDYLOID PROCESS OF MANDIBLE
CORONOID PROCESS OF MANDIBLE
MANDIBULAR NOTCH (INCISURE)
LATERAL PTERYGOID PLATE (BROKEN LINE)
PTERYGOID HAMULUS (BROKEN LINE)
STYLOMANDIBULAR LIGAMENT
PTERYGOMANDIBULAR RAPHÉ (BROKEN LINE)
MANDIBLE {RAMUS, ANGLE, BODY}
STYLOHYOID LIGAMENT
HYOID BONE {BODY, LESSER CORNU, GREATER CORNU}
MASTOID PROCESS
EXTERNAL AUDITORY MEATUS
ATLAS
STYLOID PROCESS
AXIS
3RD CERVICAL VERTEBRA
EPIGLOTTIS
THYROID CARTILAGE
CRICOID CARTILAGE
TRACHEA
7TH CERVICAL VERTEBRA
1ST THORACIC VERTEBRA
1ST RIB

Labels (lower figure):
ANGULAR SPINE
FORAMEN SPINOSUM
FORAMEN OVALE
SPHENOPALATINE FORAMEN
PTERYGOPALATINE FOSSA
CHOANAE (POSTERIOR NARES)
LATERAL LAMINA
MEDIAL LAMINA {OF PTERYGOID PROCESS}
HAMULUS
TUBEROSITY OF MAXILLA
INFRATEMPORAL FOSSA
ALVEOLAR PROCESS OF MAXILLA
PYRAMIDAL PROCESS OF PALATE BONE

F. Netter, M.D.

extensive flat portion of the bone superior to the meatus, which together with parts of the greater wing of the sphenoid, frontal and parietal bones forms the temporal fossa for the attachment of the temporalis muscle (see page 8). The petrous portion of the temporal bone extends medially and somewhat anteriorly from the meatus to insinuate itself between the basilar portion of the occipital bone and the infratemporal portion of the greater wing of the sphenoid.

The *zygomatic arch* forms a buttress over the infratemporal fossa and gives origin to the masseter muscle (see page 8). It is made up from front to back of the zygomatic process of the maxilla, the zygomatic bone and the zygomatic process of the temporal bone.

The basilar portion of the occipital bone is fused anteriorly with the body of the sphenoid bone and forms the bony framework of the roof and the upper part of the posterior wall of the pharynx. The pharyngeal tubercle on the inferior surface of the basilar portion of the occipital bone, a few millimeters anterior to the foramen magnum, is the superior attachment of the median raphé of the posterior wall of the pharynx.

The hyoid bone has a body and right and left greater and lesser cornua (see also pages 6, 11 and 22). It is a key structure in the floor of the mouth (and related tongue) and is important in the movements of these structures through the several muscles which attach to it (see page 6). The hyoid bone is also important as the origin of the middle constrictor muscle of the pharynx (see pages 21 and 22).

Supplementing the bony framework in supplying attachments to the muscles of the pharynx are the thyroid and cricoid cartilages which give origin to the inferior constrictor (see page 22) and some insertion to the stylopharyngeus muscle.

MEDIAL PTERYGOID PLATE
EUSTACHIAN TUBE (CARTILAGINOUS)
TENSOR VELI PALATINI MUSCLE
PHARYNGOBASILAR FASCIA
LEVATOR VELI PALATINI MUSCLE
TENSOR VELI PALATINI TENDON AND PALATINE APONEUROSIS
PHARYNGEAL TUBERCLE (OCCIPITAL BONE)
PHARYNGOBASILAR FASCIA
ANTERIOR LONGITUDINAL LIGAMENT
ATLANTO-OCCIPITAL MEMBRANE
APICAL LIGAMENT OF DENS
SALPINGOPHARYNGEUS MUSCLE
MUSCULATURE OF SOFT PALATE
PALATOPHARYNGEAL SPHINCTER
PTERYGOID HAMULUS
SUPERIOR CONSTRICTOR MUSCLE
PTERYGOMANDIBULAR RAPHÉ
PALATOPHARYNGEUS MUSCLE
BUCCINATOR MUSCLE
GLOSSOPHARYNGEUS MUSCLE (PART OF SUPERIOR CONSTRICTOR)
STYLOPHARYNGEUS MUSCLE
STYLOHYOID LIGAMENT
STYLOGLOSSUS MUSCLE
MIDDLE CONSTRICTOR MUSCLE
FIBERS TO PHARYNGO-EPIGLOTTIC FOLD
INTERNAL BRANCH OF SUPERIOR LARYNGEAL NERVE
LONGITUDINAL MUSCLE OF PHARYNX
INFERIOR CONSTRICTOR MUSCLE
PHARYNGEAL APONEUROSIS
CRICOPHARYNGEUS MUSCLE (PART OF INFERIOR CONSTRICTOR)
CRICOID ATTACHMENT OF ESOPHAGEAL LONGITUDINAL MUSCLE
ESOPHAGEAL CIRCULAR MUSCLE
ESOPHAGEAL LONGITUDINAL MUSCLE

C1
C2
C4

HYOGLOSSUS MUSCLE
GENIOHYOID MUSCLE
MYLOHYOID MUSCLE
HYOID BONE
THYROHYOID MEMBRANE
THYROID CARTILAGE
CRICOTHYROID MEMBRANE
ARYTENOID AND CORNICULATE CARTILAGES
CRICOID CARTILAGE
TRACHEA

F. Netter M.D.

MUSCULATURE OF PHARYNX

Much of the framework of the lateral and posterior walls of the pharynx is formed by the musculature of the pharynx which is composed of an outer and inner layer. These layers are not completely separable throughout, since in some areas they are definitely intermingled. The outer layer is more nearly arranged in a circular fashion and is made up of the three constrictor muscles of the pharynx, designated as superior, middle and inferior pharyngeal constrictors, which overlap each other from below upward. The inner layer, which falls far short of being a complete layer, is more nearly longitudinally arranged and is composed of the stylopharyngeus, the palatopharyngeus and the salpingopharyngeus plus some other variable and rather irregular bundles of muscle fibers.

The *superior pharyngeal constrictor muscle* (see also pages 7 and 11) is quadrilateral in shape, pale and somewhat thin. Its line of origin from above down is the dorsal edge of the caudal portion (lower one third or so, below the notch for the *Eustachian tube*) of the medial pterygoid plate (see page 9), the hamulus of the medial pterygoid plate, the pterygomandibular raphé, which runs from the hamulus to the lingula of the mandible (see page 4), the posterior one fifth or so of the mylohyoid line and the adjacent part of the alveolar process of the mandible, and the side of the root of the tongue (the glossopharyngeus muscle). From this line of origin, the fibers course posteriorly, with the lower fibers passing somewhat downward and then medially to meet the ones of the opposite side in the median *pharyngeal raphé*. This raphé extends most of the length of the posterior wall of the pharynx, being attached superiorly to the *basilar part of the occipital bone* at the *pharyngeal tubercle,* to which the uppermost fibers of the superior constrictor are also attached. The curved upper edge of the muscle passes under the Eustachian tube and is thus separated by a short distance from the base of the skull except at the midline posteriorly. At this gap the framework of the pharynx is formed by only the *pharyngobasilar fas-*

cia (see also page 18). The *buccinator muscle* runs anteriorly from the pterygomandibular raphé, which serves as part of its origin (see also page 9), and this muscle and the superior constrictor thus form a continuous sheet (see page 16), which is the framework of the lateral wall of the oral and oropharyngeal cavities, as they are continuous with each other. A slip of the cranial part of the superior constrictor muscle (see page 22) blends into the palatine aponeurosis, forming the so-called *palatopharyngeal sphincter,* contraction of which produces a ridge (Passavant's ridge) against which the soft palate is raised. A triangular gap filled with fibrous connective tissue can be noted between the lower border of the superior constrictor muscle, the posterior border of the *hyoglossus muscle* and the upper border of the middle constrictor muscle. Here the stylopharyngeus muscle insinuates itself between the superior and middle constrictors, and the

stylohyoid ligament and glossopharyngeal nerve cross this gap (see page 29).

The *middle pharyngeal constrictor muscle* has a V-shaped line of origin, with the V resting on its side and the angle pointing forward. The upper arm of this V is formed by the terminal portion of the stylohyoid ligament and the lesser cornu of the hyoid bone, whereas the lower arm of the V is formed by the entire length of the greater cornu of the hyoid bone. From this rather narrow origin the fibers fan out, quite widely, with the upper fibers coursing superiorly and curving posteriorly and medially, the middle fibers coursing horizontally and curving posteriorly and medially and the inferior fibers coursing inferiorly and curving posteriorly and medially. The upper fibers overlap the superior constrictor and reach almost as high as it does, and the inferior fibers

(Continued on page 22)

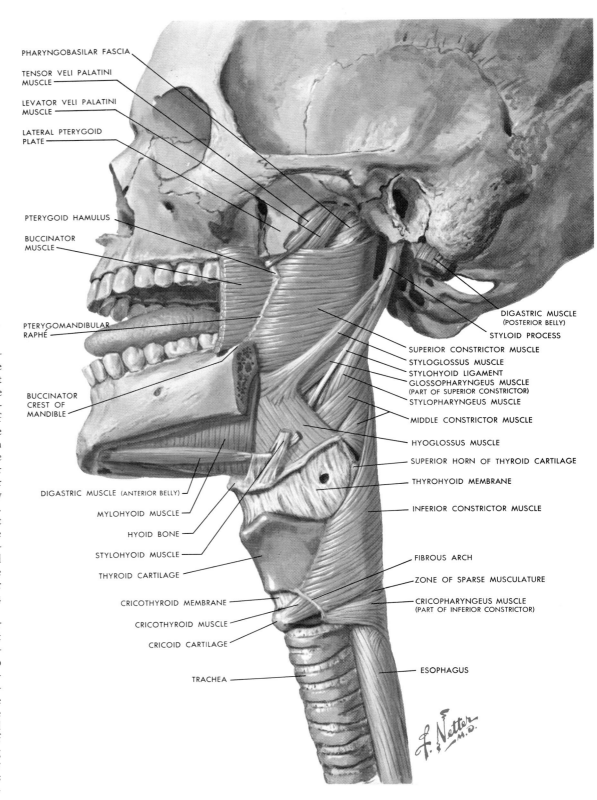

PHARYNGOBASILAR FASCIA

TENSOR VELI PALATINI MUSCLE

LEVATOR VELI PALATINI MUSCLE

LATERAL PTERYGOID PLATE

PTERYGOID HAMULUS

BUCCINATOR MUSCLE

PTERYGOMANDIBULAR RAPHÉ

BUCCINATOR CREST OF MANDIBLE

DIGASTRIC MUSCLE (ANTERIOR BELLY)

MYLOHYOID MUSCLE

HYOID BONE

STYLOHYOID MUSCLE

THYROID CARTILAGE

CRICOTHYROID MEMBRANE

CRICOTHYROID MUSCLE

CRICOID CARTILAGE

TRACHEA

DIGASTRIC MUSCLE (POSTERIOR BELLY)

STYLOID PROCESS

SUPERIOR CONSTRICTOR MUSCLE

STYLOGLOSSUS MUSCLE

STYLOHYOID LIGAMENT

GLOSSOPHARYNGEUS MUSCLE (PART OF SUPERIOR CONSTRICTOR)

STYLOPHARYNGEUS MUSCLE

MIDDLE CONSTRICTOR MUSCLE

HYOGLOSSUS MUSCLE

SUPERIOR HORN OF THYROID CARTILAGE

THYROHYOID MEMBRANE

INFERIOR CONSTRICTOR MUSCLE

FIBROUS ARCH

ZONE OF SPARSE MUSCULATURE

CRICOPHARYNGEUS MUSCLE (PART OF INFERIOR CONSTRICTOR)

ESOPHAGUS

Musculature of Pharynx

(*Continued from page 21*)

are overlapped by the inferior constrictor and reach quite far caudally in the posterior wall of the pharynx (to about the level of the superior border of the cricoid cartilage). The middle constrictor inserts by the fibers of the muscle of one side, blending with the fibers of the muscle of the other side in the median raphé. Between the lower border of the middle constrictor and the upper border of the inferior constrictor, a triangular gap is noted, which is bounded anteriorly by the thyrohyoid muscle (see page 6). This gap is occupied by the lower part of the *stylopharyngeus muscle* and the posterior part of the thyrohyoid membrane, which is pierced by the internal branch of the superior laryngeal nerve (see also page 29) and the superior laryngeal artery and vein (see pages 24 and 26).

The *inferior pharyngeal constrictor muscle* is relatively thick and strong. It arises from the oblique line of the thyroid cartilage and the area just dorsal to that line, from a tendinous arch (a thickening in the fascia covering the cricothyroid muscle) extending from the lower end of the oblique line of the thyroid cartilage to the side of the cricoid cartilage, and from the lateral surface of the cricoid cartilage. That portion arising from the cricoid cartilage is frequently referred to as the *cricopharyngeus muscle*. As do the other constrictor muscles, the inferior constrictor, in general, passes posteriorly and then medially to be inserted by blending with the muscle of the opposite side at the pharyngeal raphé. The cranial fibers pass more and more obliquely as they approach the raphé and overlap the middle constrictor, reaching almost as far superiorly as the middle constrictor does. The fibers of the cricopharyngeus portion of the muscle course horizontally and form an annular bundle (no median raphé in this region), which blends to some extent with the related circular fibers of the esophagus, thus forming an attachment of the esophagus. A zone of sparse musculature is present between the cricopharyngeus muscle and the rest of the inferior constrictor muscle, which creates a weaker

area in the posterior wall of the pharynx, where an instrument may be accidentally pushed through the wall. Spasm of the cricopharyngeus muscle may occur, and contraction of this muscle may make for difficulty in the passing of an esophagoscope. Just below the inferior border of the cricopharyngeus muscle, a triangular area (sometimes called Laimer's triangle, see also page 37) occurs in which the posterior wall of the esophagus is variably deficient, because the longitudinal muscle fibers of the esophagus tend to diverge laterally and pass around the esophagus to attach on the cricoid cartilage. It is thus seen that there is more than one weakened area in the posterior wall of the general region of the pharyngo-esophageal junction, where, theoretically, pulsion diverticula might occur (see page 143). No real agreement exists between workers in this field as to which is the most common site for this to occur or as to exactly what the

mechanism is which is involved. The recurrent laryngeal nerve (see page 29) and accompanying inferior laryngeal vessels pass under cover of the inferior constrictor muscle to travel superiorly behind the cricothyroid joint in entering the larynx.

On the basis of the several origins of each of the three constrictor muscles, each one has been described as being made up of several muscles, to which special names have been given. Much of this detail has been omitted in the present description, the palatopharyngeus and the cricopharyngeus being the only specially named parts to which reference has been made.

As their names indicate, the major action of the superior, middle and inferior constrictor muscles of the pharynx is to constrict the pharynx. They are involved, as they contract in sequence, in grasping the bolus of food as it is passed from the mouth

(*Continued on page 23*)

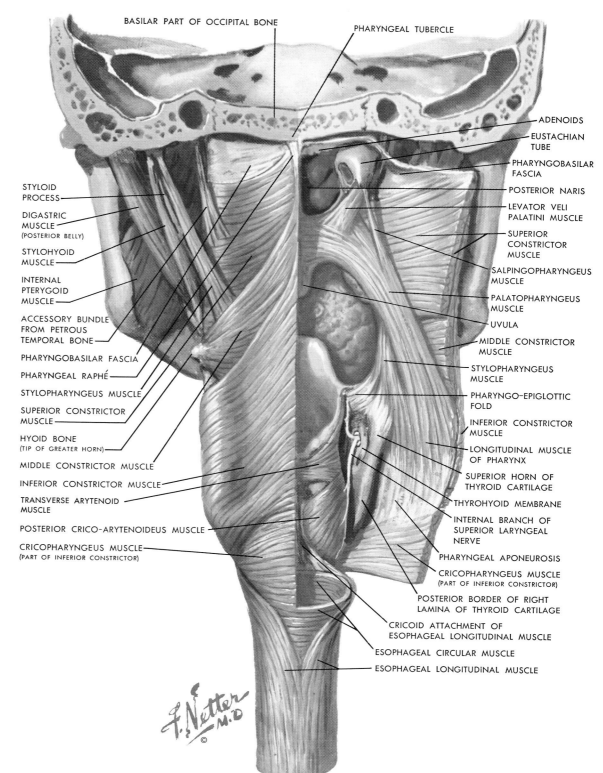

BASILAR PART OF OCCIPITAL BONE

PHARYNGEAL TUBERCLE

ADENOIDS

EUSTACHIAN TUBE

PHARYNGOBASILAR FASCIA

POSTERIOR NARIS

LEVATOR VELI PALATINI MUSCLE

SUPERIOR CONSTRICTOR MUSCLE

SALPINGOPHARYNGEUS MUSCLE

PALATOPHARYNGEUS MUSCLE

UVULA

MIDDLE CONSTRICTOR MUSCLE

STYLOPHARYNGEUS MUSCLE

PHARYNGO-EPIGLOTTIC FOLD

INFERIOR CONSTRICTOR MUSCLE

LONGITUDINAL MUSCLE OF PHARYNX

SUPERIOR HORN OF THYROID CARTILAGE

THYROHYOID MEMBRANE

INTERNAL BRANCH OF SUPERIOR LARYNGEAL NERVE

PHARYNGEAL APONEUROSIS

CRICOPHARYNGEUS MUSCLE (PART OF INFERIOR CONSTRICTOR)

POSTERIOR BORDER OF RIGHT LAMINA OF THYROID CARTILAGE

CRICOID ATTACHMENT OF ESOPHAGEAL LONGITUDINAL MUSCLE

ESOPHAGEAL CIRCULAR MUSCLE

ESOPHAGEAL LONGITUDINAL MUSCLE

STYLOID PROCESS

DIGASTRIC MUSCLE (POSTERIOR BELLY)

STYLOHYOID MUSCLE

INTERNAL PTERYGOID MUSCLE

ACCESSORY BUNDLE FROM PETROUS TEMPORAL BONE

PHARYNGOBASILAR FASCIA

PHARYNGEAL RAPHÉ

STYLOPHARYNGEUS MUSCLE

SUPERIOR CONSTRICTOR MUSCLE

HYOID BONE (TIP OF GREATER HORN)

MIDDLE CONSTRICTOR MUSCLE

INFERIOR CONSTRICTOR MUSCLE

TRANSVERSE ARYTENOID MUSCLE

POSTERIOR CRICO-ARYTENOIDEUS MUSCLE

CRICOPHARYNGEUS MUSCLE (PART OF INFERIOR CONSTRICTOR)

F. Netter M.D.

MUSCULATURE OF PHARYNX

(*Continued from page 22*)

to the pharynx and then in passing it onward into the esophagus (see pages 74 and 75).

The nerve supply of the constrictor muscles of the pharynx is derived from the pharyngeal plexus, as described on page 29.

The *stylopharyngeus muscle* is long, slender and cylindrical above but flattened below. Its origin is the medial aspect of the base or root of the *styloid process,* and from here it passes inferiorly and anteriorly, going between the external and internal carotid arteries (see page 24) and then entering the wall of the pharynx, as indicated above, in the interval between the superior and middle constrictor muscles. As it spreads out internal to the middle constrictor muscle, the *greater horn of the hyoid bone* and the *thyrohyoid membrane,* some of its fibers join the palatopharyngeus muscle and insert on the superior and dorsal borders of the thyroid cartilage. Some fibers pass into the pharyngo-epiglottic fold and are primarily responsible for the production of this fold. The remaining fibers of the stylopharyngeus muscle spread out between the constrictor muscles and the mucous membrane (blending to some extent with the constrictors) and pass caudally in the posterolateral wall of the pharynx, until they fade out and, in part, attach to the fibrous aponeurosis of the pharynx (tela submucosa of the pharynx or pharyngobasilar fascia) a short distance above the cricopharyngeus muscle. The stylopharyngeus muscle receives its nerve supply from the glossopharyngeal nerve, which curves around the posterior border of the muscle onto the lateral aspect (see page 29) in its course toward its final distribution on the posterior third of the tongue.

The *salpingopharyngeus* (see also page 16) *muscle* is made up of a slender bundle which produces the mucous membrane fold of the same name (see page 19), rather variable in its degree of distinctness. This muscle arises from the inferior part of the cartilage of the Eustachian tube near its orifice and passes into the wall of the pharynx, blending, at least in part, with the posteromedial

border of the palatopharyngeus muscle. Some authors have described this muscle as a part of the *levator veli palatini muscle,* which gives a definite clue as to what at least part of its action is. The salpingopharyngeus muscle receives its nerve supply from the pharyngeal plexus (see page 29).

The *palatopharyngeus muscle,* together with the mucous membrane covering it, forms the posterior pillar of the fauces (see page 16) or the palatopharyngeal fold (pharyngopalatine fold). This muscle takes its origin by a narrow fasciculus from the dorsal border of the thyroid cartilage near the base of the superior cornu and by a broad expansion from the *pharyngeal aponeurosis* in the area posterior to the larynx in the region just cranial to the cricopharyngeus muscle. As the fibers pass cranially from their origin, they form a rather compact muscular band which inserts into the aponeurosis of the soft palate

by two lamellae, which are separated by the insertion of the levator veli palatini and the *musculus uvulae.* As indicated above, some of the fibers of the palatopharyngeus muscle intermingle with some of those of the stylopharyngeus muscle. The actions of the palatopharyngeus muscle include constriction of the pharyngeal isthmus by approximation of the palatopharyngeal folds, depression of the soft palate and elevation of the pharynx and larynx. This muscle also receives its nerve supply from the pharyngeal plexus.

Additional muscle bundles are quite common, such as the one labeled *Accessory Bundle From Petrous Temporal Bone,* which is an example of a new muscle arising from the base of the skull. Other additional muscles are brought about by the splitting of one of the usual muscles, quite commonly the stylopharyngeus. The majority of the additional muscles tend to run longitudinally.

BLOOD SUPPLY OF MOUTH AND PHARYNX

The *external carotid artery* and its ramifications are responsible for practically the total arterial supply of the mouth and pharynx. The common carotid artery, which arises from the innominate artery (brachiocephalic trunk) on the right and the arch of the aorta on the left, bifurcates at the level of the upper border of the thyroid cartilage into the external and internal carotid arteries. From here the external carotid artery courses superiorly to a point behind the neck of the mandible, where it divides in the substance of the parotid gland into the *maxillary* (internal maxillary) and *superficial temporal arteries*.

Five of the branches of the external carotid artery are involved in the supply of the mouth and pharynx. The *superior thyroid artery* comes off the anterior aspect of the external carotid near its beginning and courses inferiorly and anteriorly on the external surface of the inferior constrictor muscle of the pharynx, passing deep to the sternohyoid and omohyoid muscles to ramify on the anterolateral surface of the thyroid gland. The *lingual artery* (see also page 11) arises from the anterior surface of the external carotid, a short distance above the superior thyroid (opposite the tip of the greater cornu of the hyoid bone). It courses anteriorly and slightly upward deep to the stylohyoid muscle, the posterior belly of the digastric muscle and the hypoglossal nerve and then passes medial to the hyoglossus muscle along the upper border of the greater cornu of the hyoid. The portion of the artery from the anterior border of the hyoglossus forward to the tip of the tongue, called either deep *lingual* or ranine *artery*, lies deep to the genioglossus muscle and is under cover of the mucous membrane on the inferior surface of the tongue (see pages 3 and 11). The *facial* (external maxillary) *artery*, coming from the anterior aspect of the external carotid a little above the lingual, is tortuous throughout its length, to allow for movements of the head and of the lower jaw. It courses forward and upward deep to the digastric and stylohyoid muscles sheltered by the mandible, lies in a groove on the submandibular gland (see page 14) and then curves upward around the lower border of the mandible near the anterior margin of the masseter muscle (see page 8). From here it runs anteriorly and superiorly across the cheek and along the side of the nose, to end as the *angular artery* at the medial angle of the eye. The *maxillary* (internal maxillary) *artery* — the larger of the two terminal branches of the external carotid—passes forward between

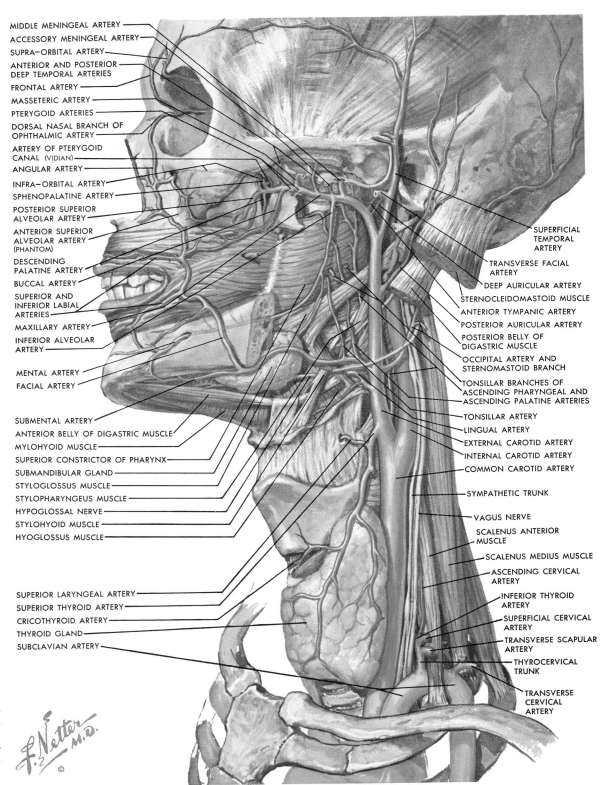

MIDDLE MENINGEAL ARTERY
ACCESSORY MENINGEAL ARTERY
SUPRA-ORBITAL ARTERY
ANTERIOR AND POSTERIOR DEEP TEMPORAL ARTERIES
FRONTAL ARTERY
MASSETERIC ARTERY
PTERYGOID ARTERIES
DORSAL NASAL BRANCH OF OPHTHALMIC ARTERY
ARTERY OF PTERYGOID CANAL (VIDIAN)
ANGULAR ARTERY
INFRA-ORBITAL ARTERY
SPHENOPALATINE ARTERY
POSTERIOR SUPERIOR ALVEOLAR ARTERY
ANTERIOR SUPERIOR ALVEOLAR ARTERY (PHANTOM)
DESCENDING PALATINE ARTERY
BUCCAL ARTERY
SUPERIOR AND INFERIOR LABIAL ARTERIES
MAXILLARY ARTERY
INFERIOR ALVEOLAR ARTERY
MENTAL ARTERY
FACIAL ARTERY
SUBMENTAL ARTERY
ANTERIOR BELLY OF DIGASTRIC MUSCLE
MYLOHYOID MUSCLE
SUPERIOR CONSTRICTOR OF PHARYNX
SUBMANDIBULAR GLAND
STYLOGLOSSUS MUSCLE
STYLOPHARYNGEUS MUSCLE
HYPOGLOSSAL NERVE
STYLOHYOID MUSCLE
HYOGLOSSUS MUSCLE
SUPERIOR LARYNGEAL ARTERY
SUPERIOR THYROID ARTERY
CRICOTHYROID ARTERY
THYROID GLAND
SUBCLAVIAN ARTERY

SUPERFICIAL TEMPORAL ARTERY
TRANSVERSE FACIAL ARTERY
DEEP AURICULAR ARTERY
STERNOCLEIDOMASTOID MUSCLE
ANTERIOR TYMPANIC ARTERY
POSTERIOR AURICULAR ARTERY
POSTERIOR BELLY OF DIGASTRIC MUSCLE
OCCIPITAL ARTERY AND STERNOMASTOID BRANCH
TONSILLAR BRANCHES OF ASCENDING PHARYNGEAL AND ASCENDING PALATINE ARTERIES
TONSILLAR ARTERY
LINGUAL ARTERY
EXTERNAL CAROTID ARTERY
INTERNAL CAROTID ARTERY
COMMON CAROTID ARTERY
SYMPATHETIC TRUNK
VAGUS NERVE
SCALENUS ANTERIOR MUSCLE
SCALENUS MEDIUS MUSCLE
ASCENDING CERVICAL ARTERY
INFERIOR THYROID ARTERY
SUPERFICIAL CERVICAL ARTERY
TRANSVERSE SCAPULAR ARTERY
THYROCERVICAL TRUNK
TRANSVERSE CERVICAL ARTERY

f. Netter M.D. ©

the ramus of the mandible and the sphenomandibular ligament (first part of the artery, see also page 5) and, continuing forward, passes superficial (sometimes deep) to the external pterygoid muscle (second part of the artery), between the two heads of which it dips to reach the pterygopalatine fossa (third part of the artery). The *infra-orbital artery,* which appears to be the continuation of the maxillary, courses through the infra-orbital canal to end in terminal branches on the face as it leaves the infra-orbital foramen. The *ascending pharyngeal artery* arises from the posteromedial aspect of the external carotid very near its beginning. From here it ascends vertically between the internal carotid artery and the posterolateral aspect of the pharynx, to go as high as the undersurface of the base of the skull.

The lips, which are very vascular, are supplied chiefly by the *superior* and *inferior labial* branches of the facial artery, each of which courses from near the angle of the mouth, where it arises, toward the midline of the respective lip to meet the one of the opposite side. In this course it lies for the most part between the orbicularis oris muscle and the mucous membrane related to its inner surface. The *mental branch of the inferior alveolar artery* anastomoses with the inferior labial artery, and the labial branch of the *infra-orbital artery* anastomoses with the superior labial artery.

The cheek receives much of its arterial supply by way of the *buccal artery,* which springs from the second part of the maxillary artery and runs downward and forward on the external surface of the buccinator muscle.

The arterial supply of the upper teeth and the related alveolar processes and gums is furnished in the

(Continued on page 25)

BLOOD SUPPLY OF MOUTH AND PHARYNX

(Continued from page 24)

molar and premolar area by the posterior superior alveolar branch of the second part of the maxillary artery. It courses inferiorly in the pterygopalatine fossa to divide into several small branches, most of which enter small foramina on the posterior aspect of the tuberosity of the maxilla. The *anterior* and less constant middle *superior alveolar branches* of the infra-orbital artery pass along the wall of the maxillary sinus to supply the rest of the upper jaw.

The lower teeth with the related bone and gums are taken care of by the inferior alveolar branch of the first part of the maxillary artery. It enters the mandibular foramen to course in the alveolar canal (see pages 6 and 15) and continues as the *mental artery* which exits through the mental foramen to supply the chin. Before leaving the bone the artery gives off an incisive branch which travels forward in the bone.

The arterial supply of the tongue is, for the most part, by way of the lingual artery (see above). The anastomoses between the branches of the right and left lingual arteries are of a small enough caliber so that ligation of one artery makes that side of the tongue sufficiently bloodless for an operative procedure. Under cover of the posterior border of the hyoglossus muscle, the lingual artery gives off dorsal lingual branches, which travel upward medial to the styloglossus muscle and supply the mucous membrane of the dorsum as far back as the epiglottis, anastomosing with other vessels supplying the tonsil.

The mucous membrane of the floor of the mouth and the sublingual gland receive blood through the sublingual artery (see page 14) which branches from the lingual near the anterior border of the hyoglossus muscle and courses forward superior to the mylohyoid muscle and lateral to the genioglossus. The muscles of the floor of the mouth are supplied by the submental branch of the facial artery and the mylohyoid branch coming off from the inferior alveolar just before it enters the mandibular foramen. These two arteries contribute some blood to the submandibular gland, which gets most of its supply from the facial artery while it is in intimate relationship with this gland.

The arterial supply of the palate (see also page 7) is chiefly from the *descending palatine branch* of the third part of the *maxillary artery,* which travels inferiorly through the *pterygopalatine canal* to emerge from the greater palatine foramen and then courses forward medial

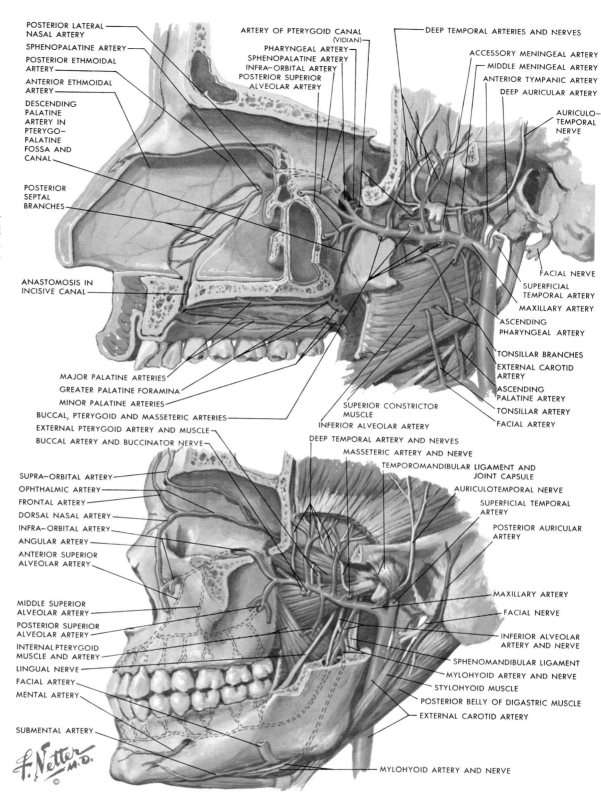

to the alveolar process to anastomose at the incisive foramen with a septal branch of the *sphenopalatine artery.* Lesser (*minor*) *palatine arteries* (see also page 16), which run posteriorly from the descending palatine at the greater palatine foramen, supply the soft palate and anastomose with other arteries which supply the tonsil. Anastomoses exist also with a palatine branch of the ascending pharyngeal artery, the dorsal lingual arteries and the ascending palatine from the facial artery.

The muscles of mastication receive arterial twigs, named according to the muscle supplied. These are branches of the second part of the maxillary artery.

The parotid gland (see page 15) surrounds part of the external carotid artery and the beginnings of its terminal branches. The gland gets many small branches from these vessels in its substance.

The pharynx receives some blood from many

sources, the amount from each source varying a great deal individually. One of the chief sources is the *ascending pharyngeal artery,* usually from the external carotid artery (described above). Other arteries which course in relation to the pharynx and can thus contribute to its supply are the ascending palatine and tonsillar branches of the facial artery, the superior thyroid artery and its superior laryngeal branch and the inferior laryngeal and ascending cervical branches of the thyrocervical trunk from the subclavian artery. The pharyngeal branch of the third part of the facial artery passes through a bony canal to reach the roof of the pharynx, and the descending palatine artery, also from the third part of the facial, contributes to the supply in the region of the tonsil by its lesser palatine branches.

The arteries which form the rich supply to the tonsil are listed and pictured on page 16.

VENOUS DRAINAGE OF MOUTH AND PHARYNX

As elsewhere in the body, the veins of this region (face, oral cavity and pharynx) are more variable than are the arteries, but the tendency of the veins to lie more superficially than do the corresponding arteries and the tendency to form plexuses substituting for single, definite venous changes are far greater than in general.

The *internal jugular vein* eventually receives almost all of the blood derived from the mouth and pharynx. This vein begins as a continuation of the sigmoid sinus at the jugular foramen and descends in the neck lateral to the internal and then the common carotid arteries to about the level of the sternoclavicular joint, where it joins the subclavian vein to form the brachiocephalic (innominate) vein.

For the most part the arteries, described on pages 24 and 25 as those going to the various structures of the mouth and the pharynx, have veins of the same name accompanying them, but the veins into which these drain differ in various ways from the branches of the external carotid artery from which those arteries spring. The *superior thyroid vein* does not differ greatly from the superior thyroid artery, but it does usually empty directly into the internal jugular vein. Frequently, one encounters a *middle thyroid vein* which has no corresponding artery and also empties into the internal jugular.

The deep *lingual (ranine) vein,* often more than one channel, accompanies the corresponding artery (see pages 3 and 24) from the tip of the tongue to the anterior border of the hyoglossus muscle, where the major vein receives the sublingual vein and then accompanies the hypoglossal nerve (often called vena comitans of the hypoglossal nerve) on the lateral surface of the hyoglossus muscle, and a smaller vein(s) runs with the lingual artery (see also page 11). Near the posterior border of the hyoglossus muscle, one of these veins receives the dorsal lingual veins, and then they either join to form a short lingual vein or continue separately to empty either into the common facial vein or directly into the internal jugular vein.

The anterior *facial vein* follows a line (not so tortuous as that of the corresponding artery) from the medial angle of the eye to the lower border of the mandible near the anterior margin of the masseter muscle. From here it courses posteriorly in the submandibular triangle (not sheltered by the mandible as the artery is) to join the anterior division of the *poste-*

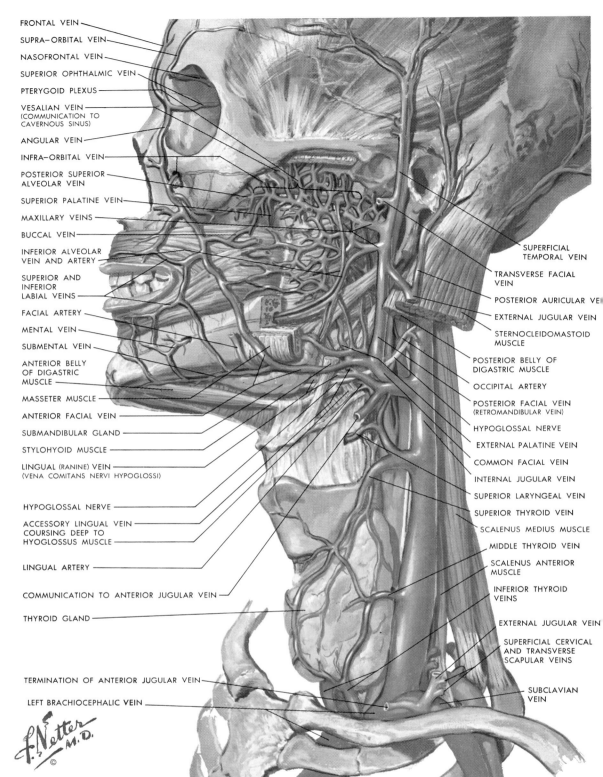

FRONTAL VEIN
SUPRA-ORBITAL VEIN
NASOFRONTAL VEIN
SUPERIOR OPHTHALMIC VEIN
PTERYGOID PLEXUS
VESALIAN VEIN (COMMUNICATION TO CAVERNOUS SINUS)
ANGULAR VEIN
INFRA-ORBITAL VEIN
POSTERIOR SUPERIOR ALVEOLAR VEIN
SUPERIOR PALATINE VEIN
MAXILLARY VEINS
BUCCAL VEIN
INFERIOR ALVEOLAR VEIN AND ARTERY
SUPERIOR AND INFERIOR LABIAL VEINS
FACIAL ARTERY
MENTAL VEIN
SUBMENTAL VEIN
ANTERIOR BELLY OF DIGASTRIC MUSCLE
MASSETER MUSCLE
ANTERIOR FACIAL VEIN
SUBMANDIBULAR GLAND
STYLOHYOID MUSCLE
LINGUAL (RANINE) VEIN (VENA COMITANS NERVI HYPOGLOSSI)
HYPOGLOSSAL NERVE
ACCESSORY LINGUAL VEIN COURSING DEEP TO HYOGLOSSUS MUSCLE
LINGUAL ARTERY
COMMUNICATION TO ANTERIOR JUGULAR VEIN
THYROID GLAND
TERMINATION OF ANTERIOR JUGULAR VEIN
LEFT BRACHIOCEPHALIC VEIN

SUPERFICIAL TEMPORAL VEIN
TRANSVERSE FACIAL VEIN
POSTERIOR AURICULAR VEIN
EXTERNAL JUGULAR VEIN
STERNOCLEIDOMASTOID MUSCLE
POSTERIOR BELLY OF DIGASTRIC MUSCLE
OCCIPITAL ARTERY
POSTERIOR FACIAL VEIN (RETROMANDIBULAR VEIN)
HYPOGLOSSAL NERVE
EXTERNAL PALATINE VEIN
COMMON FACIAL VEIN
INTERNAL JUGULAR VEIN
SUPERIOR LARYNGEAL VEIN
SUPERIOR THYROID VEIN
SCALENUS MEDIUS MUSCLE
MIDDLE THYROID VEIN
SCALENUS ANTERIOR MUSCLE
INFERIOR THYROID VEINS
EXTERNAL JUGULAR VEIN
SUPERFICIAL CERVICAL AND TRANSVERSE SCAPULAR VEINS
SUBCLAVIAN VEIN

rior facial vein in the formation of the *common facial vein* which empties into the internal jugular. The anterior facial vein receives tributaries corresponding, for the most part, to the branches of the facial artery but also has other communications, some from the *pterygoid plexus,* one of which is often called the deep facial or external palatine vein.

The *maxillary* (internal maxillary) *vein* is sometimes a distinct vein with tributaries corresponding to the artery, but, more commonly, one or more short veins drain from the pterygoid plexus, which substitutes for the maxillary vein, and join the *superficial temporal vein* in the formation of the *posterior facial (retromandibular) vein.* The pterygoid plexus is partly superficial and partly deep to the external pterygoid muscle. The tributaries are those veins which correspond to the branches of the maxillary artery, and the plexus communicates with the cavern-

ous sinus by small veins passing through the foramina in the floor of the middle cranial fossa and with the pharyngeal plexus, in addition to the other connections previously mentioned.

The bulk of a pharyngeal plexus of veins lies superficial to the constrictor muscles of the pharynx. This plexus communicates in all directions, with connections to the internal and external jugular veins, the pterygoid plexus, the common facial vein, the lingual vein, the superior thyroid vein and a submucosal plexus, which is best developed in the lower part of the posterior pharyngeal wall.

The posterior division of the retromandibular vein joins the posterior auricular vein to form the external jugular vein, and an anterior jugular vein begins in the chin superficial to the mylohyoid muscle and courses inferiorly and then laterally to empty into the external jugular.

LYMPHATIC DRAINAGE OF MOUTH AND PHARYNX

The lymph, which is picked up by the lymphatic capillaries in the tissues of the mouth and pharynx, is all eventually taken by the lymphatic vessels, either directly or with the interruption by interposed lymph nodes, to the *chain of nodes* lying along the *internal jugular vein*. The efferent vessels from these nodes enter into the formation of the jugular lymphatic trunk, which, characteristically, on the left side empties into the *thoracic duct* near its termination and on the right side into the right lymphatic duct. The thoracic duct and the right lymphatic duct pour their lymph into the blood stream at the junction of the internal jugular and subclavian veins on the respective side. On either side the *jugular trunk* may empty directly into the veins near this site.

A more specific description of the lymph nodes and groups of nodes involved in the lymphatic drainage of the mouth and pharynx is necessary because of their importance in the metastasis of cancer and the significance attached to the enlargement of a node when an infection occurs in its area of drainage. However, any specific description of lymph nodes is complicated by the facts that the lymphatics are quite variable and are difficult or impossible to see in dissection when they are not pathologically conspicuous and that the grouping of the nodes is at best arbitrary and, to quite an extent, artificial. Because of these facts, descriptions of lymphatics vary greatly, and many different names have been employed for individual nodes and groups of nodes. The number of groups of nodes described for any region can, of course, differ, depending on whether certain nodes are interpreted as forming a separate group or are considered as subsidiaries of another group.

The groups of nodes involved in the drainage of lymph from the mouth and pharynx belong, of course, to the portion of the lymphatic system designated as the lymphatic system of the head and neck. The grouping of the nodes of the head and neck can be described briefly as follows: A "collar" or "string of beads" of groups of nodes is located at the general region of the junction of the head and neck. From the midline posteriorly to the midline anteriorly, the groups encountered, in order, are *occipital, retroauricular (mastoid), parotid* (some or all of which are called pre-auricular by

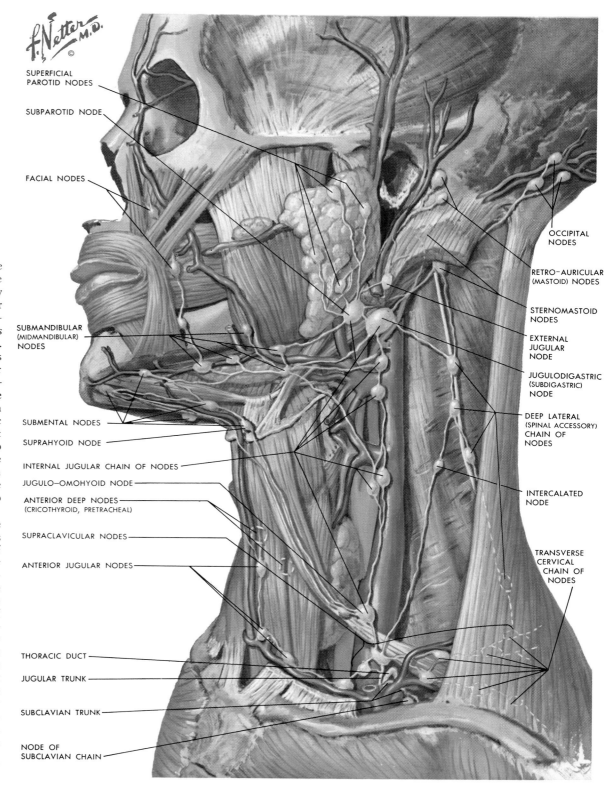

SUPERFICIAL PAROTID NODES

SUBPAROTID NODE

FACIAL NODES

SUBMANDIBULAR (MIDMANDIBULAR) NODES

SUBMENTAL NODES

SUPRAHYOID NODE

INTERNAL JUGULAR CHAIN OF NODES

JUGULO—OMOHYOID NODE

ANTERIOR DEEP NODES (CRICOTHYROID, PRETRACHEAL)

SUPRACLAVICULAR NODES

ANTERIOR JUGULAR NODES

THORACIC DUCT

JUGULAR TRUNK

SUBCLAVIAN TRUNK

NODE OF SUBCLAVIAN CHAIN

OCCIPITAL NODES

RETRO-AURICULAR (MASTOID) NODES

STERNOMASTOID NODES

EXTERNAL JUGULAR NODE

JUGULODIGASTRIC (SUBDIGASTRIC) NODE

DEEP LATERAL (SPINAL ACCESSORY) CHAIN OF NODES

INTERCALATED NODE

TRANSVERSE CERVICAL CHAIN OF NODES

some authors), *submandibular* (some or all of which are called midmandibular by some authors; extending superiorly from this group is a variable chain of *facial nodes*) and *submental* (*suprahyoid*). A group of nodes superficial to the sternomastoid muscle and in relation to the external jugular vein (*external jugular nodes*) is called by many the superficial cervical group; by others it is considered as an extension of the parotid group which is also often subdivided into superficial and deep parts. The majority of the groups of nodes not included in the "collar" just described run more or less vertically in the neck. Minor chains of *nodes* lie *along the anterior jugular vein* and the *spinal accessory nerve*, and the *major chain accompanies the internal jugular vein* throughout its full length. The latter is most commonly designated as the deep cervical group of nodes and is often divided into superior deep cervical glands superior to

the point at which the omohyoid muscle crosses the internal jugular vein and the inferior deep cervical glands inferior to this point. What is considered by some authors as an expansion of the superior portion of the superior deep cervical group and by others as a separate group are some nodes located between the superolateral part of the pharynx and the prevertebral fascia, often called the *retropharyngeal group*. Individual nodes are encountered constantly enough in two locations in the superior deep cervical chain so that they have merited special naming. A *jugulodigastric node* is located between the angle of the mandible and the anterior border of the sternomastoid muscle, at about the level of the greater cornu of the hyoid bone and between the posterior belly of the digastric muscle and the internal jugular vein. This node receives lymph from the area of the palatine

(*Continued on page 28*)

LYMPHATIC DRAINAGE OF MOUTH AND PHARYNX

(Continued from page 27)

tonsil, the tongue and the teeth. A *jugulo-omohyoid node,* usually considered as the lowest node of the superior deep cervical group, lies immediately above the intermediate tendon or the inferior belly of the omohyoid muscle and may project beyond the posterior border of the sternomastoid muscle. This node receives some vessels directly from the tongue in addition to its other afferents. A *subparotid node* just inferior to the parotid gland is specially named by some authors. The inferior deep cervical nodes, also called *supraclavicular nodes,* extend into the posterior triangle of the neck, send expansions along the transverse cervical and transverse scapular veins and intermingle with the *subclavian* (apical axillary) *nodes.* In addition to the groups of nodes described above, some scattered nodes, part of which are often called *anterior deep cervical nodes,* pertain to the larynx, trachea, esophagus and thyroid gland.

The groups of glands specifically involved in the drainage of lymph from definite portions of the mouth and pharynx are indicated briefly in the following statements: The LIPS have cutaneous and mucosal plexuses from which the lymph goes to the submandibular, submental and, to a slight extent, the superficial cervical groups, with that from the central part of the lower lip going to the submental glands. Lymph from the CHEEK travels mostly to the submandibular glands but also to superficial cervical glands and, in part, directly to superior deep cervical glands. From the anterior part of the FLOOR OF THE MOUTH, drainage is, in part, directly to the lower of the superior deep cervical group and, in part, to the submental and submandibular glands. The posterior part drains to submandibular and superior deep cervical glands. Lymph from the HARD AND SOFT PALATES may travel directly to superior deep cervical nodes (near the digastric muscle) or to submandibular nodes or, particularly from the soft palate, to *retropharyngeal nodes.* The lymphatics of the TEETH anastomose with those of the GUMS. Similar connections exist between the gums and the lingual side of the alveolar process, between the upper jaw and the lymphatics of the palate; between the lower jaw and the floor of the mouth and between the outer side of the alveolar process and the lymphatics of the lips and cheek. The jugulodigastric node, or at least a node in

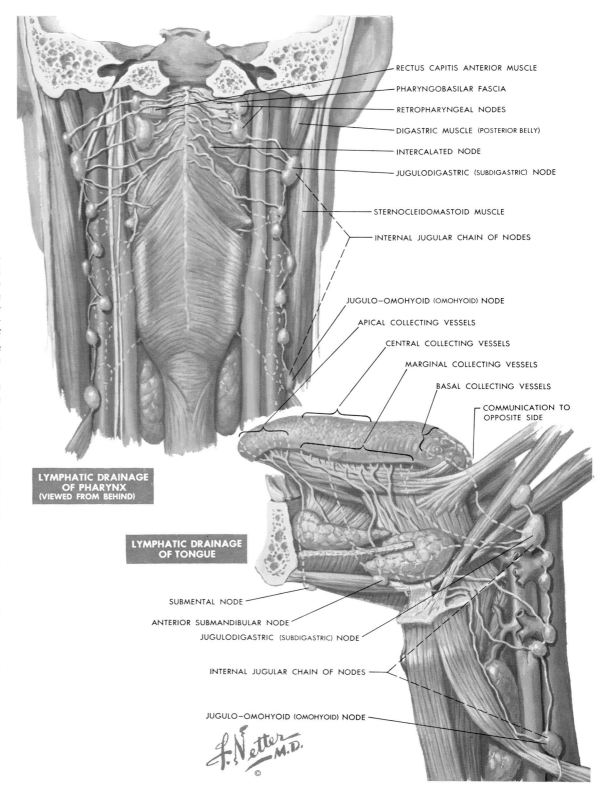

RECTUS CAPITIS ANTERIOR MUSCLE
PHARYNGOBASILAR FASCIA
RETROPHARYNGEAL NODES
DIGASTRIC MUSCLE (POSTERIOR BELLY)
INTERCALATED NODE
JUGULODIGASTRIC (SUBDIGASTRIC) NODE
STERNOCLEIDOMASTOID MUSCLE
INTERNAL JUGULAR CHAIN OF NODES
JUGULO-OMOHYOID (OMOHYOID) NODE
APICAL COLLECTING VESSELS
CENTRAL COLLECTING VESSELS
MARGINAL COLLECTING VESSELS
BASAL COLLECTING VESSELS
COMMUNICATION TO OPPOSITE SIDE

LYMPHATIC DRAINAGE OF PHARYNX (VIEWED FROM BEHIND)

LYMPHATIC DRAINAGE OF TONGUE

SUBMENTAL NODE
ANTERIOR SUBMANDIBULAR NODE
JUGULODIGASTRIC (SUBDIGASTRIC) NODE
INTERNAL JUGULAR CHAIN OF NODES
JUGULO-OMOHYOID (OMOHYOID) NODE

that area, may be enlarged when a tooth, particularly in the molar region, is infected. The lymphatic drainage of the TONGUE tends to follow the course of the blood vessels less than does drainage from other portions of the mouth and pharynx. The drainage from the tongue goes either directly or indirectly to the superior deep cervical nodes, and, in general, the farther forward the area on the tongue, the lower in the deep cervical chain is the related node. Four sets of collecting vessels of the tongue are described: *apical vessels,* which lead to submental nodes and to the jugulo-omohyoid node; *marginal vessels,* to superior deep cervical nodes and perhaps submandibular nodes; *basal vessels,* to superior deep cervical nodes (chiefly, the jugulodigastric node); and *central vessels,* mostly to superior deep cervical nodes with a few to submandibular nodes. The central vessels from each side of the tongue go to both right and left superior

deep cervical nodes. No vessels from the tongue are said to reach any of the more superficial nodes. Drainage from the LARGE SALIVARY GLANDS is much as would be expected: parotid gland, to parotid nodes (some of which are described as being in the substance of the gland); submandibular gland, in part to submandibular nodes but mostly to superior deep cervical nodes; and sublingual gland, much like that of the submandibular gland. Part of the lymph from the area of the PALATINE TONSIL goes to the superior deep cervical nodes and much of it to the jugulodigastric node or a node in that region. The mucosa of the PHARYNX is rich in lymphatics, and the drainage from the roof and upper part of the posterior wall is to the retropharyngeal nodes. The collecting vessels of the laryngeal pharynx gather in the wall of the piriform sinus, pierce the thyrohyoid membrane and then continue to nearby superior deep cervical nodes.

NERVE SUPPLY OF MOUTH AND PHARYNX

Six of the twelve pairs of cranial nerves contribute to the nerve supply of the mouth and pharynx. The trigeminal nerve (cranial V) emerges from the lateral surface of the pons (see also CIBA COLLECTION, Vol. 1, pages 42, 43, 47 and 59) by a larger sensory and a smaller motor root. A short distance from the pons the sensory root is expanded by the presence of many afferent nerve cell bodies into the semilunar ganglion which lies in a depression on the apex of the petrous portion of the temporal bone. From the anterior margin of this ganglion arise the ophthalmic, maxillary and mandibular divisions of the trigeminal nerve. The motor root courses along the medial and then the inferior side of the sensory root and ganglion and joins the *mandibular nerve* near its beginning. The *maxillary* division passes through the foramen rotundum into the pterygopalatine fossa, where it gives off the following branches: (1) two or three branches to the *sphenopalatine ganglion,* which leave the ganglion as a pharyngeal branch passing through a bony canal to the mucous membrane of the upper part of the nasal pharynx, the *palatine nerves* passing through the pterygopalatine canal to exit through the greater and lesser palatine foramina to supply the mucous membrane of the palate (see page 7), and a sphenopalatine branch, which enters the nasal cavity and sends a branch along the nasal septum to reach the palate through the incisive foramen; (2) the *posterior superior alveolar nerves,* which enter the maxilla and supply the molar teeth and related gums. The maxillary nerve continues as the *infra-orbital nerve,* which gives off the *middle and anterior superior alveolar nerves* in the infra-orbital canal and a branch to the upper lip after it reaches the face. The mandibular nerve reaches the infratemporal fossa through the foramen ovale and has the following branches: (1) nerves to each of the muscles of mastication, the one to the *internal pterygoid* also supplying the tensor veli palatini muscle; (2) the inferior alveolar, which, before entering the mandibular foramen, gives off the *mylohyoid branch* to that muscle and the anterior belly of the digastricus, courses through the alveolar canal supplying the mandibular teeth (see also page 13) and ends as the *mental nerve* which exits through the mental foramen to give sensory supply to the chin and part of the lower lip; (3) the *buccinator* (buccal) *nerve* giving sensory supply to the cheek; (4) the *lingual nerve* (see also pages 6, 11 and 15), which, after receiving the chorda tympani branch from the facial nerve, courses inferiorly and then forward on the lateral surface of the hyoglossus muscle to reach the undersurface of the tongue. The trigeminal fibers in the lingual nerve take care of the general sensation of the anterior two thirds of the tongue.

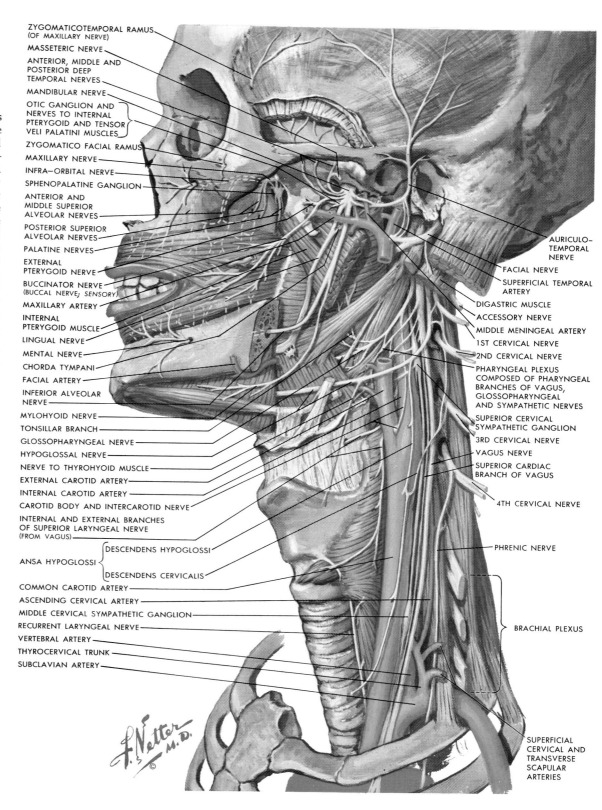

ZYGOMATICOTEMPORAL RAMUS (OF MAXILLARY NERVE)
MASSETERIC NERVE
ANTERIOR, MIDDLE AND POSTERIOR DEEP TEMPORAL NERVES
MANDIBULAR NERVE
OTIC GANGLION AND NERVES TO INTERNAL PTERYGOID AND TENSOR VELI PALATINI MUSCLES
ZYGOMATICO FACIAL RAMUS
MAXILLARY NERVE
INFRA–ORBITAL NERVE
SPHENOPALATINE GANGLION
ANTERIOR AND MIDDLE SUPERIOR ALVEOLAR NERVES
POSTERIOR SUPERIOR ALVEOLAR NERVES
PALATINE NERVES
EXTERNAL PTERYGOID NERVE
BUCCINATOR NERVE (BUCCAL NERVE; SENSORY)
MAXILLARY ARTERY
INTERNAL PTERYGOID MUSCLE
LINGUAL NERVE
MENTAL NERVE
CHORDA TYMPANI
FACIAL ARTERY
INFERIOR ALVEOLAR NERVE
MYLOHYOID NERVE
TONSILLAR BRANCH
GLOSSOPHARYNGEAL NERVE
HYPOGLOSSAL NERVE
NERVE TO THYROHYOID MUSCLE
EXTERNAL CAROTID ARTERY
INTERNAL CAROTID ARTERY
CAROTID BODY AND INTERCAROTID NERVE
INTERNAL AND EXTERNAL BRANCHES OF SUPERIOR LARYNGEAL NERVE (FROM VAGUS)
DESCENDENS HYPOGLOSSI
ANSA HYPOGLOSSI
DESCENDENS CERVICALIS
COMMON CAROTID ARTERY
ASCENDING CERVICAL ARTERY
MIDDLE CERVICAL SYMPATHETIC GANGLION
RECURRENT LARYNGEAL NERVE
VERTEBRAL ARTERY
THYROCERVICAL TRUNK
SUBCLAVIAN ARTERY

AURICULO-TEMPORAL NERVE
FACIAL NERVE
SUPERFICIAL TEMPORAL ARTERY
DIGASTRIC MUSCLE
ACCESSORY NERVE
MIDDLE MENINGEAL ARTERY
1ST CERVICAL NERVE
2ND CERVICAL NERVE
PHARYNGEAL PLEXUS COMPOSED OF PHARYNGEAL BRANCHES OF VAGUS, GLOSSOPHARYNGEAL AND SYMPATHETIC NERVES
SUPERIOR CERVICAL SYMPATHETIC GANGLION
3RD CERVICAL NERVE
VAGUS NERVE
SUPERIOR CARDIAC BRANCH OF VAGUS
4TH CERVICAL NERVE
PHRENIC NERVE
BRACHIAL PLEXUS
SUPERFICIAL CERVICAL AND TRANSVERSE SCAPULAR ARTERIES

F. Netter M.D.

The *facial nerve* (cranial VII) emerges from the lower border of the lateral aspect of the pons by a larger motor and a smaller sensory root (nervus intermedius which contains the general visceral efferent fibers of VII as well as afferent fibers) (see also CIBA COLLECTION, Vol. 1, pages 42, 43 and 47). It leaves the cranial cavity by way of the internal acoustic meatus and then follows a curving bony canal (the facial canal) to exit at the stylomastoid foramen, near which it gives off branches to the stylohyoid muscle and the posterior belly of the digastricus. From the stylomastoid foramen, the facial nerve runs forward through the substance of the parotid gland, crosses the external carotid artery and divides in the substance of the gland into branches which leave the anterior border of the gland (see page 14) and distribute to the muscles of facial expression, of which the ones surrounding the oral orifice, including the

buccinator (see page 8), are of interest in this discussion. As the facial nerve traverses the facial canal, the geniculate ganglion is present at a sharp bend in the nerve, and the nerve gives off the greater superficial petrosal nerve, which eventually reaches the sphenopalatine ganglion (see page 31 for description), and the chorda tympani branch, which eventually joins the lingual nerve. The chorda tympani contains special visceral afferent fibers, which take care of the sense of taste of the anterior two thirds of the tongue, and preganglionic general visceral efferent fibers, which go to the submandibular ganglion (see page 31 for description).

The *glossopharyngeal nerve* (cranial IX) emerges by a series of rootlets from the cranial part of the groove between the restiform body and the olivary eminence of the medulla (see CIBA COLLECTION,

(Continued on page 30)

NERVE SUPPLY OF MOUTH AND PHARYNX

(Continued from page 29)

Vol. 1, pages 42 and 47). It leaves the cranial cavity by way of the jugular foramen near which it exhibits two ganglionic swellings, courses downward along the posterior border of the stylopharyngeus muscle and disappears deep to the hyoglossus muscle to break up into its terminal branches to the tongue. The glossopharyngeal nerve branches and contributes to the nerve supply of the mouth and pharynx. The tympanic branch follows a bony canal from the margin of the jugular foramen to the tympanic cavity, where it helps to form the tympanic plexus and then continues as the lesser superficial petrosal nerve which eventually brings preganglionic general visceral efferent fibers to the otic ganglion. The pharyngeal branches, for the most part, join with the pharyngeal branches of the vagus and branches of the superior cervical ganglion to form the pharyngeal plexus, which supplies the muscles of the pharynx except the stylopharyngeus, the muscles of the soft palate except the tensor veli palatini and the mucous membrane of the pharynx. Probably the muscles are mostly innervated by the vagus and the mucous membrane by the glossopharyngeal. A muscular branch of the glossopharyngeal goes to the stylopharyngeus muscle. The *tonsillar branches* (see also page 16) arise near the base of the tongue and supply also the soft palate and the faucial pillars. The *lingual* and terminal *branches* of IX take care of both the general sense and the sense of taste of the posterior one third of the tongue and also supply, at least in part, the glosso-epiglottic and the pharyngo-epiglottic folds.

The *vagus nerve* (cranial X) emerges from the medulla at the sulcus between the olivary eminence and the restiform body. It leaves the cranial cavity by way of the jugular foramen and has two ganglionic (afferent) swellings in this region, one at the foramen and one below the foramen. Entering the carotid sheath, the vagus courses caudally in the neck behind and between the internal jugular vein and the internal and then common carotid artery. Some branches of the vagus contribute to the supply of the mouth and pharynx. The *pharyngeal branches* (variable in number) enter into the formation of the pharyngeal plexus (see above and CIBA COLLECTION, Vol. 1, page 86). It is probable that the branchial (special visceral) efferent fibers of the vagus, which go to the muscles supplied by the pharyngeal plexus, come, to quite an extent, from the internal ramus of the accessory nerve (XI). The *superior laryngeal nerve* divides into an external and an internal branch. The external branch runs downward and forward on the external surface of the inferior constrictor to which it gives some supply. The internal branch pierces the thyrohyoid membrane and divides into an

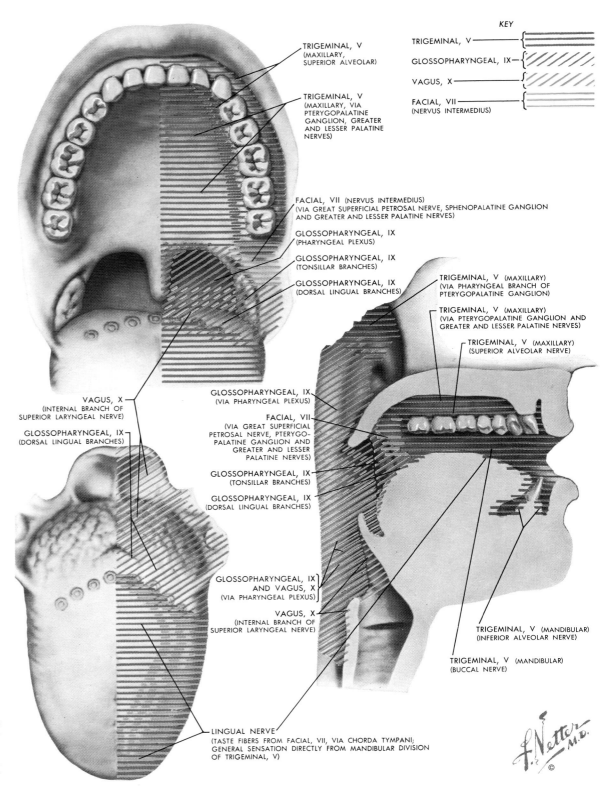

ascending and a descending branch, the former going to the mucous membrane covering the epiglottis and a small adjacent part of the tongue, the latter supplying the mucous membrane on the pharyngeal surface of the larynx in addition to its laryngeal distribution. The recurrent laryngeal branch of the vagus gives some supply to the inferior constrictor muscle as it passes under the inferior border of this muscle in entering the larynx.

The internal ramus (cranial part) of the accessory (spinal accessory) nerve (cranial XI) emerges from the caudal part of the sulcus between the olivary eminence of the medulla and the restiform body. It becomes an integral part of the vagus nerve and, as such, is described above.

The *hypoglossal nerve* (cranial XII) emerges by a series of rootlets from the sulcus between the olivary eminence and the pyramid of the medulla (see CIBA

COLLECTION, Vol. 1, pages 42 and 43). It leaves the cranial cavity by way of the hypoglossal canal and runs downward and forward between the internal carotid artery and the internal jugular vein, becoming superficial to them near the angle of the mandible, where it passes forward across the external carotid and lingual arteries deep to the digastricus. From here it continues forward between the mylohyoid and hyoglossus muscles and on toward the tip of the tongue. The hypoglossal nerve supplies the intrinsic muscles of the tongue and the styloglossus, hyoglossus and genioglossus muscles. Fibers from the first and second cervical nerves run with the hypoglossal to supply the geniohyoid muscle.

The areas of sensory supply of the mucous membrane of the oral cavity and pharynx, shown diagrammatically, are only approximations because no complete agreement as to their limits exists.

AUTONOMIC INNERVATION OF MOUTH AND PHARYNX

Autonomic (general visceral efferent) innervation goes to the glands and the smooth muscle. The smooth muscle of the mouth and pharynx is, for the most part, in blood vessel walls and erector pili muscles in the related skin. The glands receive both sympathetic (thoracolumbar general visceral efferent) and parasympathetic (craniosacral general visceral efferent) supply. The typical pattern for these innervations is a two-neuron chain with the cell body of the first neuron in the central nervous system and the cell body of the second neuron in a visceral ganglion (see CIBA COLLECTION, Vol. 1, page 81).

For the innervation of the palatine glands, the cell body of the first-order parasympathetic neuron is located in the superior salivary nucleus of the pons, and the axon of this neuron follows the nervus intermedius root of VII, the greater superficial petrosal branch of VII and then the Vidian nerve (nerve of the pterygoid canal) to reach the *sphenopalatine ganglion* (see also page 29), where it synapses with the cell body of the second-order neuron. The axon of this second-order neuron follows the palatine nerves and their branches to be distributed as shown on page 7. In the sympathetic pathway to the palatine glands, the first-order neuron cell body is located in the intermediolateral cell column of the upper thoracic segments of the spinal cord. The axon of this neuron follows the ventral root of the related thoracic nerve, the common trunk of this nerve and then the anterior primary division of the nerve to the white ramus communicans, along which it goes to the chain ganglion of the level. From here, the axon of the first-order neuron travels up the sympathetic trunk to synapse with the second-order neuron cell body in the *superior cervical ganglion*. The axon of this second-order neuron enters the periarterial plexus around the nearby internal carotid artery and, from here, may take two courses. One course follows the plexus up to the carotid canal and then leaves the plexus in the deep petrosal nerve which joins the *greater superficial petrosal nerve* in the foramen lacerum to form the Vidian nerve. The sympathetic fibers pass through the sphenopalatine ganglion without synapse and follow the palatine nerves to their distribution. The other course follows periarterial plexuses all of the way to the distribution.

For the innervation of the submandibular and sublingual glands (see also page 71), the first-order parasympathetic neuron reaches the facial nerve, as described above for the innervation of the palatine glands, and then follows the *chorda tympani* branch to the lingual nerve (see also page 29). The axon then accompanies the lingual nerve until it leaves by a

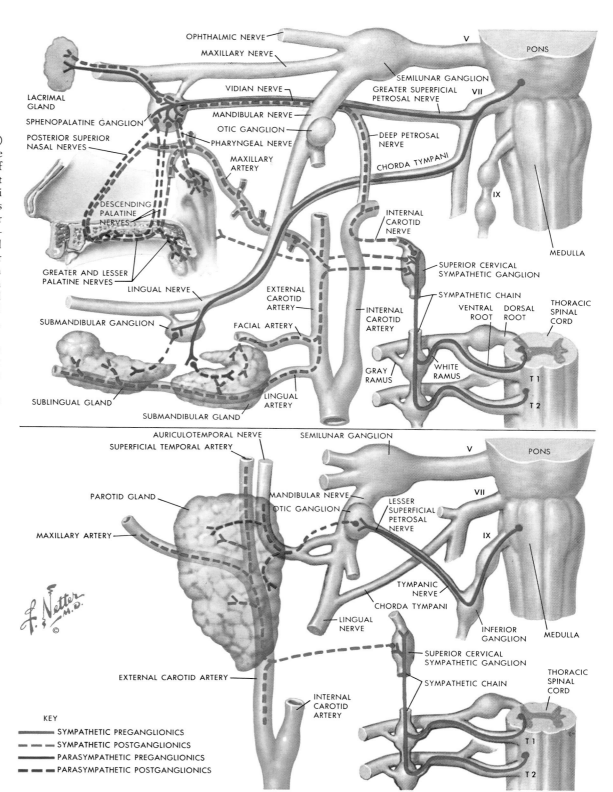

KEY
—— SYMPATHETIC PREGANGLIONICS
- - - SYMPATHETIC POSTGANGLIONICS
━━ PARASYMPATHETIC PREGANGLIONICS
━ ━ PARASYMPATHETIC POSTGANGLIONICS

branch to the *submandibular ganglion* (see also pages 6, 14 and 29), where the pathway to the sublingual gland synapses. Many of the fibers carrying impulses to the submandibular gland pass through this ganglion without synapse, to synapse in small ganglia on the surface of the submandibular gland. The axons of the second-order neurons go to the submandibular and sublingual glands. Those destined for the latter may follow the lingual nerve on their way. The sympathetic supply to these two glands follows the course described above for palatine gland innervation as far as the periarterial plexus around the internal carotid artery. From here, the fibers follow the blood vessels leading to the submandibular and sublingual glands (see pages 24 and 25).

For the innervation of the parotid gland, the first-order parasympathetic neuron has its cell body in the inferior salivary nucleus of the medulla, and the

axon of this neuron follows the glossopharyngeal nerve, its *tympanic branch* and then the *lesser superficial petrosal nerve* (see also page 29) to the *otic ganglion* (see page 9), where it synapses with the second-order neuron cell body. The axon of this neuron follows the *auriculotemporal nerve* to the parotid gland. The sympathetic innervation is similar to that described above for the submandibular and sublingual glands.

For parasympathetic supply of small glands not discussed, one must assume that axons of second-order neurons with cell bodies in the parasympathetic ganglia, described above, follow nerves going to the area, or that the parasympathetic fibers in IX or X synapse in small ganglia in the area. For the sympathetic supply, second-order neuron cell bodies in the superior cervical ganglion can send axons by any convenient nerve or periarterial plexus.

Section II

ANATOMY OF THE ESOPHAGUS

by

FRANK H. NETTER, M.D.

in collaboration with

NICHOLAS A. MICHELS, M.A., D.Sc.
Plates 8 and 9

PROF. G. A. G. MITCHELL, O.B.E., T.D., M.B., Ch.M., D.Sc.
Plates 11-13

MAX L. SOM, M.D., F.A.C.S.
Plates 1-7, 10

TOPOGRAPHIC RELATIONSHIPS, CONTOURS AND NORMAL CONSTRICTIONS OF ESOPHAGUS

The esophagus commences in the neck as a downward continuation of the pharynx (*cervical esophagus*). This point of origin corresponds to the caudal border of the *cricoid cartilage* and the lower margin of the cricopharyngeus muscle at about the level of the sixth cervical vertebra. The esophagus extends downward through the lower portion of the neck and the superior and posterior mediastina of the thorax. It then passes through the esophageal hiatus of the *diaphragm* to join the cardia of the stomach at about the level of the tenth thoracic vertebra. (The esophagogastric junction is described on page 38.)

The esophagus follows generally the anteroposterior curvature of the vertebral column, except in the lower portion (see below). It also forms two lateral curvatures, so that actually, when viewed from the front, it assumes the form of a gentle reversed "S". The upper of the two lateral curvatures is convex toward the left. The lower curvature, in the lower thorax and abdomen, is convex toward the right. From its commencement at the lower margin of the cricoid cartilage, the esophagus inclines slightly to the left until its left border projects approximately ¼" to the left of the tracheal margin. It then swings somewhat to the right, reaching the midline at about the level of the fourth thoracic vertebra behind the aortic arch. It continues its inclination to the right until about the level of the seventh thoracic vertebra, where it again turns left somewhat more sharply than in its previous curves, and in this direction it passes through the esophageal hiatus.

The esophagus comprises the cervical, thoracic and abdominal portions. Anterior to the cervical portion lies the membranous wall of the trachea, to which it is rather loosely connected by areolar tissue (see page 37) and some muscular strands, so that the anterior esophageal and the posterior tracheal walls are occasionally referred to as the "common party wall". In the grooves on each side between the trachea and the esophagus ascend the *recurrent laryngeal nerves*. Posteriorly, the esophagus lies here upon the vertebral bodies and the *longus colli*

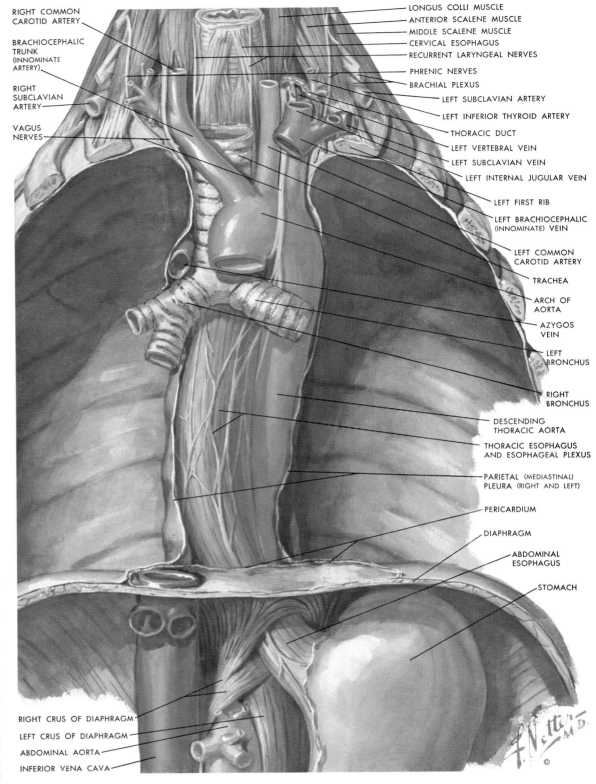

muscles, with the prevertebral fascia intervening. On each side the carotid sheath and the structures it contains accompany the cervical esophagus. Owing to the afore-mentioned curvature of the esophageal tube to the left in this region, it is closer to the carotid sheath on this side than it is on the right. The lobes of the thyroid gland partially overlap the esophagus on each side. The *thoracic duct* ascends in the root of the neck on the left side of the esophagus and then arches laterally behind the carotid sheath and anterior to the vertebral vessels to enter the left brachiocephalic or left subclavian vein at the medial margin of the anterior scalenus muscle.

The *thoracic esophagus* continues to lie posterior to the trachea as far as the level of the fifth thoracic vertebral body, where the trachea bifurcates. The *trachea* deviates slightly to the right at its lower end, so that the *left main bronchus* crosses in front of the

esophagus. Below this point the esophagus is separated anteriorly from the left atrium of the heart by the pericardium. In the very lowest portion of its thoracic course, the esophagus passes behind the diaphragm to reach the esophageal hiatus. On the left side the esophageal wall in the upper thoracic region is the ascending portion of the left subclavian artery and the *parietal pleura;* at about the level of the fourth thoracic vertebra, the *arch of the aorta* passes backward and alongside the esophagus. Below this point the *descending aorta* lies to the left, but when that vessel passes behind the esophagus, the left mediastinal pleura again comes to adjoin the esophageal wall. On the right side the right *parietal pleura* is intimately applied to the esophagus, except when, at about the level of the fourth thoracic vertebra, the azygos vein intervenes as it turns forward. In the

(Continued on page 35)

Labels on illustration:
RIGHT COMMON CAROTID ARTERY
BRACHIOCEPHALIC TRUNK (INNOMINATE ARTERY)
RIGHT SUBCLAVIAN ARTERY
VAGUS NERVES
RIGHT CRUS OF DIAPHRAGM
LEFT CRUS OF DIAPHRAGM
ABDOMINAL AORTA
INFERIOR VENA CAVA
LONGUS COLLI MUSCLE
ANTERIOR SCALENE MUSCLE
MIDDLE SCALENE MUSCLE
CERVICAL ESOPHAGUS
RECURRENT LARYNGEAL NERVES
PHRENIC NERVES
BRACHIAL PLEXUS
LEFT SUBCLAVIAN ARTERY
LEFT INFERIOR THYROID ARTERY
THORACIC DUCT
LEFT VERTEBRAL VEIN
LEFT SUBCLAVIAN VEIN
LEFT INTERNAL JUGULAR VEIN
LEFT FIRST RIB
LEFT BRACHIOCEPHALIC (INNOMINATE) VEIN
LEFT COMMON CAROTID ARTERY
TRACHEA
ARCH OF AORTA
AZYGOS VEIN
LEFT BRONCHUS
RIGHT BRONCHUS
DESCENDING THORACIC AORTA
THORACIC ESOPHAGUS AND ESOPHAGEAL PLEXUS
PARIETAL (MEDIASTINAL) PLEURA (RIGHT AND LEFT)
PERICARDIUM
DIAPHRAGM
ABDOMINAL ESOPHAGUS
STOMACH

TOPOGRAPHIC RELATIONSHIPS, CONTOURS AND NORMAL CONSTRICTIONS OF ESOPHAGUS

(Continued from page 34)

upper part of its thoracic course, the esophagus continues to lie upon the longus colli muscle and the vertebral bodies, with the prevertebral fascia intervening. At about the level of the eighth thoracic vertebra, however, the aorta comes to lie behind the esophagus. The azygos vein ascends behind and to the right of the esophagus as far as the level of the fourth vertebral body, where it turns forward. The hemiazygos vein (see page 42) also crosses from left to right behind the esophagus, as do the upper five right intercostal arteries. The thoracic duct, ascending first to the right of the esophagus, inclines to the left behind it at about the level of the fifth vertebral body, to continue its ascent on the left side of the esophagus.

In its short *abdominal portion* the esophagus lies upon the diaphragm, with the esophageal impression of the liver (see CIBA COLLECTION, Vol. 3/III, page 5) applied tunnellike to its anterior aspect.

Below the tracheal bifurcation the *esophageal plexus* of nerves and the anterior and posterior vagal trunks are closely applied to the esophagus (see page 44).

The course of the esophagus is marked by several indentations and constrictions:

1. The first narrowing of the esophagus is found at its commencement, caused by the *cricopharyngeus muscle* and the cricoid cartilage.

2. The esophagus is indented on its left side by the arch of the aorta (*aortic constriction*), and at this level the aortic pulsations may often be observed through the esophagoscope.

3. Just below this point the left main bronchus causes, generally, an impression on the left anterior aspect of the esophagus.

4. At its lower end the esophagus is narrowed by the *inferior esophageal sphincter* and the *esophagogastric vestibule* (see pages 38, 76 and 77).

The over-all length of the esophagus varies to some extent, generally, in accordance with the length of the trunk of the individual. Thus, the average dis-

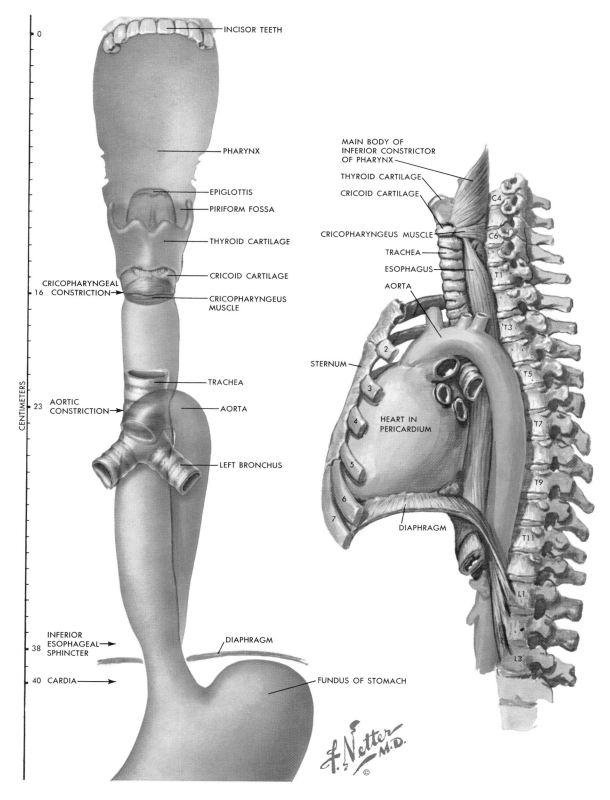

tance of the cardia from the upper incisor teeth is approximately 40 cm., but in some "long" individuals this distance may be as much as 42 or 43 cm. This average distance of 40 cm. from incisor teeth to cardia may be subdivided as follows: The distance from the incisor teeth to the lower border of the cricopharyngeus muscle, which corresponds to the commencement of the esophagus, averages 16 cm. It is thus apparent that the average length of the esophagus itself is 40 cm. minus 16 cm., or 24 cm., which is approximately 10 inches. At about 23 cm. from the incisor teeth, the arch of the aorta crosses the esophagus on its left side. This crossing is obviously, therefore, about 7 cm. below the cricopharyngeus. A few centimeters below this point the left main bronchus passes in front of the esophagus. The inferior esophageal sphincter (see pages 76 and 77), or commencement of the esophagogastric vestibule, is

located at about 37 to 38 cm. from the incisor teeth (see also page 38). It is of considerable significance to note that the esophageal hiatus of the diaphragm is slightly below (approximately 1 cm.) this point, and the cardia is at a still slightly lower level.

The figures given above are for adults; in children the dimensions are proportionately smaller. At birth the distance from the incisor teeth to the cardia is usually only 18 cm., at 3 years approximately 22 cm. and at 10 years approximately 27 cm.

Although the esophagus is usually described as tubelike, it is, in general, flattened anteroposteriorly, so that the transverse axis is somewhat larger than its anteroposterior axis. In the resting state the esophageal walls are in approximation. The width or diameter of the esophagus varies considerably with its state of tonus, but the average resting width is given as approximately 2 cm.

MUSCULATURE OF ESOPHAGUS

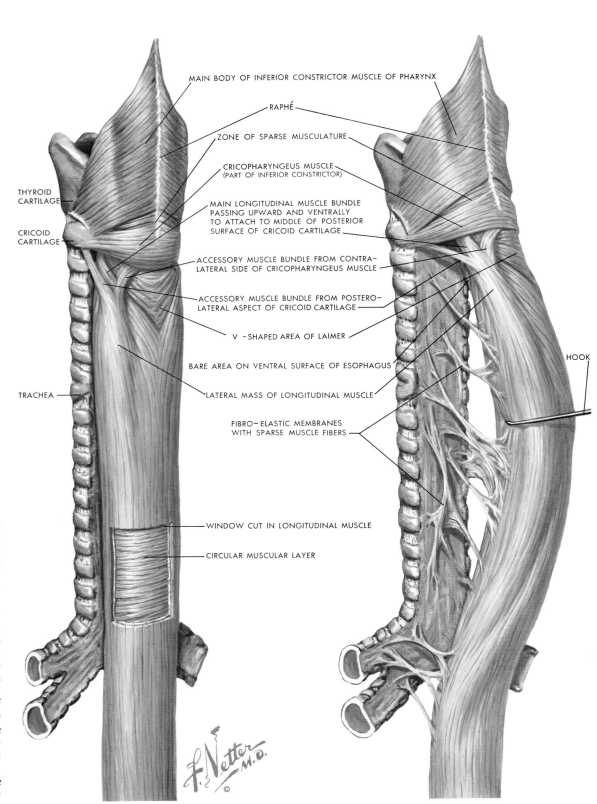

MAIN BODY OF INFERIOR CONSTRICTOR MUSCLE OF PHARYNX

RAPHÉ

ZONE OF SPARSE MUSCULATURE

CRICOPHARYNGEUS MUSCLE (PART OF INFERIOR CONSTRICTOR)

MAIN LONGITUDINAL MUSCLE BUNDLE PASSING UPWARD AND VENTRALLY TO ATTACH TO MIDDLE OF POSTERIOR SURFACE OF CRICOID CARTILAGE

ACCESSORY MUSCLE BUNDLE FROM CONTRA-LATERAL SIDE OF CRICOPHARYNGEUS MUSCLE

ACCESSORY MUSCLE BUNDLE FROM POSTERO-LATERAL ASPECT OF CRICOID CARTILAGE

V-SHAPED AREA OF LAIMER

BARE AREA ON VENTRAL SURFACE OF ESOPHAGUS

LATERAL MASS OF LONGITUDINAL MUSCLE

FIBRO-ELASTIC MEMBRANES WITH SPARSE MUSCLE FIBERS

WINDOW CUT IN LONGITUDINAL MUSCLE

CIRCULAR MUSCULAR LAYER

THYROID CARTILAGE

CRICOID CARTILAGE

TRACHEA

HOOK

F. Netter M.D.

The musculature of the esophagus consists of an outer *longitudinal muscle* layer and an inner muscular layer, generally described for convenience as the *circular muscle layer,* although, strictly speaking, the term "circular" is not properly descriptive, as will be seen below. The outer longitudinal muscle layer originates principally from a stout tendinous band which is attached to the upper part of the vertical ridge on the dorsal aspect of the cricoid cartilage. From this tendon two muscle bands take origin and diverge as they descend and sweep around the respective sides of the esophagus to its dorsal aspect. They meet and interdigitate somewhat in the dorsal midline, leaving a V-shaped gap above and between them. This gap is known as the *V-shaped area of Laimer,* who first described it. The base of the area is formed by the underlying circular muscle. Above, it is delimited by the *cricopharyngeus muscle.* A few sparse fibers of the longitudinal muscle spread over this area, as do also some accessory fibers from the lower margin of the cricopharyngeus. The longitudinal muscle fibers in their descent are not uniformly distributed over the surface of the esophagus in its upper part. Instead, the fibers gather into thick *lateral longitudinal muscle masses* on each side of the esophagus, while they remain considerably thinner over other parts of the tube. The muscle is thinnest on the anterior wall, *i.e.,* the wall which is applied to the posterior tendinous surface of the trachea. Indeed, high up on the ventral surface, the longitudinal muscle is said to be entirely lacking, and this portion of the esophagus is designated as the *"bare" area.* The longitudi-

nal muscle of the esophagus also usually receives additional contributions by way of *accessory muscle* slips on each side, which originate from the posterolateral aspect of the cricoid cartilage and also from the contralateral side of the deep portion of the cricopharyngeus muscle. As the longitudinal muscle descends, it progressively forms a more uniform sheath over the entire circumference of the esophagus.

The anterior wall of the esophagus is firmly applied to the posterior tendinous wall of the trachea in its upper portion (see also page 21), where the two organs are attached to each other by *fibro-elastic membranous tissue* containing some muscle fibers.

The inner, so-called *circular, muscle layer* of the esophagus underlies the longitudinal muscle layer. Although a definite layer, it is slightly thinner than is the longitudinal coat. This ratio of longitudinal and circular muscle coat is unique for the esophagus

and is reversed in all other parts of the alimentary tract. Whether or not the inner circular layer receives contributions of muscle fibers from the cricopharyngeus above it is a matter of controversial opinion. It has been claimed (Lerche) that the circular fibers commence at their upper end independently of any other group of muscle fibers and that they receive no contribution from the cricopharyngeus muscle. In any event, at this level the esophageal circular muscle is in very close proximity to the encircling lower fibers of the cricopharyngeus. The fibers in the upper esophageal portion are not truly circular but rather elliptical, with the anterior part of the ellipse at a lower level than the posterior part. The inclination of the ellipses becomes less as one descends the esophagus, until, at about the junction of the upper and middle thirds, the fibers run in a truly horizontal plane.

(Continued on page 37)

36

MUSCULATURE OF ESOPHAGUS

(Continued from page 36)

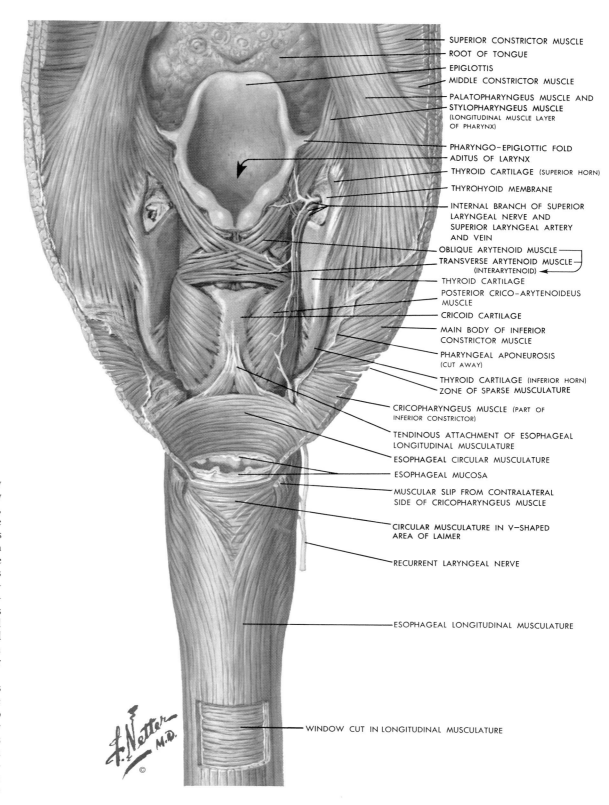

SUPERIOR CONSTRICTOR MUSCLE
ROOT OF TONGUE
EPIGLOTTIS
MIDDLE CONSTRICTOR MUSCLE
PALATOPHARYNGEUS MUSCLE AND
STYLOPHARYNGEUS MUSCLE
(LONGITUDINAL MUSCLE LAYER
OF PHARYNX)
PHARYNGO-EPIGLOTTIC FOLD
ADITUS OF LARYNX
THYROID CARTILAGE (SUPERIOR HORN)
THYROHYOID MEMBRANE
INTERNAL BRANCH OF SUPERIOR
LARYNGEAL NERVE AND
SUPERIOR LARYNGEAL ARTERY
AND VEIN
OBLIQUE ARYTENOID MUSCLE
TRANSVERSE ARYTENOID MUSCLE
(INTERARYTENOID)
THYROID CARTILAGE
POSTERIOR CRICO-ARYTENOIDEUS
MUSCLE
CRICOID CARTILAGE
MAIN BODY OF INFERIOR
CONSTRICTOR MUSCLE
PHARYNGEAL APONEUROSIS
(CUT AWAY)
THYROID CARTILAGE (INFERIOR HORN)
ZONE OF SPARSE MUSCULATURE
CRICOPHARYNGEUS MUSCLE (PART OF
INFERIOR CONSTRICTOR)
TENDINOUS ATTACHMENT OF ESOPHAGEAL
LONGITUDINAL MUSCULATURE
ESOPHAGEAL CIRCULAR MUSCULATURE
ESOPHAGEAL MUCOSA
MUSCULAR SLIP FROM CONTRALATERAL
SIDE OF CRICOPHARYNGEUS MUSCLE
CIRCULAR MUSCULATURE IN V-SHAPED
AREA OF LAIMER
RECURRENT LARYNGEAL NERVE
ESOPHAGEAL LONGITUDINAL MUSCULATURE
WINDOW CUT IN LONGITUDINAL MUSCULATURE

Here, for a segment of about 1 cm., they may be said to be truly circular. Below this point they again become elliptical, but with a reverse inclination; *i.e.*, the posterior part of the ellipse now assumes a lower level than the anterior part. In the lower third of the esophagus, the course of the fibers again changes (Laimer). Here they follow a screwshaped or spiral course, winding progressively on downward as they pass around the esophagus. It should be noted also that the elliptical, circular and spiral fibers of this layer are not truly uniform and parallel but may overlap and cross or even have clefts between them.

Some fibers in the lower two thirds of the esophagus occasionally leave the elliptical or spiral fibers at one level, to pass diagonally or even perpendicularly upward and downward to join the fibers at another level, but they never form a continuous layer. They may be threadlike or 2 to 3 mm. in width and from 1 to 5 cm. in length; they are usually branched.

Spontaneous rupture of the esophagus almost invariably occurs in the lower 2 cm. of the esophagus. A linear tear occurs through the entire thickness of the esophageal wall. Severe vomiting predisposes to rupture of the gullet, with escape of gastric juice into the mediastinum.

The musculature of the esophagogastric vestibule is discussed on page 38.

The *cricopharyngeus muscle,* although strictly speaking a muscle of the pharyngeal wall, being the lowermost portion of the *inferior constrictor of the pharynx* (see pages 21 and 22), is nevertheless of great importance in the function and malfunction of the esophagus. This narrow band of muscle fibers originates on each side from the posterolateral mar-

gin of the cricoid cartilage and passes slinglike around the dorsal aspect of the pharyngo-esophageal junction. Its uppermost fibers ascend to join the median *raphé* of the inferior constrictor muscle posteriorly. The lower fibers do not have any median raphé but pass continuously around the dorsal aspect of the pharyngo-esophageal junction, and a few of its fibers pass on down over the esophagus itself (see above). The cricopharyngeus is believed to act somewhat as a sphincter of the upper end of the esophagus, and, indeed, the term "cricopharyngeal pinchcock" has been applied to it for this reason. The cricopharyngeal constriction is felt when the esophagoscope is introduced, because even at rest the muscular tonus felt within the esophageal lumen is greater at the level of the cricopharyngeus than in other parts of the esophagus, and the relaxation of this muscle is an integral part of the act of swallowing (see pages 76 and 77).

Above the cricopharyngeus, *i.e.,* between this muscle and the main part of the inferior constrictor, the musculature is somewhat weaker and sparser posteriorly. It is through this sparse area that most pulsion diverticula are believed to originate (see page 143).

The musculature of the upper portion of the esophagus is striated, whereas that of the lower portion belongs to the smooth variety, but the level at which this transition takes place varies. In general, it may be said that the upper fourth of the esophagus contains purely striated muscle, the second fourth is a transitional zone in which both striated and smooth muscle are present and the lower half contains purely smooth muscle.

Between the two muscle coats of the esophagus, a narrow layer of connective tissue is inserted, which accommodates the myenteric plexus of Auerbach (see pages 45 and 46).

ESOPHAGOGASTRIC JUNCTION

The structure as well as the function of the lower end of the esophagus and its junction with the stomach have been the subject of much investigation and conjecture, and with good reason, because an improved knowledge of this region is bound to achieve a better understanding not only of the function of the normal esophagus but also of such ailments as achalasia (see page 145), hiatal hernia (see page 158), esophagitis and peptic ulcer of the esophagus (see pages 146, 147 and 148).

The longitudinal muscle coat of the esophagus extends downward and continues over the surface of the stomach in the form of the outer longitudinal muscle of the stomach (see page 53). The so-called inner circular layer of esophageal musculature, which at this point is spiral in character (see page 37), also continues over the stomach but divides, in the region of the cardia, into the middle circular layer of the gastric musculature and the inner oblique layer. The inner oblique muscle fibers pass slinglike across the cardiac incisura, whereas the middle circular fibers pass more or less horizontally around the stomach. These two layers of muscle fibers thus cross each other at an angle, forming a muscular ring, which became known as *collare Helvetii*, and to which a sphincteric action has been ascribed by some.

No structures, either in the lower esophagus or at the cardia, satisfying the anatomic concept of a sphincter, have, however, been definitely established. The existence of a functional or physiologic sphincter in this region, nevertheless, can scarcely be doubted, because of the many observations of the normal process of deglutition (see pages 76 and 77) and because, obviously, some mechanism seems to be present which prevents regurgitation under normal conditions.

A gradual but moderate thickening of both the so-called *circular and longitudinal muscles* takes place in the lower end of the esophagus, commencing about 1 or 2 cm. above the diaphragmatic hiatus and extending to the cardia. This region has been termed by Lerche the "esophagogastric vestibule". A distinguishable group of muscle fibers at the upper end of the esophagogastric vestibule has been described (Laimer, Lerche) to which the term "inferior esophageal sphincter" has been applied. Whether

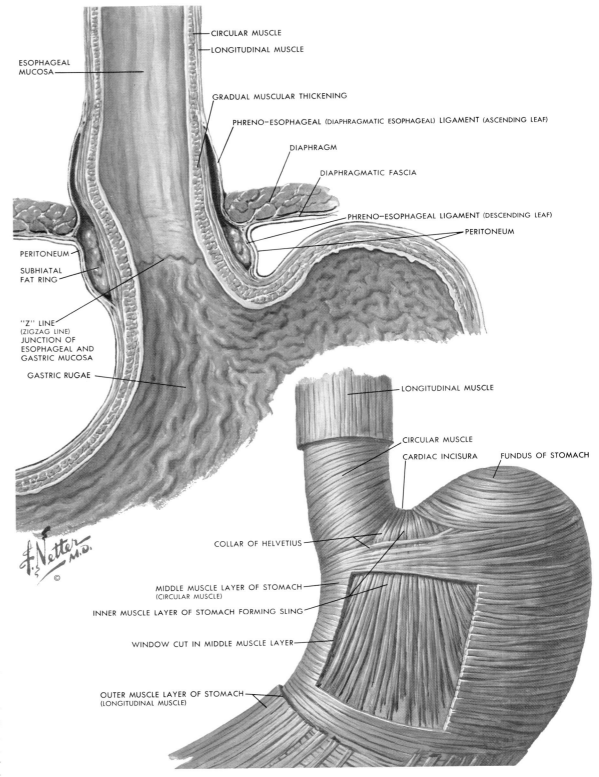

or not such a specialized group of muscle fibers really exists, it is now coming to be recognized that the vestibule contracts and relaxes as a unit (see pages 76 and 77). Thus, the term "inferior esophageal sphincter" has some functional justification and has remained and is accepted as a means of designating the upper end of the vestibule. It is believed that the bolus is transiently arrested just above the diaphragmatic hiatus by the tonicity of the entire vestibule and, contrariwise, that its passage into the stomach is made possible by the relaxation of the entire vestibule working as an integrated or co-ordinated unit. It is likewise believed that the contraction of the esophagogastric vestibule is one of the important factors in the prevention of regurgitation from the stomach. Other factors in the prevention of regurgitation are believed to be the angulation of the esophagus as it passes through the diaphragm while passing over into the

stomach and a rosettelike formation of loose gastric mucosa at the cardia. The possibility of sphincteric action of the diaphragm is debated, although it is recognized that in deep inspiration, when the diaphragm is in strong contraction, passage into the stomach may be impeded.

The mucosa of the esophagus (see also page 40) is smooth and rather pale in color. When the esophagus is contracted, the mucosa is gathered up into irregular longitudinal folds. The gastric mucosa, on the other hand, is a much deeper red in color and definitely rugous in character. The transition from esophageal to gastric mucosa, easily recognizable by this color change, takes place along an irregular dentate or zigzag line, known as the "Z-Z" line or simply as the *"Z" line*. The position of the "Z-Z" line or of the transition from squamous to columnar epithelium

(Continued on page 39)

ESOPHAGOGASTRIC JUNCTION

(Continued from page 38)

usually does not coincide with the anatomic border of the cardia but slightly above it, somewhere between that level and the hiatus of the diaphragm. In some instances the gastric mucosa may extend for a considerable distance proximally into the esophagus (see page 139).

In its passage through the esophageal hiatus of the diaphragm, the esophagus is surrounded by the *phreno-esophageal ligament,* also known as phrenico-esophageal ligament and diaphragmatico-esophageal ligament. The phreno-esophageal ligament arises from the circumference of the hiatus as an extension of the inferior fascia of the diaphragm, which is continuous with the transversalis fascia. At the margin of the hiatus, it divides into an *ascending leaf* and a *descending leaf.* The ascending leaf passes upward through the hiatus and surrounds the esophagus in a tentlike fashion. It extends for several centimeters above the hiatus, where it is inserted circumferentially into the adventitia of the esophagus. The descending leaf passes downward and is inserted around the cardia deep to the *peritoneum.* Within the cavity thus formed by the phreno-esophageal ligament and below the diaphragmatic hiatus lies a ring of rather dense fat. The function of the phreno-esophageal ligament has been the subject of much speculation. From its structure it certainly would seem to play a part as a fixation mechanism, which still permits the limited excursion required for respiration, deglutition and postural changes. It also serves as an additional means of preventing pressure transmission through the hiatus. The possibility that it also may in some manner take part in the closure or sphincteric mechanism of the esophagus in connection with diaphragmatic action cannot be denied.

The formation and configuration of the esophageal hiatus of the diaphragm are of considerable interest in view of the current discussion as to whether or not the diaphragm plays a part in the gastro-esophageal sphincteric mechanism. According to the standard description (given by Low in 1907), the left crus of the diaphragm plays no part in the formation of the esophageal hiatus. One band of muscle fibers, originating from the right crus, ascends and passes to the right of the esophagus. Another band of muscle fibers, originating also from the

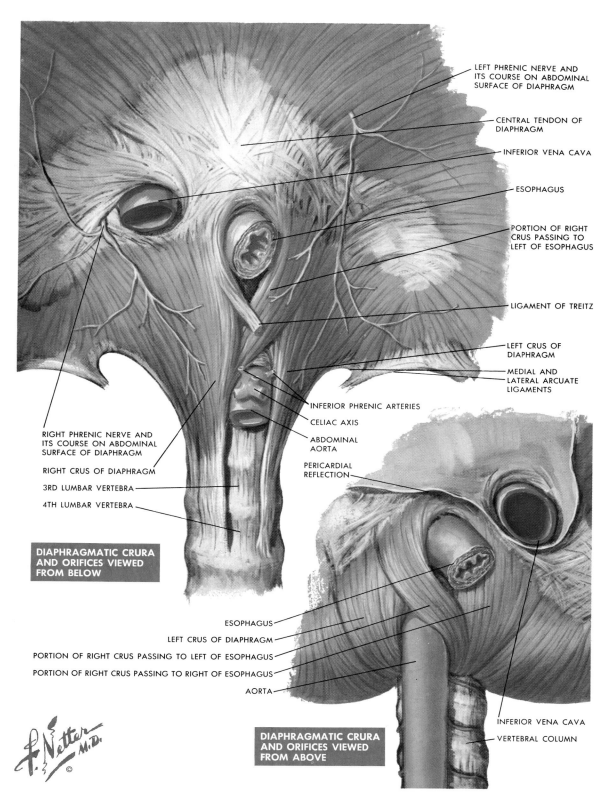

LEFT PHRENIC NERVE AND ITS COURSE ON ABDOMINAL SURFACE OF DIAPHRAGM

CENTRAL TENDON OF DIAPHRAGM

INFERIOR VENA CAVA

ESOPHAGUS

PORTION OF RIGHT CRUS PASSING TO LEFT OF ESOPHAGUS

LIGAMENT OF TREITZ

LEFT CRUS OF DIAPHRAGM

MEDIAL AND LATERAL ARCUATE LIGAMENTS

INFERIOR PHRENIC ARTERIES

CELIAC AXIS

ABDOMINAL AORTA

PERICARDIAL REFLECTION

RIGHT PHRENIC NERVE AND ITS COURSE ON ABDOMINAL SURFACE OF DIAPHRAGM

RIGHT CRUS OF DIAPHRAGM

3RD LUMBAR VERTEBRA

4TH LUMBAR VERTEBRA

DIAPHRAGMATIC CRURA AND ORIFICES VIEWED FROM BELOW

ESOPHAGUS

LEFT CRUS OF DIAPHRAGM

PORTION OF RIGHT CRUS PASSING TO LEFT OF ESOPHAGUS

PORTION OF RIGHT CRUS PASSING TO RIGHT OF ESOPHAGUS

AORTA

INFERIOR VENA CAVA

VERTEBRAL COLUMN

DIAPHRAGMATIC CRURA AND ORIFICES VIEWED FROM ABOVE

right crus but more deeply, ascends and passes to the left of the esophagus. These muscle bands overlap scissorwise and are inserted into the central tendon of the diaphragm. Thus, all the muscle fibers about the esophageal hiatus arise from the right crus of the diaphragm. It is interesting to note that those fibers of the right crus which pass to the right of the esophagus are innervated by the *right phrenic nerve,* whereas those which pass to the left of the esophageal hiatus appear to be innervated by a branch of the *left phrenic nerve,* as is also the left crus itself. The *right crus* of the diaphragm is usually considerably larger than is the left crus.

This standard pattern varies considerably (Collis, Kelly and Wiley). Occasionally, one may find what has come to be known as the "muscle of Low". This is a small band of muscle fibers which originates from the left crus and crosses over to the right, passing

between the muscle fibers of the right crus to reach the central tendon in the region of the foramen of the *inferior vena cava.* Somewhat more frequently, a similar muscle bundle appears on the superior surface of the diaphragm.

More significant is the fact that, in a considerable number of individuals, an anatomic variation may be found that has been described as a "shift to the left". In such cases fibers from the left crus of the diaphragm enter into formation of the right side of the esophageal hiatus. In some instances the muscle to the right of the esophageal hiatus may take origin entirely from the left crus and those to the left of the hiatus entirely from the right crus. The *ligament of Treitz* (see also page 51), or the suspensory muscle of the duodenum, takes origin usually from the fibers of the right crus of the diaphragm which pass to the right of the esophagus.

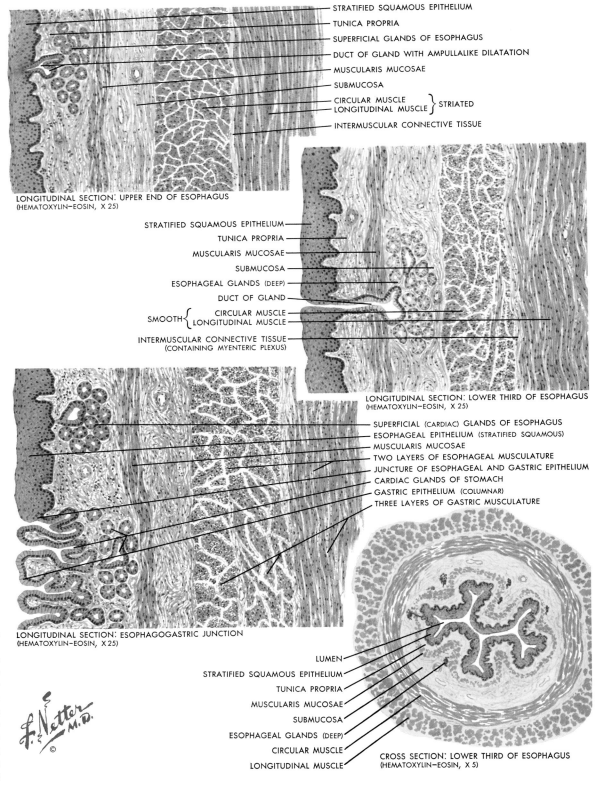

STRATIFIED SQUAMOUS EPITHELIUM
TUNICA PROPRIA
SUPERFICIAL GLANDS OF ESOPHAGUS
DUCT OF GLAND WITH AMPULLALIKE DILATATION
MUSCULARIS MUCOSAE
SUBMUCOSA
CIRCULAR MUSCLE
LONGITUDINAL MUSCLE } STRIATED
INTERMUSCULAR CONNECTIVE TISSUE

LONGITUDINAL SECTION: UPPER END OF ESOPHAGUS
(HEMATOXYLIN–EOSIN, X 25)

STRATIFIED SQUAMOUS EPITHELIUM
TUNICA PROPRIA
MUSCULARIS MUCOSAE
SUBMUCOSA
ESOPHAGEAL GLANDS (DEEP)
DUCT OF GLAND
SMOOTH { CIRCULAR MUSCLE
LONGITUDINAL MUSCLE
INTERMUSCULAR CONNECTIVE TISSUE
(CONTAINING MYENTERIC PLEXUS)

LONGITUDINAL SECTION: LOWER THIRD OF ESOPHAGUS
(HEMATOXYLIN–EOSIN, X 25)

SUPERFICIAL (CARDIAC) GLANDS OF ESOPHAGUS
ESOPHAGEAL EPITHELIUM (STRATIFIED SQUAMOUS)
MUSCULARIS MUCOSAE
TWO LAYERS OF ESOPHAGEAL MUSCULATURE
JUNCTURE OF ESOPHAGEAL AND GASTRIC EPITHELIUM
CARDIAC GLANDS OF STOMACH
GASTRIC EPITHELIUM (COLUMNAR)
THREE LAYERS OF GASTRIC MUSCULATURE

HISTOLOGY OF
ESOPHAGUS

LONGITUDINAL SECTION: ESOPHAGOGASTRIC JUNCTION
(HEMATOXYLIN–EOSIN, X 25)

LUMEN
STRATIFIED SQUAMOUS EPITHELIUM
TUNICA PROPRIA
MUSCULARIS MUCOSAE
SUBMUCOSA
ESOPHAGEAL GLANDS (DEEP)
CIRCULAR MUSCLE
LONGITUDINAL MUSCLE

CROSS SECTION: LOWER THIRD OF ESOPHAGUS
(HEMATOXYLIN–EOSIN, X 5)

The esophagus, like other parts of the alimentary canal, is comprised of a mucosa, a submucosa, a muscularis and an adventitia. The mucosa is made up of epithelium, the lamina propria and a muscularis mucosae. The esophagus is lined by *stratified squamous epithelium,* which is a continuation from the pharyngeal lining. The surface cells of this epithelium are flattened and contain a few keratohyalin granules, but are not cornified. An abrupt transition takes place between the stratified squamous epithelium of the esophagus and the columnar epithelium of the stomach along an irregular zigzag line, also known as the "Z-Z" line, situated usually just a little above the cardia (see page 38). The lamina propria consists of loose connective tissue, with papillae projecting into the epithelium. The *muscularis mucosae* appears to be a continuation downward from the pharyngeal aponeurosis, plainly visible in the pictures on pages 21 and 23. A transition to muscular tissue takes place in this aponeurosis at about the level of the cricoid cartilage. It comprises both *longitudinal smooth muscle fibers* and some elastic tissue and is thicker at the lower end of the esophagus.

The *submucosa* is quite dense and contains both elastic and collagen fibers. A moderate number of lymphocytes is scattered through both the lamina propria and the submucosa, and occasionally these may be found in isolated concentric

groups. In its contracted state the esophageal mucosa is thrown into irregular longitudinal folds. The submucosa extends into these folds, but the true muscular layer does not.

The muscular coat consists of an inner layer, called the circular layer, and an outer longitudinal layer (see pages 36 and 37). A thin layer of connective tissue, in which is embedded the myenteric plexus of Auerbach (see pages 45 and 46), is spread between the two muscular layers. The submucosa contains Meissner's plexus and also some blood vessels. The musculature of the upper one fourth of the esophagus is generally striated in character, the second fourth contains both striated and smooth muscle and the lower half is composed entirely of smooth muscle (see also pages 36 and 37). The adventitia consists of loose connective tissue, connecting the esophagus to its surrounding structure.

Two types of glands can be recognized in the esophagus. One of them, the *esophageal glands* proper, or deep glands, are irregularly distributed throughout the entire length of the tube. They are small, compound racemose glands of the mucous type. Their ducts penetrate the muscularis mucosae, and their branched tubules lie in the submucosa. The glands of the other type are known as the *cardiac glands,* or *superficial glands,* because they closely resemble or are identical with the cardiac glands of the stomach (see page 52). They are found at both ends of the esophagus, *i.e.,* for a few centimeters below the level of the cricopharyngeus muscle and also just above the cardia. They differ from the esophageal glands proper in that their ducts do not penetrate the muscularis mucosae and their branched and coiled tubules are located in the lamina propria, NOT in the submucosa.

BLOOD SUPPLY OF ESOPHAGUS

RIGHT COMMON CAROTID ARTERY

RIGHT SUBCLAVIAN ARTERY

ESOPHAGEAL BRANCHES OF INFERIOR THYROID ARTERIES

SUPERFICIAL CERVICAL ARTERY (LEFT)
TRANSVERSE SCAPULAR ARTERY (LEFT)
THYROCERVICAL TRUNK (LEFT)

LEFT SUBCLAVIAN ARTERY

INTERNAL MAMMARY ARTERY (LEFT)

VERTEBRAL ARTERY (LEFT)

LEFT COMMON CAROTID ARTERY

BRACHIOCEPHALIC TRUNK (INNOMINATE ARTERY)

TRACHEA

3RD RIGHT INTERCOSTAL ARTERY

RIGHT BRONCHIAL ARTERY

SUPERIOR LEFT BRONCHIAL ARTERY

ESOPHAGEAL BRANCH OF RIGHT BRONCHIAL ARTERY

INFERIOR LEFT BRONCHIAL ARTERY

THORACIC AORTA

AORTIC ESOPHAGEAL ARTERIES

ESOPHAGUS

DIAPHRAGM

STOMACH

ESOPHAGEAL ARTERY
INFERIOR PHRENIC ARTERIES
LEFT GASTRIC ARTERY
CELIAC AXIS
SPLENIC ARTERY
HEPATIC ARTERY

FREQUENT VARIATIONS: ESOPHAGEAL ARTERY ORIGINATING FROM CELIAC AXIS, FIRST PART OF SPLENIC, SHORT GASTRICS, SUPERIOR SPLENIC POLAR AND PREVALENT LARGE OR SMALL POSTERIOR GASTRO-ESOPHAGEAL BRANCH FROM SPLENIC. LEFT INFERIOR PHRENIC ARTERY VIA ITS RECURRENT BRANCH TO ABDOMINAL ESOPHAGUS OFTEN AFFORDS LIFE-SUSTAINING BLOOD SUPPLY TO THIS ENTERIC SEGMENT

In accord with recent anatomic investigations (Shapiro and Robillard, Anson et al., Michels), the blood supply of the esophagus is extremely varied. The main supply of the cervical portion is derived from the *inferior thyroid artery.* While the majority of *esophageal branches* arise from the terminal branches of this artery, its ascending and descending portions frequently give rise to one or more esophageal branches. The anterior cervical esophageal arteries give twiglike branches to both esophagus and trachea. Accessory arteries to the cervical esophagus derive frequently from the *subclavian, common carotid,* vertebral, ascending pharyngeal, *superficial cervical* and costocervical *trunk.*

The thoracic segment of the esophagus is supplied by branches from (1) bronchial arteries, (2) *aorta* and (3) *right intercostals.* The bronchial arteries give off esophageal twigs at or below the tracheal bifurcation, those from the *left inferior bronchial artery* being the most common. Patterns of the bronchial arteries vary markedly. The standard textbook type (two left, one right) occurs only in about one half of the population. Aberrant types comprise one right and one left (25 per cent), two right and two left (15 per cent), one left and two right (8 per cent) and, in some instances, three right or three left. Near the bifurcation point of the trachea, the esophagus may receive additional twigs from the aorta, aortic arch, uppermost intercostals, internal mammary and carotid. The *aortic branches to the thoracic esophagus* are not segmentally arranged; nor are they four in number, as commonly taught, but comprise only two unpaired vessels. The upper or superior one is small (3 to 4 cm.) and, usually, arises at the level of T6 to 7. The lower or inferior is longer (6 to 7 cm.) and arises at T7 to 8 disk level. Both arteries pass behind the esophagus and divide into ascending and descending branches that anastomose longitudinally, with descending branches from the inferior thyroid and bronchial arteries and with ascending branches from the left gastric and left inferior phrenic. Right intercostal arteries, mainly the fifth, give rise to esophageal branches in about 20 per cent of the population.

The abdominal esophagus receives its blood supply primarily through branches from the *left gastric,* short gastrics (see page 57) and from the *recurrent branch of the left inferior phrenic,* given off by the latter after it has passed under the esophagus in its course to the diaphragm. The left gastric supplies cardio-esophageal branches, either via a single vessel which subdivides or via several branches (two to five), given off in seriation before its division into an anterior and a posterior primary gastric branch. Other arterial sources to the abdominal esophagus comprise branches from (1) an aberrant left hepatic from the left gastric, an accessory left gastric from the left hepatic, or branches from a persistent primitive gastrohepatic arterial arc; (2) cardio-esophageal branches from the splenic trunk, its superior polar, terminal divisions (short gastrics) and its occasional large posterior gastric artery; (3) a direct, slender cardio-esophageal branch from the aorta, celiac or first part of the splenic artery.

With every resectional operation, areas of devascularization may be induced by (1) a too low resection of the cervical segment, which should always have a supply from the inferior thyroid; (2) excessive mobilization of the esophagus at the tracheal bifurcation and laceration of the bronchial arteries; (3) excessive sacrifice of the left gastric and the *recurrent branch of the left inferior phrenic* to facilitate gastric mobilization. The anastomosis about the abdominal esophagus is usually very copious (see page 57), but, in some instances, it may be extremely meager.

VENOUS DRAINAGE OF ESOPHAGUS

The venous drainage of the esophagus is effected by tributaries that empty into various single veins and into the azygos and hemiazygos systems. Drainage begins in a *submucosal venous plexus,* branches of which, after piercing the muscle layers, form a venous plexus on the external surface of the esophagus. Tributaries from the cervical *periesophageal venous plexus* drain into the *inferior thyroid vein,* which empties into the right or left *brachiocephalic* (innominate) *vein,* or into both. Tributaries from the thoracic periesophageal plexus, on the right side, join the *azygos, right brachiocephalic* and, occasionally, the *vertebral vein;* on the left side they join the *hemiazygos, accessory hemiazygos, left brachiocephalic* and, occasionally, the vertebral vein. Tributaries from the short abdominal esophagus drain mostly into the *left gastric (coronary) vein* of the stomach; others are in continuity with the *short gastric veins* and thereby also with the *splenic* and *left gastro-epiploic veins* or with branches of the *left inferior phrenic,* the latter joining the inferior vena cava directly or the suprarenal before it enters the renal vein.

The composition and arrangement of the azygos system of veins are extremely variable (Adachi). The *azygos vein* arises in the abdomen from the ascending right lumbar vein that receives the first and second lumbar and the subcostal veins. It may arise directly from the inferior vena cava or have connections with the right common iliac, or renal, vein. In the thorax it receives the right posterior intercostal veins from the fourth to the eleventh spaces and terminates in the superior vena cava. The highest intercostal vein from the first space drains into the right brachiocephalic or, occasionally, into the vertebral vein. The veins from the second and third spaces unite in a common trunk (*right superior intercostal*) that ends in the terminal arched portion of the azygos. The *hemiazygos* arises as a continuation of the left ascending lumbar or from the left renal vein. It receives the left subcostal vein and the intercostal veins from the eighth or ninth to the eleventh spaces, then crosses the vertebral column posterior to the esophagus to join the azygos. The *accessory hemiazygos* receives the intercostal veins from the fourth to the seventh or eighth

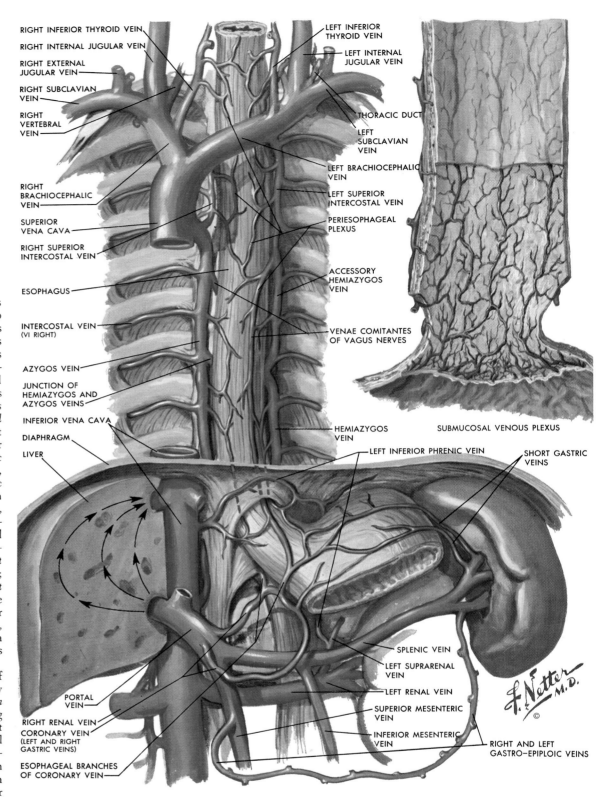

spaces, then crosses the spine posterior to the esophagus to join the hemiazygos or to end separately in the azygos. Above, it may communicate with the left superior intercostal that drains the second and third spaces and ends in the left brachiocephalic. Drainage of the first space is into the left brachiocephalic or vertebral vein.

Often the hemiazygos, accessory hemiazygos and superior intercostal trunk form a continuous longitudinal channel, with no connections with the azygos. Communications of the left azygos system with that of the right may be so numerous (three to five) that a hemiazygos or accessory hemiazygos is not formed. The left azygos system may be reduced to a slender channel, the main left venous drainage of the esophagus and the intercostal spaces then being in the veins of the respective vertebrae. Interruptions in the left azygos system by crossing to the right azygos usually

occur between the seventh and ninth intercostal veins, the most common vertebral level of crossing being T8.

At the cardio-esophageal end of the stomach, branches from the left gastric (coronary) vein are in continuity with the lower esophageal branches through which blood may be shunted into the superior vena cava via the azygos and hemiazygos veins. From this same cardio-esophageal region, blood may be shunted into the splenic vein, retroperitoneal veins and inferior phrenic vein of the diaphragm, through which communication is established with the caval system. Backflow of the venous blood through the esophageal veins leads to their dilatation, with formation of varicosities (see CIBA COLLECTION, Vol. 3/III, page 69). Since short gastrics pass up from the splenic to the cardio-esophageal end of the stomach, thrombosis of the splenic vein may readily lead to esophageal varices and fatal hemorrhages.

LYMPHATIC DRAINAGE OF ESOPHAGUS

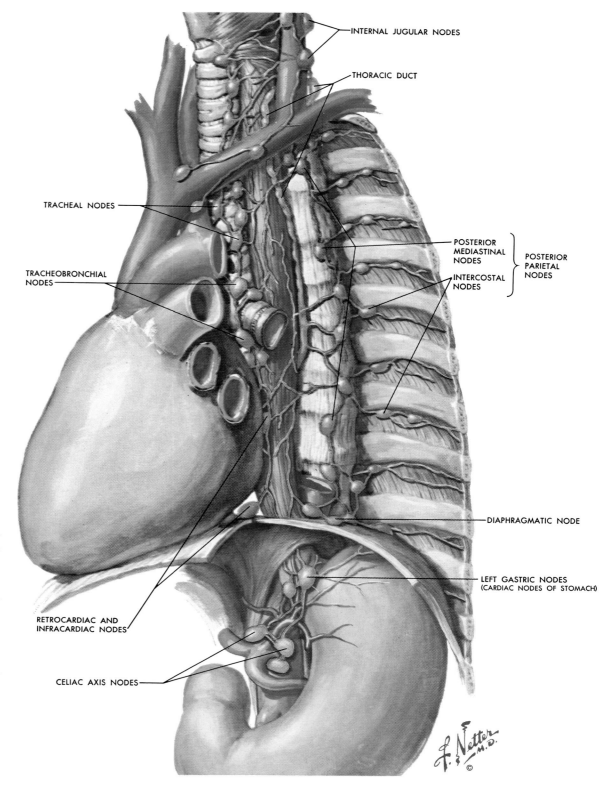

INTERNAL JUGULAR NODES

THORACIC DUCT

TRACHEAL NODES

TRACHEOBRONCHIAL NODES

POSTERIOR MEDIASTINAL NODES

POSTERIOR PARIETAL NODES

INTERCOSTAL NODES

DIAPHRAGMATIC NODE

LEFT GASTRIC NODES (CARDIAC NODES OF STOMACH)

RETROCARDIAC AND INFRACARDIAC NODES

CELIAC AXIS NODES

The esophagus contains a rich network of lymphatic vessels, largely in the lamina propria of the mucosa but also in the other layers.

From the cervical esophagus, lymph vessels course chiefly to the lower *internal jugular nodes* and possibly also to the upper *tracheal nodes* situated in the groove between the esophagus and trachea.

From the thoracic esophagus, the lymphatics drain posteriorly to the *posterior parietal nodes,* and in the more distal parts to the *diaphragmatic nodes.* Anteriorly, the thoracic esophagus drains in its upper part to the *tracheal* and *tracheobronchial nodes,* and lower down to the *retrocardiac* and *infracardiac nodes.*

From the short abdominal portion of the esophagus, the drainage is similar to that from the upper portion of the lesser curvature of the stomach, *i.e.,* chiefly to the paracardial nodes (also known as the "cardiac nodes") which are a subdivision of the upper left gastric group (see page 63). From here, in turn, drainage is to the celiac nodes. Some lymph vessels from this region also pass upward through the esophageal hiatus of the diaphragm and connect with the vessels and nodes above the diaphragm.

The *internal jugular chain* of nodes, a subdivision of the deep cervical nodes, lies along the internal jugular vein from the parotid gland to the clavicle (see page 27). They drain on the left side to the thoracic duct and on the right to the short right lymph duct, which opens into the right subclavian vein at the angle

formed by the latter with the internal jugular vein.

The *posterior parietal nodes* comprise both the *posterior mediastinal* and the *intercostal nodes.* The posterior mediastinal nodes lie alongside the vertebral column, and the intercostal nodes are in the intercostal spaces close by. Both these groups drain generally upward and, eventually, empty into the thoracic duct or into the right lymph duct, which terminates at the right subclavian vein, where it joins the right jugular vein. Of the diaphragmatic nodes it is chiefly the posterior group that is related to the esophagus, and these are closely associated with the posterior parietal nodes, to which they drain.

The *tracheal nodes,* sometimes referred to as the paratracheal nodes, form a chain on each side alongside the trachea along the course of the recurrent nerves. The tracheobronchial nodes are that group which is situated about the bifurcation of the trachea

and in the angle formed by the bifurcation. This is the group of nodes which may be responsible for the formation of traction diverticula when they become fibrosed as a result usually of tuberculous involvement (see page 143). The tracheal and tracheobronchial nodes drain upward and usually form on each side a bronchomediastinal trunk, which, in turn, joins either the thoracic duct or the right lymph duct. They may, however, also have independent openings into the veins or may unite with the internal mammary chain or a low node of the internal jugular chain. The *retrocardiac* and *infracardiac nodes* also drain upward with the tracheal and tracheobronchial nodes.

Drainage from the left gastric nodes is along the course of the left gastric artery and coronary vein to the celiac nodes situated on the aorta in relation to the root of the celiac trunk. These nodes, in turn, empty into the cisterna chyli or the thoracic duct.

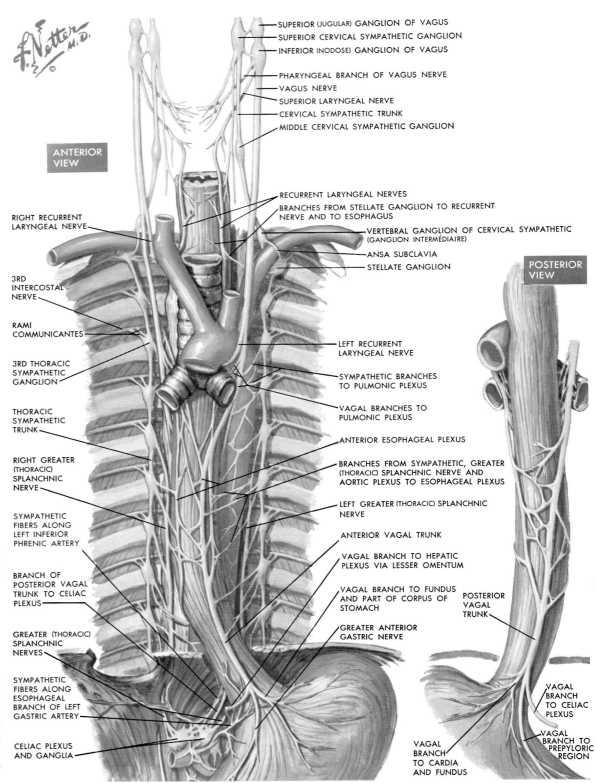

ANTERIOR VIEW

SUPERIOR (JUGULAR) GANGLION OF VAGUS
SUPERIOR CERVICAL SYMPATHETIC GANGLION
INFERIOR (NODOSE) GANGLION OF VAGUS
PHARYNGEAL BRANCH OF VAGUS NERVE
VAGUS NERVE
SUPERIOR LARYNGEAL NERVE
CERVICAL SYMPATHETIC TRUNK
MIDDLE CERVICAL SYMPATHETIC GANGLION

RIGHT RECURRENT LARYNGEAL NERVE

RECURRENT LARYNGEAL NERVES
BRANCHES FROM STELLATE GANGLION TO RECURRENT NERVE AND TO ESOPHAGUS
VERTEBRAL GANGLION OF CERVICAL SYMPATHETIC (GANGLION INTERMÉDIAIRE)
ANSA SUBCLAVIA
STELLATE GANGLION

3RD INTERCOSTAL NERVE

RAMI COMMUNICANTES

3RD THORACIC SYMPATHETIC GANGLION

THORACIC SYMPATHETIC TRUNK

RIGHT GREATER (THORACIC) SPLANCHNIC NERVE

SYMPATHETIC FIBERS ALONG LEFT INFERIOR PHRENIC ARTERY

BRANCH OF POSTERIOR VAGAL TRUNK TO CELIAC PLEXUS

GREATER (THORACIC) SPLANCHNIC NERVES

SYMPATHETIC FIBERS ALONG ESOPHAGEAL BRANCH OF LEFT GASTRIC ARTERY

CELIAC PLEXUS AND GANGLIA

LEFT RECURRENT LARYNGEAL NERVE
SYMPATHETIC BRANCHES TO PULMONIC PLEXUS
VAGAL BRANCHES TO PULMONIC PLEXUS
ANTERIOR ESOPHAGEAL PLEXUS
BRANCHES FROM SYMPATHETIC, GREATER (THORACIC) SPLANCHNIC NERVE AND AORTIC PLEXUS TO ESOPHAGEAL PLEXUS
LEFT GREATER (THORACIC) SPLANCHNIC NERVE
ANTERIOR VAGAL TRUNK
VAGAL BRANCH TO HEPATIC PLEXUS VIA LESSER OMENTUM
VAGAL BRANCH TO FUNDUS AND PART OF CORPUS OF STOMACH
GREATER ANTERIOR GASTRIC NERVE

POSTERIOR VIEW

POSTERIOR VAGAL TRUNK

VAGAL BRANCH TO CELIAC PLEXUS

VAGAL BRANCH TO PREPYLORIC REGION

VAGAL BRANCH TO CARDIA AND FUNDUS

INNERVATION OF ESOPHAGUS

The esophagus is supplied by the vagus (parasympathetic) and sympathetic nerves, which contain efferent and afferent fibers and which convey impulses to and from the vessels, glands and muscular and mucous coats of the viscus (see also CIBA COLLECTION, Vol. 1, pages 81, 83, 84, 85 and 93).

Parasympathetic Supply

The parasympathetic efferent and afferent fibers are carried in the *vagus nerves* and end in the dorsal vagal nucleus which contains both visceral efferent and afferent cells. The fibers supplying the striated musculature in the pharynx and upper part of the esophagus arise in the nucleus ambiguus.

The vagi intercommunicate with filaments from the paravertebral sympathetic trunks and their branches, so that, from the neck downward, they are really mixed parasympathetic-sympathetic nerves.

In the neck the esophagus receives twigs from the *recurrent laryngeal nerves* which run upward on each side in the grooves between the esophagus and trachea, and inconstant filaments pass to the esophagus from the main vagus nerves which lie in the carotid sheath behind and between the common carotid artery and internal jugular vein. On the right side the recurrent laryngeal nerve arises from the vagus nerve at the root of

the neck and winds below the corresponding subclavian artery. On the left side the recurrent nerve arises from the left vagus nerve opposite the aortic arch and curves beneath the arch to reach the groove between the trachea and esophagus (see page 29).

In the thorax the part of the esophagus in the superior mediastinum receives filaments from the left recurrent laryngeal nerve and from both vagus nerves. The vagus nerves descend posterior to the lung roots, giving off branches which unite with filaments from the sympathetic trunks to form the smaller anterior and larger posterior pulmonary plexuses. Below the lung roots the vagi usually break up into two to four branches, which become closely apposed to the esophagus in the posterior mediastinum. The branches from the right and left nerves incline, respectively,

posteriorly and anteriorly, and they divide and reunite to form an open-meshed *esophageal plexus* containing small ganglia. At a variable distance above the esophageal hiatus in the diaphragm, the meshes of the plexus become reconstituted into one or, less often, into two or more vagal trunks, which are located anterior and posterior to the lowest part of the esophagus, lying on the surface or partially embedded in the wall. Offshoots from the esophageal plexus and from the *anterior and posterior vagal trunks* sink into the esophageal wall. Common variations in the plexus and in the vagal trunks (see opposite page) are of especial significance to anyone performing vagotomy, and the surgeon should remember that there may be more than one anterior

(Continued on page 45)

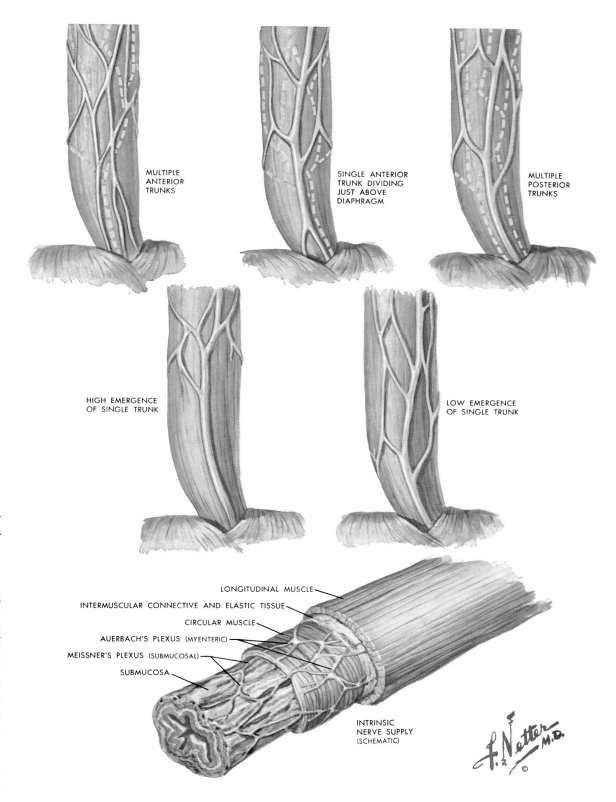

MULTIPLE ANTERIOR TRUNKS

SINGLE ANTERIOR TRUNK DIVIDING JUST ABOVE DIAPHRAGM

MULTIPLE POSTERIOR TRUNKS

HIGH EMERGENCE OF SINGLE TRUNK

LOW EMERGENCE OF SINGLE TRUNK

LONGITUDINAL MUSCLE
INTERMUSCULAR CONNECTIVE AND ELASTIC TISSUE
CIRCULAR MUSCLE
AUERBACH'S PLEXUS (MYENTERIC)
MEISSNER'S PLEXUS (SUBMUCOSAL)
SUBMUCOSA

INTRINSIC NERVE SUPPLY (SCHEMATIC)

Innervation of Esophagus

(Continued from page 44)

or posterior vagal trunk. (For further distribution of the vagal trunks, see pages 64 and 65.)

Sympathetic Supply

The sympathetic preganglionic fibers are the axons of lateral (intermediolateral) cornual cells, located mainly in the fourth to the sixth thoracic segments of the spinal cord. These preganglionic fibers emerge in the anterior spinal nerve roots corresponding to the segments containing their parent cells. They leave the spinal nerves in white or mixed *rami communicantes* and pass to the paravertebral *sympathetic* ganglionated *trunks*. Some fibers form synapses with cells in the midthoracic ganglia, but others pass to higher and lower ganglia in the trunks before relaying. The axons of the ganglionic cells, the postganglionic fibers, reach the esophagus through filaments from the sympathetic trunks or their branches. The afferent impulses are conveyed in fibers which pursue a route reverse to that just described, but they do not relay in the sympathetic trunks, and they enter the cord via the posterior spinal nerve roots; their cytons are located in the posterior spinal nerve root ganglia.

The uppermost part of the esophagus is supplied by offshoots from the pharyngeal plexus; lower down, it receives filaments from the cardiac branches of the *superior cervical ganglia* and, occasionally, from the *middle cervical* or *verte-*

bral ganglia of the sympathetic trunks. Other fibers reach the esophagus in the delicate nerve plexuses accompanying its fine arteries of supply.

In the upper thorax esophageal filaments are supplied by the *stellate ganglia* or *ansae subclaviae,* and the delicate thoracic cardiac nerves (not illustrated) are often associated with fibers for the esophagus, trachea, aorta and pulmonary structures.

In the lower thorax twigs pass from the *greater (superior thoracic) splanchnic nerves* to the nearby esophageal plexus (vide supra). The greater splanchnic nerves arise by three or four larger roots and an inconstant number of smaller rootlets from the fifth or sixth to the ninth or tenth thoracic ganglia, inclusive of the sympathetic trunks. The roots and rootlets pass obliquely forward, inward and downward across

the sides of the thoracic vertebral bodies and intervertebral disks and coalesce to form a nerve of considerable size. On each side the nerve enters the abdomen by piercing the homolateral diaphragmatic crus or, less often, by passing between the lateral margins of the crura and the fibers arising from the medial arcuate ligament. The intra-abdominal course is short, and each nerve breaks up into branches which end mainly in the celiac plexus (see also pages 64 and 65). The lesser and least thoracic splanchnic nerves end, respectively, mainly in the aorticorenal ganglia and renal plexuses (see page 65).

Filaments from the terminal part of the left greater splanchnic nerve and from the right inferior phrenic plexus reach the abdominal part of the esophagus (see page 65).

INTRINSIC INNERVATION OF ALIMENTARY TRACT

From the esophagus (see page 45) to the rectum, the intrinsic innervation is effected through the enteric plexuses. These are composed of numerous groups of ganglion cells interconnected by networks of fibers which lie between the layers of the muscular coats (Auerbach's plexus) and in the submucosa (Meissner's plexus). The former is relatively coarse, and its meshes consist of thick, medium and thin bundles of fibers, which are described as its primary, secondary and tertiary parts. Meissner's plexus is more delicate. Other subsidiary plexuses have been described, such as a rarefied subserous plexus in those parts of the alimentary canal covered by peritoneum, but minute details of these need not be given.

The *enteric plexuses* vary in pattern in different parts of the alimentary tract and in different species of animals. They are well developed in the regions from the stomach to the lower end of the rectum and are less well formed in the esophagus, particularly in its upper half. The ganglion cells are also not distributed uniformly; thus, the density of cell distribution in Auerbach's plexus is lowest in the esophagus, rises steeply in the stomach until it reaches its peak at the pylorus, falls to an intermediate level throughout the small intestine and then increases again along the colon and especially in the rectum. The density of cell population in Meissner's plexus seems to run roughly parallel to that in Auerbach's plexus.

The enteric plexuses contain postganglionic sympathetic and pre- and postganglionic parasympathetic fibers, afferent fibers, and the intrinsic ganglion cells and their processes. Vagal preganglionic fibers form synapses with the ganglion cells whose axons are the postganglionic parasympathetic fibers. The sympathetic preganglionic fibers have already relayed in paravertebral or prevertebral ganglia, and so the sympathetic fibers in the plexuses are postganglionic and pass through them to their terminations without synaptic interruptions. The afferent fibers from the esophagus, stomach and duodenum are carried to the brain stem and cord through the vagal and sympathetic nerves supplying these parts, but they form no synaptic connections with the ganglion cells in the enteric plexuses (see also CIBA COLLECTION, Vol. 1, pages 82, 83, 93, 94 and 95).

Two chief forms of nerve cells, Types I and II, occur in the enteric plexuses, excluding the *"interstitial cells"* of Cajal, which are found associated with the terminal networks (ground plexuses) of all autonomic nerves and which have been the subject of much controversy, many investigators regarding them as primitive ganglion cells and others as connective tissue or microglial elements. *Type I* cells are *multipolar* and confined to Auerbach's plexus, and their dendrites branch close to the parent cells. Their axons run for varying distances through

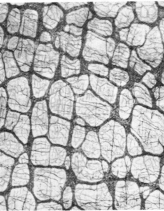

1. MYENTERIC PLEXUS (AUERBACH'S) LYING ON LONGITUDINAL MUSCLE COAT. FINE TERTIARY BUNDLES CROSSING MESHES (DUODENUM OF GUINEA PIG. CHAMPY-COUJARD, OSMIC STAIN, X 20)

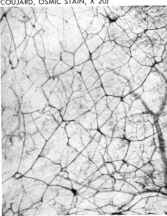

2. SUBMUCOUS PLEXUS (MEISSNER'S) (ASCENDING COLON OF GUINEA PIG. STAINED BY GOLD IMPREGNATION, X 20)

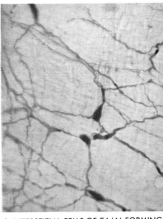

3. INTERSTITIAL CELLS OF CAJAL FORMING PART OF DENSE NETWORK BETWEEN MUSCLE LAYERS (DESCENDING COLON OF GUINEA PIG. METHYLENE BLUE, X 375)

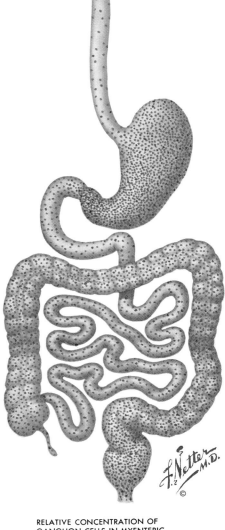

RELATIVE CONCENTRATION OF GANGLION CELLS IN MYENTERIC (AUERBACH'S) PLEXUS AND IN SUBMUCOUS (MEISSNER'S) PLEXUS IN VARIOUS PARTS OF ALIMENTARY TRACT (MYENTERIC PLEXUS CELLS REPRESENTED BY MAROON, SUBMUCOUS BY BLUE DOTS)

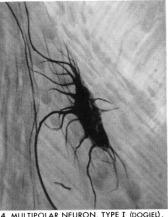

4. MULTIPOLAR NEURON, TYPE I (DOGIEL), LYING IN GANGLION OF MYENTERIC (AUERBACH'S) PLEXUS (ILEUM OF MONKEY. BIELSCHOWSKY, SILVER STAIN, X 375)

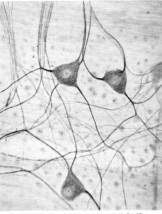

5. GROUP OF MULTIPOLAR NEURONS, TYPE II, IN GANGLION OF MYENTERIC (AUERBACH'S) PLEXUS (ILEUM OF CAT. BIELSCHOWSKY, SILVER STAIN, X 200)

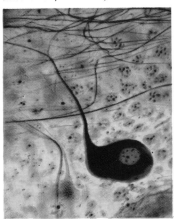

6. PSEUDO-UNIPOLAR NEURON WITHIN GANGLION OF MYENTERIC PLEXUS (ILEUM OF CAT. BIELSCHOWSKY, SILVER STAIN X 375)

the plexuses to establish synapses with *cells of Type II*, which are more numerous and are found in both Auerbach's and Meissner's plexuses. Most Type II cells are multipolar, and their longer dendrites proceed in bundles for variable distances before ramifying in other cell clusters. Many of their axons pass outward to end in the muscle coats, and others proceed inward to supply the muscularis mucosae and to ramify around vessels and between epithelial secretory cells; their distribution suggests that they are motor or secretomotor in nature.

Under experimental conditions peristaltic movements occur in isolated portions of the gut, indicating the importance of the intrinsic neuromuscular mechanism, but the extrinsic nerves are probably essential for the co-ordinated regulation of all activities. Some authorities believe that local reflex arcs exist in the enteric plexuses; others maintain that the effects pro-

duced are explainable on the basis of axon reflexes. It is interesting and possibly significant, however, that in addition to the Types I and II multipolar cells, much smaller numbers of pseudo-unipolar and bipolar cells can be detected in the submucosa and, occasionally, elsewhere; they could be the afferent links in local reflex arcs.

In megacolon (Hirschsprung's disease), and possibly also in achalasia (see page 98), the enteric plexuses are apparently undeveloped or degenerated over a segment of the alimentary tract, although the extrinsic nerves are intact. Peristaltic movements are defective or absent in the affected segment, and this also indicates the importance of the intrinsic neuromuscular mechanism.

Photomicrographs kindly provided by Dr. J. R. Rintoul and Mr. P. Howarth, Manchester University, England.

Section III

ANATOMY OF THE STOMACH AND DUODENUM

by

FRANK H. NETTER, M.D.

in collaboration with

NICHOLAS A. MICHELS, M.A., D.Sc.
Plates 8-14

PROF. G. A. G. MITCHELL, O.B.E., T.D., M.B., Ch.M., D.Sc.
Plates 16 and 17

PROF. GERHARD WOLF-HEIDEGGER, M.D., Ph.D.
Plates 1-7, 15

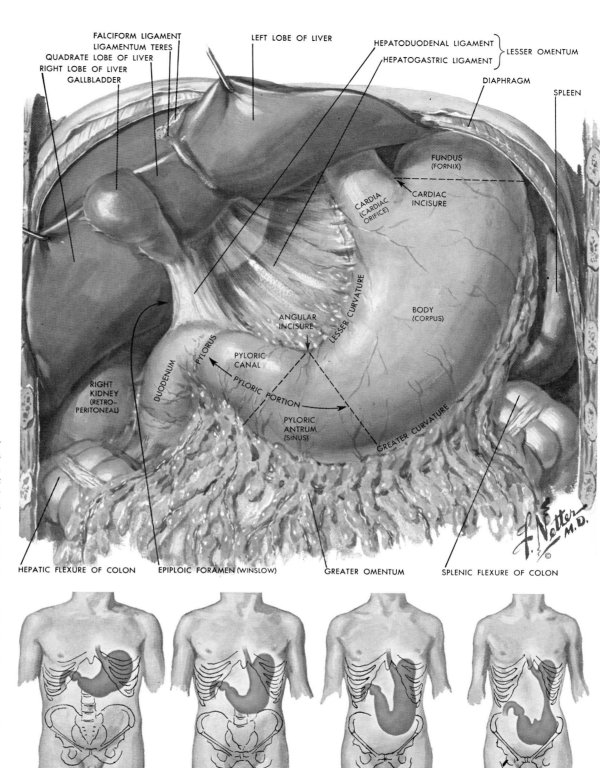

FALCIFORM LIGAMENT
LIGAMENTUM TERES
QUADRATE LOBE OF LIVER
RIGHT LOBE OF LIVER
GALLBLADDER
LEFT LOBE OF LIVER
HEPATODUODENAL LIGAMENT
HEPATOGASTRIC LIGAMENT
LESSER OMENTUM
DIAPHRAGM
SPLEEN
FUNDUS (FORNIX)
CARDIA (CARDIAC ORIFICE)
CARDIAC INCISURE
LESSER CURVATURE
BODY (CORPUS)
ANGULAR INCISURE
PYLORUS
PYLORIC CANAL
PYLORIC PORTION
DUODENUM
RIGHT KIDNEY (RETRO-PERITONEAL)
PYLORIC ANTRUM (SINUS)
GREATER CURVATURE
HEPATIC FLEXURE OF COLON
EPIPLOIC FORAMEN (WINSLOW)
GREATER OMENTUM
SPLENIC FLEXURE OF COLON

HYPERTONIC STOMACH   ORTHOTONIC STOMACH   HYPOTONIC STOMACH   ATONIC STOMACH

ANATOMY, NORMAL VARIATIONS AND RELATIONS OF STOMACH

The stomach is a retort-shaped reservoir of the digestive tract, in which ingested food is soaked in gastric juice, containing enzymes and hydrochloric acid, and then released spasmodically into the duodenum by gastric peristalsis (see also pages 52, 80-84). The form and size of the stomach vary considerably, depending on the position of the body and the degree of filling. Special functional configurations of the stomach (see below) are of interest to the clinician and radiologist.

The stomach has a ventral and a dorsal surface, which may be vaulted or flattened and which practically touch when the organ is empty. It also has two borders, *i.e.*, the concave *lesser curvature* above on the right and the convex *greater curvature* below on the left; the two join at the cardia, where the esophagus enters. The cardia, which is not the uppermost part of the organ, constitutes the point of demarcation between both curvatures. Whereas on the right the esophagus continues smoothly into the lesser curvature, on the left there is a definite indentation (*cardiac incisure*), which becomes most obvious when the uppermost hoodlike portion of the stomach (the *fundus* or *fornix*) is full and bulges upward. The major portion of the stomach (the *body* or *corpus*) blends imperceptibly into the *pyloric portion*, except along the lesser curvature, where a notch (the *angular incisure*) marks the boundary between the corpus and the pyloric portion. The latter is divided into the *pyloric antrum*, or vestibule, which narrows into the *pyloric canal*, terminating at the *pyloric valve*. External landmarks of the pylorus are a circular ridge of sphincter muscle and the subserosal pyloric vein (see page 53).

The stomach is entirely covered with peritoneum. A double layer of peritoneum, deriving from the embryonal ventral mesogastrium, extends on the lesser

curvature beyond the stomach; known as the *lesser omentum*, it passes over to the porta hepatis and may be divided into a larger, thinner and proximal portion (the *hepatogastric ligament*) and a smaller, thicker and distal portion (the *hepatoduodenal ligament*), which attaches to the pyloric region and to the upper horizontal portion of the duodenum. The free edge of the hepatoduodenal ligament, through which run the portal vein, hepatic artery and common bile duct (see page 50 and CIBA COLLECTION, Vol. 3/III, page 6), forms the ventral margin of the *epiploic foramen of Winslow*, which gives access to the lesser peritoneal sac (bursa omentalis). The *greater omentum*, a derivative of the embryonal dorsal mesogastrium, passes caudally from the greater curvature and contains, between its two frontal and two dorsal sheets, the inferior recess of the bursa omentalis.

The anterior surface of the stomach abuts against

the anterior abdominal wall, against the inferior surface of the left lobe of the liver and, to some extent in the pyloric region, against the quadrate lobe of the liver and the gallbladder. Its posterior surface is in apposition with retroperitoneal structures (pancreas, splenic vessels, left kidney and adrenal) from which, however, it is separated by the bursa omentalis. The fundus bulges against the left diaphragmatic dome. On the left, adjacent to the fundus, is the spleen, which is connected with the stomach by the gastrosplenic ligament (also derived from the dorsal mesogastrium).

The four principal functional types of stomach (see also page 86) recognized are known as *orthotonic, hypertonic, hypotonic* and *atonic*. In the hypotonic and atonic types, the axis of the stomach is more longitudinal, whereas in the orthotonic and, particularly, the hypertonic types, it is more transverse.

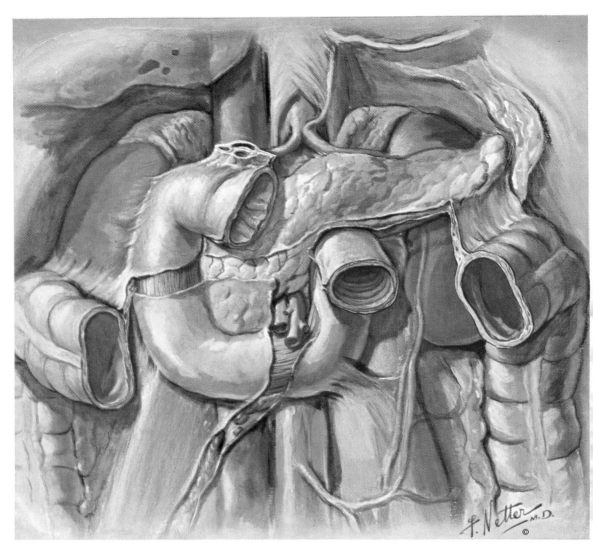

ANATOMY AND RELATIONS OF DUODENUM

The duodenum, the first part of the small intestine, has a total length of about 25 to 30 cm. It is shaped like a horseshoe, the open end facing to the left.

The *pars superior,* lying at the level of the first lumbar vertebra, extends almost horizontally from the pylorus to the first flexure (flexura duodeni superior). As a result of its intraperitoneal position, this first duodenal portion is freely movable and can adapt its course according to the filling condition of the stomach. The anterior and superior surfaces of the first half of this duodenal segment are in close relation to the inferior surface of the liver (lobus quadratus; see CIBA COLLECTION, Vol. 3/III, page 5) and the gallbladder. The roentgenologic designation "duodenal bulb" refers to the most proximal end of the pars superior duodeni, which is slightly dilated when the organ is filled and then more sharply separated from the stomach because of the pyloric contraction.

The two layers of peritoneum which cover the anterosuperior and postero-inferior surfaces, respectively, join together on the upper border of the superior portion of the duodenum and move as the hepatoduodenal ligament cranially toward the liver, forming the right, free edge of the lesser omentum (see also page 49). This ligament contains the important triad — the portal vein, the hepatic artery and the common bile duct (see CIBA COLLECTION, Vol. 3/III, page 3). Dorsal to the first portion of the duodenum lies the head of the pancreas, both organs being separated by a peritoneal fold of the bursa omentalis. In the pyloric region the gastroduodenal artery crosses underneath the duodenum.

The second, or *descending, part of the duodenum* extends vertically from the first to the second duodenal flexure, the latter lying approximately at the level of the third lumbar vertebra. The upper part of this portion rests laterally upon the structures constituting the hilus of the right kidney, while medially its whole length is attached by connective

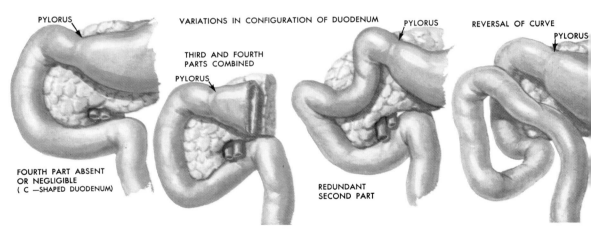

PYLORUS   VARIATIONS IN CONFIGURATION OF DUODENUM   PYLORUS   REVERSAL OF CURVE

THIRD AND FOURTH PARTS COMBINED

PYLORUS

PYLORUS

FOURTH PART ABSENT OR NEGLIGIBLE (C —SHAPED DUODENUM)

REDUNDANT SECOND PART

tissue to the duodenal margin of the caput pancreatis. About halfway, the descending portion is crossed anteriorly by the parietal line of attachment of the transverse mesocolon. The common bile duct, which, together with the portal vein, occupies, at the commencement of the hepatoduodenal ligament, a position dorsal to the superior duodenal portion, continues its course between the descending portion and the head of the pancreas to its opening at the major papilla (Vateri); this topographic relationship explains the danger of an obstruction of the duct in the presence of a tumor of the caput pancreatis.

The third, or *inferior, portion* begins at the second flexure. It runs, first, almost horizontally (*horizontal part*) or sometimes in a slightly ascending direction until it reaches the region of the left border of the aorta, where, curving cranially, it changes direction to pass into the terminal duodenal segment, or *ascend-*

ing portion. Whereas the caudal part of the second portion and the second flexure lie over the psoas major of the right side of the body, the third duodenal portion, with its horizontal segment, passes over the vena cava and the abdominal aorta. The superior mesenteric vessels, before entering the root of the mesentery (see pages 57 and 58), cross over the horizontal part of the third portion near its transition to the ascending part. During its course the third portion is increasingly covered by the peritoneum, and a complete intraperitoneal situation is attained at the duodenojejunal flexure, which is located caudal to the mesocolon transversum at the level of the second lumbar vertebra or of the disk between L1 and L2.

In X-ray pictures the duodenum usually takes on the form of a C (usual duodenal curve), although not infrequently it shows individual variations such as a redundant second part.

DUODENAL FOSSAE AND LIGAMENT OF TREITZ

The duodenojejunal flexure lies left of the midline at the level of the first and second lumbar vertebrae. The suspensory ligament of the duodenum (*ligament of Treitz, suspensory muscle of the duodenum*) is a flat, fibromuscular ligament arising at the right crus of the diaphragm, near the aortic hiatus; it passes, with some individual variations, downward left of both the celiac trunk and superior mesenteric artery dorsal to the pancreas, and fans out into the duodenal wall in the region of the duodenojejunal flexure, which it helps to keep in position. The smooth muscle cells of the ligament are largely continuous with the musculature of the two above-mentioned arteries; at the intestinal attachment they are connected with the longitudinal muscular layer of the gut, some extending as far as the mesentery of the small intestine. The attachment of the ligament to the duodenum may be quite narrow or it may extend over a considerable portion of the third part of the duodenum. If the ligament of Treitz is short, the duodenojejunal flexure is high; if the ligament is long, the flexure may lie so low that the terminal duodenal segment does not take the usual ascending course (see page 50).

Several peritoneal recesses exist to the left of the ascending portion of the duodenum and the duodenojejunal flexure. These result from secondary fixation of the mesentery of the descending colon to the posterior abdominal wall; they vary greatly in depth and size from individual to individual. The most important are those arising from the *superior duodenomesocolic fold* and the *inferior duodenomesocolic fold*. These originate from the point of attachment of descending mesocolon and run archlike from left to right, the superior to the duodenojejunal flexure and the inferior to the ascending portion of the duodenum. The superior fold is caudally concave and forms the aperture of the so-called *fossa of Broesike* (superior duodenal fossa — S.D.F.), whereas the inferior fold is cranially concave and forms the aperture of the *fossa of Treitz* (inferior duodenal fossa — I.D.F.). These fossae may be clinically significant as

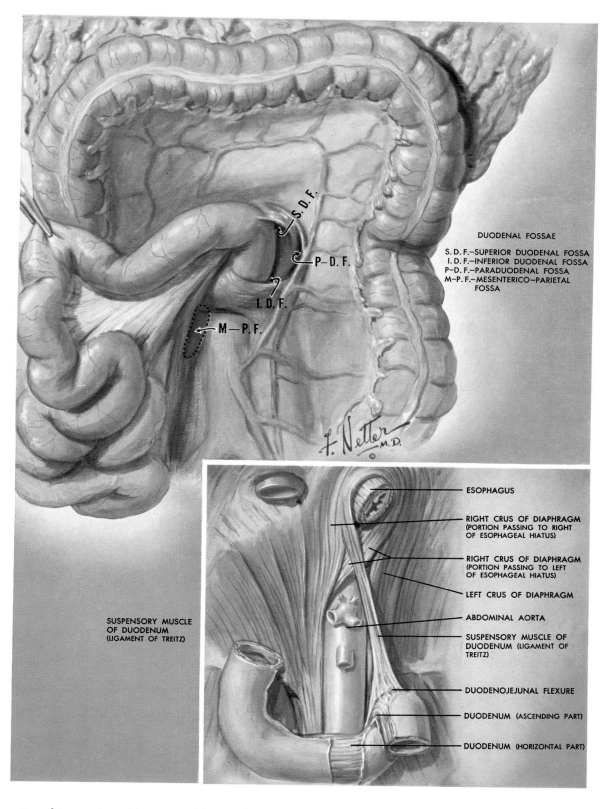

DUODENAL FOSSAE

S. D. F.—SUPERIOR DUODENAL FOSSA
I. D. F.—INFERIOR DUODENAL FOSSA
P-D. F.—PARADUODENAL FOSSA
M-P. F.—MESENTERICO-PARIETAL FOSSA

SUSPENSORY MUSCLE OF DUODENUM (LIGAMENT OF TREITZ)

ESOPHAGUS
RIGHT CRUS OF DIAPHRAGM (PORTION PASSING TO RIGHT OF ESOPHAGEAL HIATUS)
RIGHT CRUS OF DIAPHRAGM (PORTION PASSING TO LEFT OF ESOPHAGEAL HIATUS)
LEFT CRUS OF DIAPHRAGM
ABDOMINAL AORTA
SUSPENSORY MUSCLE OF DUODENUM (LIGAMENT OF TREITZ)
DUODENOJEJUNAL FLEXURE
DUODENUM (ASCENDING PART)
DUODENUM (HORIZONTAL PART)

sites of intraperitoneal herniation. They are bounded ventrally by the superior and inferior duodenomesocolic folds, respectively, and on the left by the ascending portion of the duodenum or the duodenojejunal flexure. Both fossae are bounded on the right by the parietal peritoneum and extend behind the dorsal duodenal wall, which is covered by visceral peritoneum. In or near the insertion of the superior fold is situated the ascending inferior mesenteric vein, and at the corresponding position in the inferior fold the ascending branch of the left colic artery. The left ureter arises immediately dorsal to the inferior duodenal fossa.

Several much rarer types of fossae are to be found, *e.g.*, the *paraduodenal fossa* (of Landzert) (P-D.F.) bounded by the two ascending blood vessels, already mentioned. Here, a somewhat longitudinal peritoneal fold, slightly concave to the right, occasionally gives

rise to a so-called left duodenal hernia (Moynihan). This fossa can sometimes be separated into two partial folds, of which the more ventral and superficial rises above the ascending branch of the left colic artery, whereas the deeper or more dorsal fold is bordered by the inferior mesenteric vein.

On very rare occasions a duodenojejunal fossa (not illustrated) extends cranially from the duodenojejunal flexure under the root of the transverse mesocolon, or a retroduodenal fossa runs cranially between the aorta and the ascending portion of the duodenum. The *mesenterico-parietal fossa* of Waldeyer (M-P.F.), invariably present in the fetus, occasionally forms the enclosing sac for a right paraduodenal hernia. It is bounded ventrally by the superior mesenteric vessels as they enter the mesentery of the small intestine, and dorsally by the parietal peritoneum over the right side of the aorta.

MUCOUS MEMBRANE OF STOMACH

The reddish-gray mucous membrane of the stomach, composed of a single surface layer of epithelial cells, the tunica propria and the submucosa, commences at the cardia along an irregular or zigzag line (often referred to as the "Z" line or "Z-Z" line, see page 38). The mucosa is thrown into a more or less marked relief of folds or rugae, which flatten considerably when the stomach is distended. In the region of the lesser curvature, where the mucosa is more strongly fixed to the muscular layer, the folds take a longitudinal course, forming what has been called the "Magenstrasse". The rugae are generally smaller in the fundus and become larger as they approach the antrum, where they show a tendency to run diagonally across the stomach toward the greater curvature. Besides these broad folds, the gastric mucosa is further characterized by numerous shallow invaginations, which divide the mucosal surface into a mosaic of elevated areas varying in shape. When viewed under magnification with a lens, these areae gastricae reveal several delicate ledges and depressions, the latter known as gastric pits or foveolae gastricae. In the depth of these pits, the width and length of which vary, the glands of the stomach open.

The gastric epithelium, a single layer of columnar cells, is, at the gastro-esophageal junction (cardiac orifice), sharply demarcated from the stratified and thicker esophageal mucosa. The *epithelial cells* are of the mucoid type and contain mucigen granules in their outer portions and a single ovoid nucleus at their base.

The glands of the stomach are tubular, and three kinds can be differentiated:

1. The *cardiac glands* are confined to a narrow zone, 0.5 to 4 cm. in width, around the cardiac orifice. They are coiled and are lined by mucus-producing cells.

2. The gastric or *fundic glands* (glandulae gastricae propriae) are located in the fundus and over the greater part of the body of the stomach. They are fairly straight, simply branched tubules, with a narrow lumen reaching down almost to the muscularis mucosae. They are lined by three types of cells: (a) The *mucoid cells* are present in the neck and

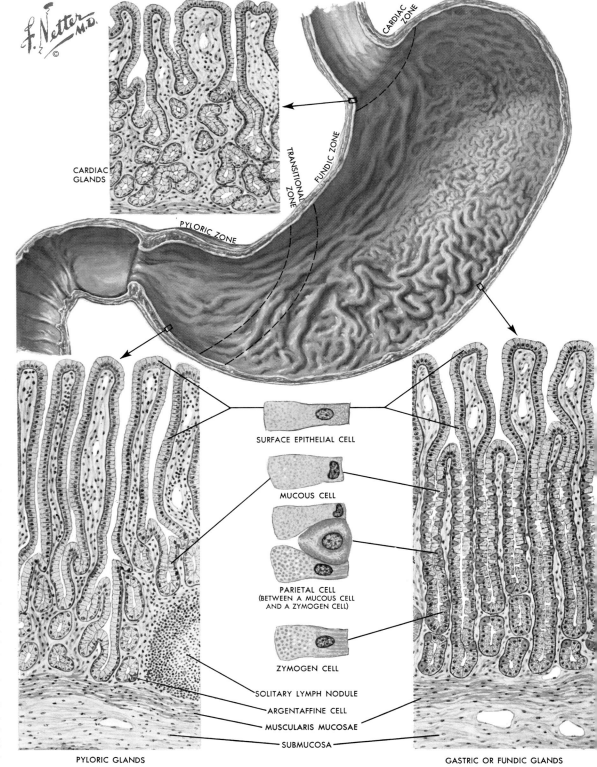

CARDIAC GLANDS

CARDIAC ZONE

TRANSITIONAL ZONE

FUNDIC ZONE

PYLORIC ZONE

SURFACE EPITHELIAL CELL

MUCOUS CELL

PARIETAL CELL (BETWEEN A MUCOUS CELL AND A ZYMOGEN CELL)

ZYMOGEN CELL

SOLITARY LYMPH NODULE

ARGENTAFFINE CELL

MUSCULARIS MUCOSAE

SUBMUCOSA

PYLORIC GLANDS

GASTRIC OR FUNDIC GLANDS

differ from the cells of the surface epithelium in that their mucigen granules have slightly different staining qualities and their nuclei tend to be flattened or concave (rather than oval) at the base of the cells. (b) The cells of the second type, the chief or *zymogenic cells*, line the lower half of the glandular tubules. They have a spheric nucleus and contain strongly light-refracting granules and a Golgi apparatus, the size and form of which vary with the state of secretory activity. They are thought to produce pepsinogen, the precursor of pepsin (see page 84). (c) The cells of the third type, the *parietal cells*, are larger and usually crowded away from the lumen, to which they connect by extracellular capillaries, stemming from intracellular canaliculi. Their intraplasmatic granules are strongly eosinophilic and less light-refracting than those of the chief cells. From recent histochemical studies it has been concluded

that the parietal cells produce the gastric hydrochloric acid, in line with the original concept of Heidenhain.

3. The *pyloric glands* are located in the *pyloric region* but also spread into a *transitional zone,* in which both gastric and pyloric glands are found and which extends diagonally and distally from the lesser to the greater curvature. The tubes of the pyloric glands are shorter, more tortuous and less densely packed, and their ends are more branched than is the case with the fundic glands. The pits are markedly deeper in the region of the pyloric glands. These glands are lined by a single type of cell, which resembles, and, indeed, may be identical with, the mucous neck cells of the fundic glands.

A fifth type of cell, the *argentaffine cell,* lies scattered on the basement membrane of the pyloric glands but may occasionally be found also in the gastric glands. Its function has thus far remained obscure.

MUSCULATURE OF STOMACH

The musculature of the gastric wall consists solely of smooth muscle fibers, which, in contrast to the arrangement in the esophagus and in the small and large intestine, are arranged in three layers instead of two. However, only one of these — the middle circular layer — covers the wall completely, whereas the other two — the superficial longitudinal and deeper oblique layers — are present as incomplete coats. Noteworthy, furthermore, is the fact that the longitudinal and circular layers, as well as the latter and the oblique muscular coats, are interconnected by continuous fibers.

The *longitudinal muscle fibers* of the stomach are continuous with the longitudinal muscle layer of the esophagus, which divides at the cardia, tapelike, into two stripes. The stronger of these muscle bands follows the lesser curvature. The other, somewhat broader but thinner, set of fibers courses along the greater curvature toward the pylorus. Thus, the middle areas of the anterior and posterior surfaces of the stomach remain free of longitudinal muscle fibers. The marginal fibers of the upper longitudinal muscle stripe radiate obliquely toward the anterior and posterior surfaces of the fundus and corpus to unite with fibers of the circular layer. In the pyloric area the two bands of longitudinal fibers converge again to form a uniform layer, which, to a great extent at least, passes over directly into the longitudinal muscular layer of the duodenum. It is the increased thickness of the longitudinal muscle layer in the ventral and dorsal parts of the pylorus which is responsible for the so-called "pyloric ligaments" (anterior and posterior pyloric ligaments, respectively).

The *middle or circular muscular coat*, which is not only the most continuous but also the strongest of the three layers, also begins at the cardia, as the continuation of the more superficial fibers of the circular esophageal muscle. The circular fibers become markedly more numerous as they approach the pylorus, where they form the pyloric sphincter (see below).

The innermost, *oblique muscular layer* (made visible in the illustration by fenestration of the circular layer) is most strongly developed in the region of the fundus and becomes progressively weaker

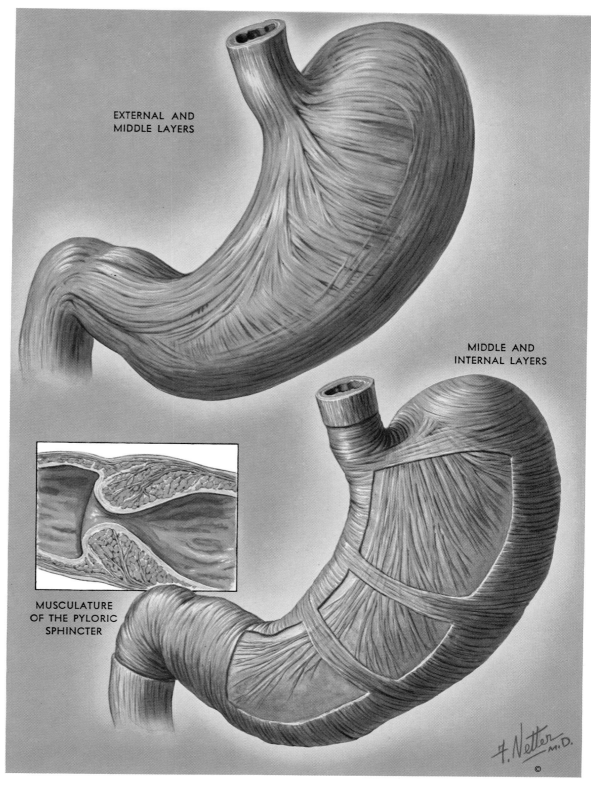

EXTERNAL AND MIDDLE LAYERS

MIDDLE AND INTERNAL LAYERS

MUSCULATURE OF THE PYLORIC SPHINCTER

H. Netter M.D.

as it approaches the pylorus. At the cardia, its fibers connect with the deeper circular layers of the esophageal muscle (see also page 38). No oblique fibers exist at the lesser curvature or in the adjacent areas of the frontal and dorsal walls. The fibers closest to the lesser curvature arise from a point to the left of the cardia and run parallel to the lesser curvature. The longitudinal furrows in the lesser curvature, caused by the absence of this innermost layer, have been called the "Magenstrasse". The oblique layer bundles, following these first more or less longitudinal fibers, bend farther and farther to the left and, finally, become practically circular in the region of the fundus, where their continuity with the fibers of the circular layer is clearly evident. Since the oblique fibers of the frontal and dorsal walls merge into one another in the region of the fundus, the oblique layer as a whole consists of U-shaped loops. The oblique

fibers never reach the greater curvature in the region of the corpus but fan out and gradually disappear in the walls of the stomach.

Musculature of Pyloric Sphincter

The middle circular layer thickens considerably at the pylorus, thus forming a muscular ring which acts as a sphincter. This pyloric sphincter is not continuous with the circular musculature of the duodenum but is separated from it by a thin, fibrous septum of connective tissue. A few fibers of the longitudinal muscle layer, the greater mass of which, as mentioned above, is continuous with the corresponding layer of the duodenum, contribute also to the muscle mass of the pyloric sphincter; they may even find their way through the network of the sphincter bundles and penetrate as far as the submucosa.

Duodenal Bulb and Mucosal Surface of Duodenum

The mucosa of the widened first portion of the duodenum, known also as the *bulbus duodeni* (see also page 50), is, except for a few not very prominent longitudinal folds, somewhat flat and smooth, in contrast to the more distal duodenal part, which, like the entire small intestine, displays the circular mucosal *folds of Kerckring*. These folds, which considerably augment the absorption surface of the intestine, begin in the region of the first flexure, increasing in number and elevation in the more distal parts of the duodenum. They do not always form complete circles along the entire intestinal wall, since some are semicircular or crescent-shaped, whereas others branch out to connect with adjacent folds. Very often they deviate from their circular pattern and pursue a more spiral course. Both the mucosa and submucosa participate in the structure of these plicae, whereas all the other layers of the small intestine, including especially its two muscular coats, are flat and smooth.

Approximately halfway down the posteromedial aspect of the descending portion of the duodenum, at a distance of 8.5 to 10 cm. from the pylorus, is located the *papilla duodeni major,* known as the *papilla of Vater.* Here the common bile duct (ductus choledochus) and the major pancreatic duct of Wirsung open into the duodenum. The common bile duct approaches the duodenum within the enfolding hepatoduodenal ligament of the lesser omentum (see page 49) and continues caudally in the groove between the descending portion of the duodenum and the pancreas (see also CIBA COLLECTION, Vol. 3/III, page 22). The terminal part of the ductus choledochus produces in the posteromedial duodenal wall a slight but perceptible longitudinal impression known as the plica longitudinalis duodeni. This fold usually ends at the papilla but may occasionally continue for a short distance beyond the papilla in the form of the so-called frenulum. Small hoodlike folds at the top of the papilla protect the mouth of the combined bile duct and pancreatic duct.

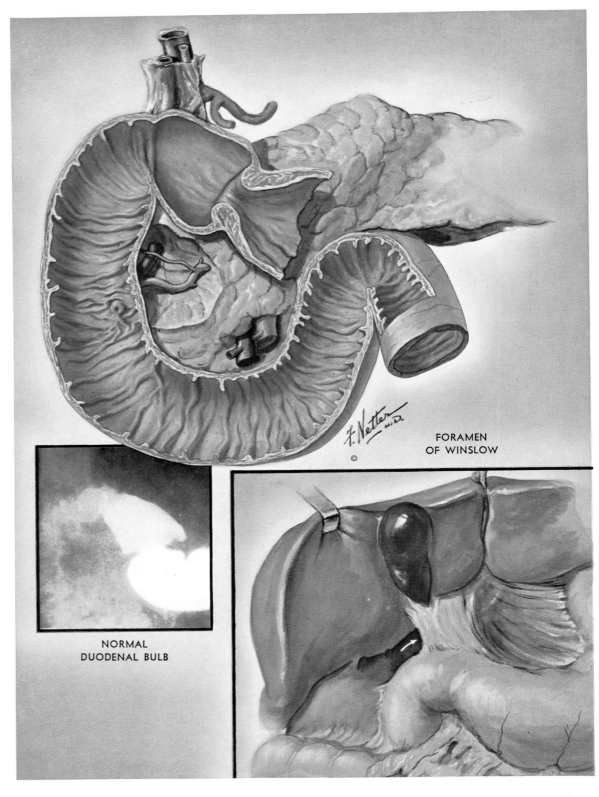

FORAMEN OF WINSLOW

NORMAL DUODENAL BULB

The various types of union of the bile and pancreatic ducts are illustrated and discussed on page 24 of Vol. 3/III, CIBA COLLECTION. A small, wartlike and generally less distinct second papilla, the papilla duodeni minor, is situated about 2.5 cm. above and slightly farther medially of the major papilla. It serves as an opening for the minor pancreatic duct or duct of Santorini, which, despite great variations in development, is almost always present (see also CIBA COLLECTION, Vol. 3/III, page 27).

Except for the first portion of the duodenum, the mucosal surface, which in living subjects is reddish in color, is lined with villi (see page 55); these account for its typical velvetlike appearance.

The duodenal bulb, varying in form, size, position and orientation, appears in the anteroposterior roentgen projection as a triangle, with its base at the pylorus and its tip pointing toward the superior flexure or the transitional region of the first and second portions of the duodenum. Certain relationships between the form of the bulb and the habitus have been postulated, and in roentgenologic nomenclature a number of different terms are used to describe the various forms of the duodenal bulb. Its longitudinal folds, as well as the circular folds of Kerckring in the lower parts of the duodenum, can, like the pattern of the gastric mucosa, be seen fairly clearly in an X-ray picture if a barium meal of appropriate quantity and consistency is given. In such a relief picture of the mucosa, the region of the papilla major occasionally appears as a small, roundish filling defect. Where the papilla is enlarged in the form of a small diverticulum, the contrast medium may sometimes enter the terminal portions of the bile and pancreatic ducts, with the result that the X-ray picture simulates the shape of a molar tooth with two roots.

STRUCTURES OF DUODENUM

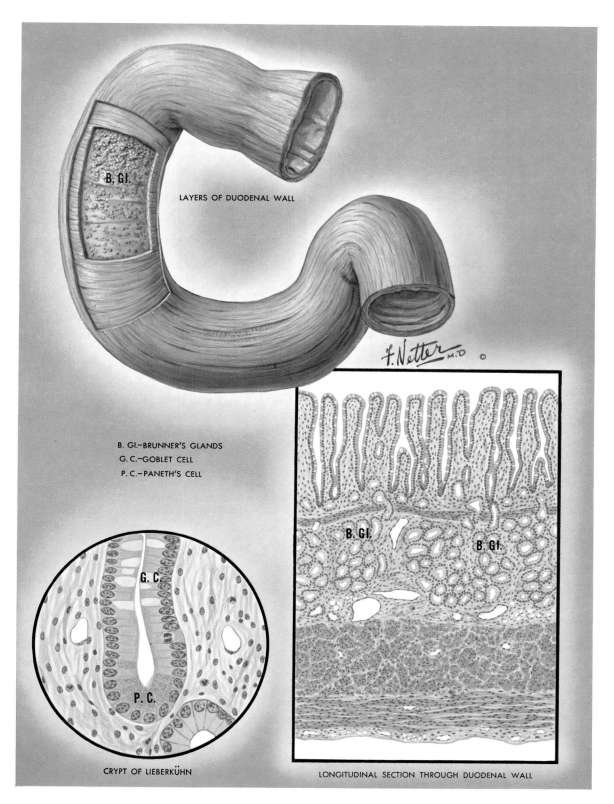

LAYERS OF DUODENAL WALL

B. Gl.–BRUNNER'S GLANDS
G. C.–GOBLET CELL
P. C.–PANETH'S CELL

CRYPT OF LIEBERKÜHN

LONGITUDINAL SECTION THROUGH DUODENAL WALL

The wall of the duodenum, like the wall of the whole intestinal tract, is made up of a mucosal, a submucosal and two muscular layers, and of an adventitia or a subserosa and serosa, wherever the duodenum is covered by peritoneum. From the embryologic, morphologic and functional aspects, the duodenum is a specially differentiated part of the small intestine. Accordingly, the duodenal mucosa displays the macroscopically visible transverse folds of the circular plicae of Kerckring (see page 54), presenting permanent duplications of the mucosa and submucosa. The surface area of the mucosa is also extensively increased on the one hand by the villi, forming a great number of prominences projecting into the lumen, and on the other hand by the valleys known as the *crypts of Lieberkühn*. The villi of the duodenum are very dense, large and, in some areas, leaflike. The epithelium of the duodenal mucosa consists of a single layer of high columnar cells with a marked cuticular border. Between these, *goblet cells* are dispersed. In the fundus of the crypts, there are cells filled with eosinophilic granules (*cells of Paneth*) and, in addition, some cells with yellow granules, which have a strong affinity to chromates. The tunica or lamina propria of the mucosa consists of loose connective tissue. Between the mucosa and submucosa is stretched a double layer of smooth muscle cells, the fibers of which enter the tunica propria and continue to the tips of the villi, enabling the latter to perform a sucking and pumping function by their own motility.

The submucosa, lying between the mucosal and the muscular layers, makes it possible for these two layers to shift in relation to each other. It is made up of collagenous connective tissue, the fibers of which are arranged in the form of a mesh. In this network are embedded the duodenal *glands of Brunner,* characteristic of the duodenum. These are tortuous acinotubular glands with multiple branches at their ends; breaking through the muscularis mucosae, they open into the crypts. Brunner's glands are more numerous and more dense in the proximal parts of the duodenum and diminish in size and density as the duodenum approaches the duodenojejunal junction, but both the extension and the density of the glands are subject to great individual variations. The number of glands is said to be much smaller in older than in younger individuals. The secretion of the duodenal glands provides an essential part of the succus enteri-

cus (see CIBA COLLECTION, Vol. 3/II, page 89) and is a clear fluid which contains mucus and, besides other components, a relatively weak proteolytic enzyme acting in an acid milieu.

The structural arrangement of the muscular coat of the duodenum is the same as in the lower intestinal tract. An inner circular layer is covered by a thinner outer longitudinal layer. The subserosa and the adventitia are composed of fine collagenous fibrils, which form a delicate lattice. The peritoneum of the duodenum consists, as do all serous membranes of the body, of a single layer of flattened mesothelial cells.

As elsewhere in the small intestine, the intramural nervous plexuses are found in the submucosa (Meissner's plexus) and in the muscularis (myenteric or Auerbach's plexus, between the circular and longitudinal layers). Their distribution and function are discussed on page 46.

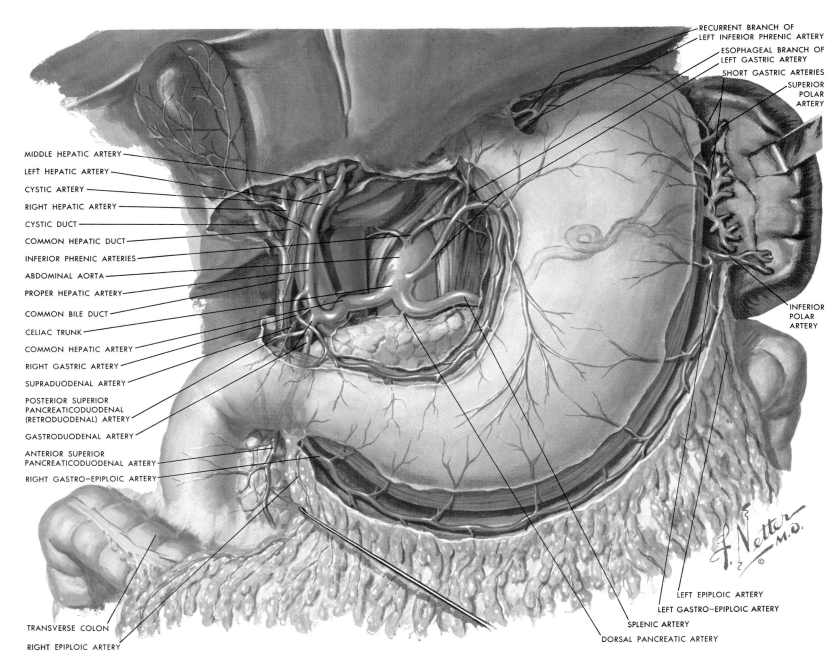

MIDDLE HEPATIC ARTERY
LEFT HEPATIC ARTERY
CYSTIC ARTERY
RIGHT HEPATIC ARTERY
CYSTIC DUCT
COMMON HEPATIC DUCT
INFERIOR PHRENIC ARTERIES
ABDOMINAL AORTA
PROPER HEPATIC ARTERY
COMMON BILE DUCT
CELIAC TRUNK
COMMON HEPATIC ARTERY
RIGHT GASTRIC ARTERY
SUPRADUODENAL ARTERY
POSTERIOR SUPERIOR PANCREATICODUODENAL (RETRODUODENAL) ARTERY
GASTRODUODENAL ARTERY
ANTERIOR SUPERIOR PANCREATICODUODENAL ARTERY
RIGHT GASTRO-EPIPLOIC ARTERY

TRANSVERSE COLON
RIGHT EPIPLOIC ARTERY

RECURRENT BRANCH OF LEFT INFERIOR PHRENIC ARTERY
ESOPHAGEAL BRANCH OF LEFT GASTRIC ARTERY
SHORT GASTRIC ARTERIES
SUPERIOR POLAR ARTERY

INFERIOR POLAR ARTERY

LEFT EPIPLOIC ARTERY
LEFT GASTRO-EPIPLOIC ARTERY
SPLENIC ARTERY
DORSAL PANCREATIC ARTERY

BLOOD SUPPLY OF STOMACH AND DUODENUM

The conventional textbook description of the blood supply of the stomach, duodenum and organs related to them (spleen and pancreas) has established the misleading concept that the vascular patterns of these organs are relatively simple and uniform, whereas, on the contrary, they are indeed always unpredictable and vary in every instance. In the following account, emphasis will be placed on the major arterial variations that may be encountered in surgical resections.

Typically, the entire blood supply of the supra-mesocolonic organs (liver, gallbladder, stomach, duodenum, pancreas and spleen) is derived from the *celiac artery* (trunk), a supplementary small portion being supplied by the superior mesenteric artery via its *inferior pancreaticoduodenal branch*. The caliber of the celiac varies from 8 to 40 mm. in width. When typical and complete, it gives off three branches, the *hepatic, splenic* (lienal) and *left gastric*, thus constituting a complete hepatolienogastric trunk, which frequently has the form of a tripod (25 per cent).

This conventional description of the celiac with its three branches occurs in only 55 per cent of the population, for the celiac often lacks one or more of its typical branches. It may be incomplete (see page 60) when the right, middle or left hepatic arises from some other source (right hepatic from superior mesenteric [12 per cent], left hepatic from left gastric [25 per cent]), thus constituting an incomplete hepatolienogastric trunk. In a complete or incomplete form, a hepatolienogastric trunk occurs in about 90 per cent. The celiac may omit the left gastric, forming a hepatolienal trunk (3.5 per cent), or the hepatic, forming a lienogastric trunk (5.5 per cent), or the splenic, forming a hepatogastric trunk (1.5 per cent). Additive branches of the celiac comprise the dorsal pancreatic (22 per cent), the inferior phrenic (74 per cent) and, occasionally, even the middle colic or an accessory middle colic. In many instances the celiac hepatic is absent, being replaced from the superior mesenteric, aorta or left gastric.

The blood supply of the stomach and abdominal esophagus is accomplished by six primary and six secondary arteries. The primary arteries comprise (1) *right gastric* and (2) *left gastric*, coursing along the lesser curvature; (3) *right gastro-epiploic* and (4) *left gastro-epiploic*, coursing along the greater curvature (each of these

four vessels giving off branches to the anterior and posterior surfaces of the stomach, where they anastomose); (5) *splenic*, which gives off in its distal third a variable number (two to ten) of short gastric and fundic branches, and from its superior or inferior terminal division the left gastro-epiploic; (6) *gastroduodenal*, by direct small branches (one to three) and, frequently, by a large pyloric branch.

The secondary arteries comprise (7) *superior pancreaticoduodenal* (end branch of gastroduodenal) by short twigs and, frequently, by a large pyloric branch; (8) *supraduodenal artery* of varied origin (gastroduodenal, retroduodenal, hepatic, right gastric) which, in addition to supplying the first inch of the duodenum, often sends one or more branches to the pylorus; (9) *retroduodenal* (posterior superior pancreaticoduodenal), predominantly the first collateral of the gastroduodenal, which, in its tortuous descent along the left side of the common bile duct to reach the back of the pancreas and duodenum, frequently gives off one or more pyloric branches, the latter, in some instances, uniting with the supraduodenal and right gastric; (10) *transverse pancreatic* (usually the left branch of the dorsal pancreatic), which, when it arises from the gastroduodenal, superior pan-

(Continued on page 57)

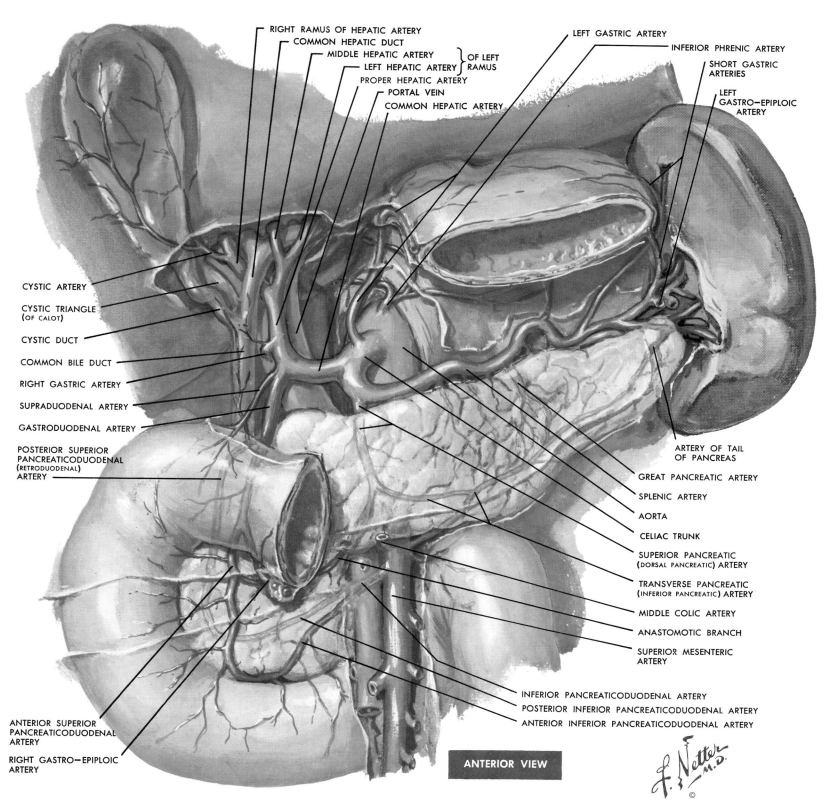

RIGHT RAMUS OF HEPATIC ARTERY
COMMON HEPATIC DUCT
MIDDLE HEPATIC ARTERY } OF LEFT
LEFT HEPATIC ARTERY } RAMUS
PROPER HEPATIC ARTERY
PORTAL VEIN
COMMON HEPATIC ARTERY

LEFT GASTRIC ARTERY
INFERIOR PHRENIC ARTERY
SHORT GASTRIC ARTERIES
LEFT GASTRO-EPIPLOIC ARTERY

CYSTIC ARTERY
CYSTIC TRIANGLE (OF CALOT)
CYSTIC DUCT
COMMON BILE DUCT
RIGHT GASTRIC ARTERY
SUPRADUODENAL ARTERY
GASTRODUODENAL ARTERY
POSTERIOR SUPERIOR PANCREATICODUODENAL (RETRODUODENAL) ARTERY

ARTERY OF TAIL OF PANCREAS
GREAT PANCREATIC ARTERY
SPLENIC ARTERY
AORTA
CELIAC TRUNK
SUPERIOR PANCREATIC (DORSAL PANCREATIC) ARTERY
TRANSVERSE PANCREATIC (INFERIOR PANCREATIC) ARTERY
MIDDLE COLIC ARTERY
ANASTOMOTIC BRANCH
SUPERIOR MESENTERIC ARTERY

ANTERIOR SUPERIOR PANCREATICODUODENAL ARTERY
RIGHT GASTRO-EPIPLOIC ARTERY

INFERIOR PANCREATICODUODENAL ARTERY
POSTERIOR INFERIOR PANCREATICODUODENAL ARTERY
ANTERIOR INFERIOR PANCREATICODUODENAL ARTERY

ANTERIOR VIEW

F. Netter M.D. ©

(Continued from page 56)

creaticoduodenal or right gastro-epiploic (10 per cent), nearly invariably gives off one or more branches to the pylorus; (11) *dorsal pancreatic* of varied origin (splenic, hepatic, celiac, superior mesenteric), the right branch of which anastomoses with the superior pancreaticoduodenal, gastroduodenal and right gastro-epiploic and, in so doing, sends small branches to the pylorus; (12) *left inferior phrenic*, which, after passing under the esophagus in its course to the diaphragm, in most instances gives off a large recurrent branch to the cardio-esophageal end of the stomach posteriorly, where its terminals anastomose with other cardio-esophageal branches

derived from the left gastric, splenic terminals, aberrant left hepatic from the left gastric and descending thoracic esophageal branches.

Typically, the *left gastric artery* arises from the celiac (90 per cent), most commonly as its first branch. In remaining cases it arises from the aorta, splenic or hepatic or from a replaced hepatic trunk. Varying in width from 2 to 8 mm., it is considerably larger than the right gastric, with which it anastomoses along the lesser curvature. Before its division into an anterior and posterior gastric branch, the left gastric supplies the cardio-esophageal end of the stomach, either by a single ramus which subdivides or by two to four rami given off in seriation by the main trunk. Accessory left gastrics occur frequently. They comprise (1) a large left gastric from the left hepatic; (2) a large ascending posterior gas-

tro-esophageal ramus from the splenic trunk or from the superior splenic polar; (3) a slender, threadlike cardio-esophageal branch from the celiac, aorta, first part of the splenic or inferior phrenic.

The terminal branches of the left gastric anastomose with (1) branches of the right gastric; (2) short gastrics from the splenic terminals or splenic superior polar or left gastro-epiploic; (3) cardio-esophageal branches from the left inferior phrenic (via its recurrent branch), the aberrant left hepatic (from left gastric), the accessory left gastric (from left hepatic) and from descending rami of thoracic esophageal branches. The degree of anastomoses about the cardio-esophageal end of the stomach is variable; it may be very extensive or very sparse.

(Continued on page 58)

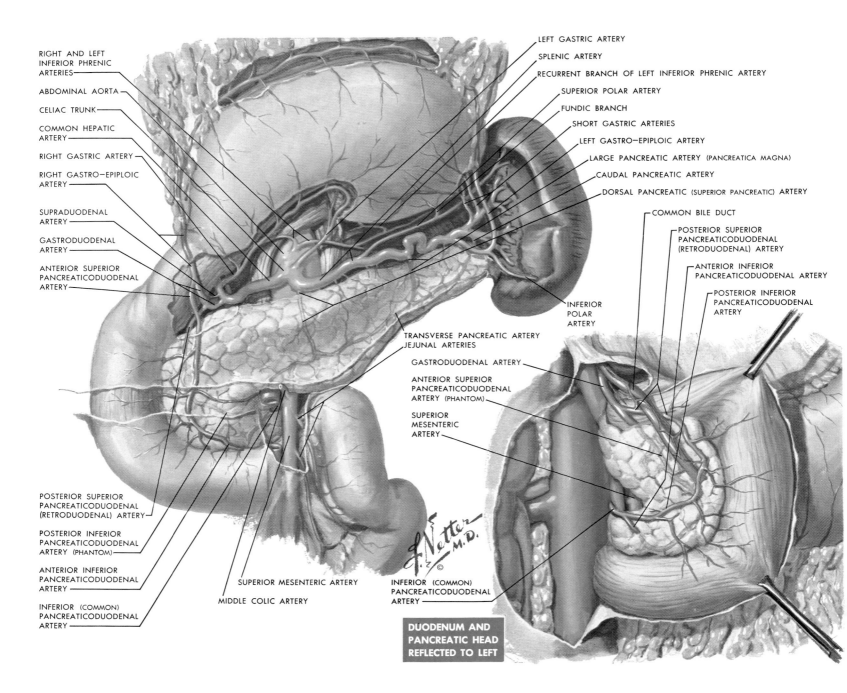

RIGHT AND LEFT INFERIOR PHRENIC ARTERIES

ABDOMINAL AORTA

CELIAC TRUNK

COMMON HEPATIC ARTERY

RIGHT GASTRIC ARTERY

RIGHT GASTRO—EPIPLOIC ARTERY

SUPRADUODENAL ARTERY

GASTRODUODENAL ARTERY

ANTERIOR SUPERIOR PANCREATICODUODENAL ARTERY

POSTERIOR SUPERIOR PANCREATICODUODENAL (RETRODUODENAL) ARTERY

POSTERIOR INFERIOR PANCREATICODUODENAL ARTERY (PHANTOM)

ANTERIOR INFERIOR PANCREATICODUODENAL ARTERY

INFERIOR (COMMON) PANCREATICODUODENAL ARTERY

SUPERIOR MESENTERIC ARTERY

MIDDLE COLIC ARTERY

LEFT GASTRIC ARTERY

SPLENIC ARTERY

RECURRENT BRANCH OF LEFT INFERIOR PHRENIC ARTERY

SUPERIOR POLAR ARTERY

FUNDIC BRANCH

SHORT GASTRIC ARTERIES

LEFT GASTRO—EPIPLOIC ARTERY

LARGE PANCREATIC ARTERY (PANCREATICA MAGNA)

CAUDAL PANCREATIC ARTERY

DORSAL PANCREATIC (SUPERIOR PANCREATIC) ARTERY

INFERIOR POLAR ARTERY

TRANSVERSE PANCREATIC ARTERY
JEJUNAL ARTERIES

GASTRODUODENAL ARTERY

ANTERIOR SUPERIOR PANCREATICODUODENAL ARTERY (PHANTOM)

SUPERIOR MESENTERIC ARTERY

INFERIOR (COMMON) PANCREATICODUODENAL ARTERY

COMMON BILE DUCT

POSTERIOR SUPERIOR PANCREATICODUODENAL (RETRODUODENAL) ARTERY

ANTERIOR INFERIOR PANCREATICODUODENAL ARTERY

POSTERIOR INFERIOR PANCREATICODUODENAL ARTERY

DUODENUM AND PANCREATIC HEAD REFLECTED TO LEFT

SECTION III—PLATE 10

(Continued from page 57)

In about one fourth of the population, the left gastric gives off a large left hepatic artery (2 to 5 mm. wide, 5 cm. long) to the left lobe of the liver. Such a left hepatic may be either replaced or accessory. In the replaced type (12 per cent) no celiac left hepatic is present, the entire blood supply to the lateral segment of the left lobe being derived from the left gastric. The accessory left hepatic is an additive vessel that supplies a region of the left lobe of the liver (either the superior or inferior area of the lateral segment) not supplied by the incomplete celiac left hepatic. If the middle hepatic is a branch of the aberrant left hepatic, then severance of the latter will devascularize the medial segment of the left lobe of the liver as well. From the functional point of view, none of the hepatic arteries is ever "accessory", because every hepatic artery supplies a definite region of the liver, as demonstrated in 150 plastic casts made by Healey and Schroy (1952) in their pioneering statistical analysis of the segmentation of the liver (see Ciba Collection, Vol. 3/III, page 13). In view of prevalent anatomic variations, every gastric resection should

be preceded by an exploratory examination to determine what type of left gastric is present, for severance of a left hepatic derived from the left gastric results in ischemia and fatal necrosis (seventh to sixteenth day) of the left lobe of the liver, as repeatedly evidenced in postmortem examinations. Quite frequently, the left gastric gives off an accessory left inferior phrenic and, in some instances, the left inferior phrenic itself.

Invariably, the *right gastric artery* is much smaller (2 mm.) than the left gastric (4 to 5 mm.), with which it anastomoses, predominantly with the latter's posterior branch. On many occasions (8 per cent) it gives off the supraduodenal or a spray of twigs to the first part of the duodenum. When the right and left hepatics are replaced from some other source, they give rise to the middle hepatic supplying the medial segment of the left lobe.

Predominantly, the *gastroduodenal artery* arises from the common hepatic (75 per cent), but, in many instances, especially with a split celiac trunk, it arises from the left hepatic (10 per cent), right hepatic (7 per cent), middle hepatic (1 per cent), replaced hepatic trunk from the superior mesenteric or aorta (3.5 per cent) and even directly from the celiac or superior mesenteric (2.5 per cent). These atypical origins

are correlated with the mode of branching of the celiac artery, for the common hepatic may divide only into the gastroduodenal and right hepatic (leaving the left hepatic to be replaced from the left gastric) or into the gastroduodenal and left hepatic with replacement of the right hepatic from the superior mesenteric. Typical branches of the gastroduodenal comprise (1) the retroduodenal, as its first collateral (90 per cent); (2) the superior pancreaticoduodenal, as an end branch; (3) the right gastro-epiploic, also an end branch. Inconstant branches are (1) the right gastric (8 per cent); (2) the supraduodenal (25 per cent); (3) the transverse pancreatic (10 per cent); (4) a cystic artery, either the superficial branch or the entire cystic (3 per cent); (5) an accessory right hepatic (occasionally); (6) the middle colic or an accessory middle colic (rarely).

In current texts the relatively large *retroduodenal artery* (1 to 3 mm. in width) is termed the posterior superior pancreaticoduodenal, in view of the fact that it forms an arcade on the back of the head of the pancreas, with branches to the duodenum. The term *retroduodenal* is preferable for, in many instances (10 per cent), the artery arises from a source other than the gastroduodenal and, when it arises from the lat-

(Continued on page 59)

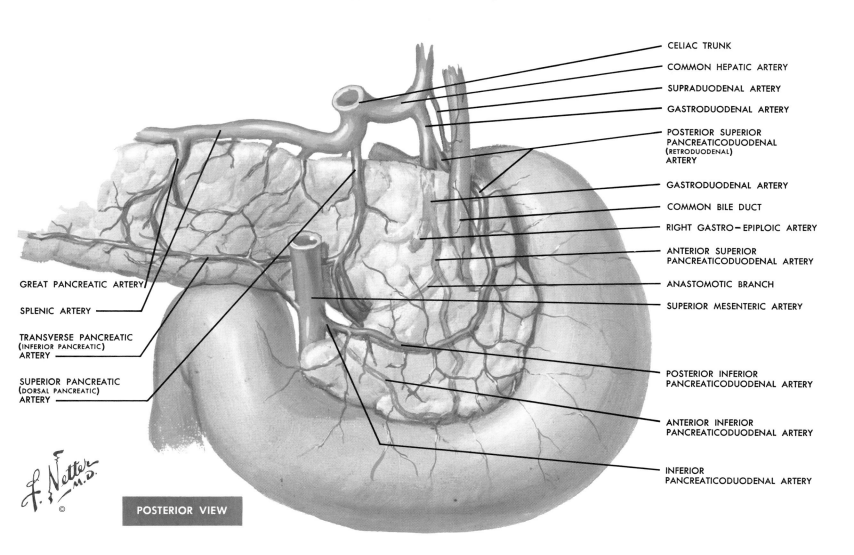

CELIAC TRUNK
COMMON HEPATIC ARTERY
SUPRADUODENAL ARTERY
GASTRODUODENAL ARTERY
POSTERIOR SUPERIOR PANCREATICODUODENAL (RETRODUODENAL) ARTERY
GASTRODUODENAL ARTERY
COMMON BILE DUCT
RIGHT GASTRO–EPIPLOIC ARTERY
ANTERIOR SUPERIOR PANCREATICODUODENAL ARTERY
ANASTOMOTIC BRANCH
SUPERIOR MESENTERIC ARTERY
POSTERIOR INFERIOR PANCREATICODUODENAL ARTERY
ANTERIOR INFERIOR PANCREATICODUODENAL ARTERY
INFERIOR PANCREATICODUODENAL ARTERY

GREAT PANCREATIC ARTERY
SPLENIC ARTERY
TRANSVERSE PANCREATIC (INFERIOR PANCREATIC) ARTERY
SUPERIOR PANCREATIC (DORSAL PANCREATIC) ARTERY

POSTERIOR VIEW

SECTION III—PLATE II

(Continued from page 58)

ter, it does so as its uppermost collateral branch and not as an end branch, as is the case with the superior pancreaticoduodenal. In contrast to the latter, the retroduodenal gives very few branches to the pancreas, its rami being primarily vasa recta to the duodenum. (The retroduodenal and superior pancreaticoduodenal will be described more fully in connection with the blood supply of the duodenum; see below.)

The *right gastro-epiploic artery* is considerably larger than the left gastro-epiploic and, in its course, extends far beyond the midline of the greater curvature of the stomach, where it anastomoses with the *left gastro-epiploic*. Of great surgical import is the fact that, in many instances (10 per cent), this anastomosis is not grossly visible, it being absent or reduced to small arterial twigs that peter out before the left gastroepiploic is reached. The infragastric omental arc, formed by the right and left gastro-epiploics, gives off a large pyloric branch, then a variable number of ascending gastric and descending omental or anterior epiploic branches. The omental branches descend between the two anterior layers of the great omentum. The short ones anastomose with neighboring vessels, the long ones proceed to the distal free edge of the great omentum, where they turn upward to become the posterior epiploic arteries. Many of these join the large epiploic arc of Barkow situated in the posterior layer of the great omentum below the transverse colon. The arc is usually formed by the right epiploic (first branch of the right gastroepiploic) and the left epiploic, a branch of the

left gastro-epiploic. Slender arteries ascend from the arc and anastomose with similar branches (posterior epiploics) given off from the middle colic or left colic and from the transverse pancreatic coursing along the inferior surface of the pancreas. The ultimate and penultimate branches of the posterior epiploics anastomose with the vasa recta of the middle colic but, apparently, are not of sufficient caliber to take over the blood supply, once the middle colic has been rendered functionless (see page 61 and Michels, 1955, Fig. 100). Aberrancies of the right gastroepiploic comprise (1) origin from the superior mesenteric (1.5 per cent) or with the middle colic and superior pancreaticoduodenal (1 per cent); (2) anastomoses with the middle colic, via a large vessel (1 per cent); (3) origin from a gastroduodenal derived from the superior mesenteric.

Usually, the left gastro-epiploic arises from the distal end of the splenic trunk (75 per cent). Next in frequency (25 per cent) is its origin from the inferior splenic terminal or from one of its lienal branches. The artery may be replaced by two to three vessels, the main artery coming from the splenic trunk, the others from an inferior splenic polar artery. Branches of the left gastro-epiploic comprise (1) short fundic branches (two to four); (2) a variable number of ascending short gastrics; (3) several short and long descending omental (epiploic) branches, some of which communicate with similar branches from the right gastro-epiploic; (4) pancreatic rami to the tail of the pancreas, one of which, when large, is termed the arteria caudae pancreatis; (5) inferior splenic polar artery; (6) the left epiploic artery, which descends in the great omentum to form the left limb of the arcus epiploicus magnus

of Barkow, the right limb being formed by the right epiploic from the right gastro-epiploic or transverse pancreatic. The epiploic arc constitutes an excellent widespread collateral pathway for all of the supramesocolonic organs, there being twenty-six different possible collateral routes of arterial blood supply to the liver.

The *blood supply of the duodenum* and *head of the pancreas* is one of the most variant in the body and, surgically considered, one of the most difficult to manipulate. The first inch of the duodenum is a critical transition zone. Paucity or insufficiency of its blood supply has repeatedly been correlated causatively with the tendency of ulcers to perforate the upper part of the duodenum just beyond the pylorus (Wilkie). Typically, the upper, anterior and posterior surfaces of the first inch of the duodenum are supplied by the *supraduodenal artery*, which predominantly is derived from the retroduodenal (50 per cent) or gastroduodenal (25 per cent) and, in the remaining cases, from the right gastric, hepatic or right hepatic. It has been claimed that the supraduodenal is an end artery, but it is not, for it frequently communicates with branches of the *right gastric, gastroduodenal, superior pancreaticoduodenal* and *retroduodenal*. The first inch of the duodenum, in the majority of cases, has a very copious blood supply. The remaining portions of the duodenum are supplied by branches from two pancreaticoduodenal arcades, one being anterior, the other posterior to the head of the pancreas. It is by virtue of these two arcades that THE DUODENUM IS THE ONLY SECTION OF THE GUT THAT HAS A DOUBLE BLOOD SUPPLY, ONE TO ITS ANTERIOR, THE OTHER TO ITS POSTERIOR SURFACE.

(Continued on page 60)

(Continued from page 59)

The anterior pancreaticoduodenal arcade is formed by the (anterior) *superior pancreaticoduodenal,* the smaller of the two end branches of the gastroduodenal artery. After making a loop of a half circle or less on the anterior surface of the pancreas, medial to the groove between the pancreas and duodenum, it sinks into the pancreas, turns to the left, ascends and, upon reaching the posterior surface of the head of the pancreas, joins the *inferior pancreaticoduodenal,* descending from the *superior mesenteric.* The arcade gives off eight to ten relatively large branches (vasa recta) to the anterior surface of all three portions of the duodenum and, in many instances, from one to three branches to the first part of the jejunum, which they reach by passing under the superior mesenteric. The arc also supplies numerous pancreatic branches, some of which are arranged in arcade fashion and anastomose with branches given off by the uncinate branch of the dorsal pancreatic, derived from the first part of the splenic or hepatic.

The *posterior pancreaticoduodenal arcade* is made by the retroduodenal artery (posterior superior pancreaticoduodenal of Woodburne and Olsen), which, as a rule, is the first branch of the gastroduodenal given off by the latter above the duodenum and, often, above the upper border of the head of the pancreas, where it may be cryptically hidden by connective tissue. The term "retroduodenal" is justifiable, for in about 10 per cent of the cases it has a decidedly different origin, being derived from the hepatic (4 per cent), right hepatic (2 per cent), aberrant right hepatic from the superior mesenteric (3 per cent) or dorsal pancreatic (1 per cent). After its typical origin from the gastroduodenal, the artery (1 to 3 mm. in width) descends for 1 cm. or more on the left side of the common bile duct and then, after crossing the latter anteriorly, descends for several centimeters along its right side before swinging to the left and downward to form the posterior arcade.

The major portion of the U- or V-shaped posterior arcade lies behind the center of the head of the pancreas, at a level cephalad to that of the anterior arcade. It comes into full view when the duodenum is mobilized, *i.e.,* turned forward to expose its dorsal surface. It is covered by a fold of connective tissue (Toldt's fascia, primitive mesoduodenum) sufficiently thin that the arc and its branches can be seen. It is accompanied by a venous arcade that lies superficial to the arterial arcade and that empties directly into the portal vein. The arcade crosses the intra-(retro-) pancreatic part of the common bile duct (which it supplies) posteriorly, thereby placing the latter in an arterial circle, for at its origin it crosses it anteriorly. Ultimately, the retroduodenal unites with an inferior pancreaticoduodenal derived from the superior mesenteric at a higher level than that of the anterior arcade (40 per cent),

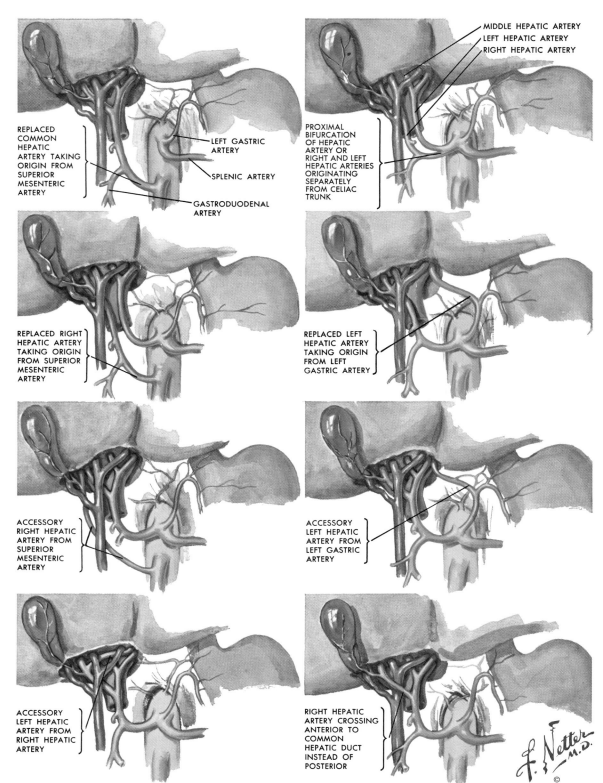

REPLACED COMMON HEPATIC ARTERY TAKING ORIGIN FROM SUPERIOR MESENTERIC ARTERY

LEFT GASTRIC ARTERY

SPLENIC ARTERY

GASTRODUODENAL ARTERY

MIDDLE HEPATIC ARTERY
LEFT HEPATIC ARTERY
RIGHT HEPATIC ARTERY

PROXIMAL BIFURCATION OF HEPATIC ARTERY OR RIGHT AND LEFT HEPATIC ARTERIES ORIGINATING SEPARATELY FROM CELIAC TRUNK

REPLACED RIGHT HEPATIC ARTERY TAKING ORIGIN FROM SUPERIOR MESENTERIC ARTERY

REPLACED LEFT HEPATIC ARTERY TAKING ORIGIN FROM LEFT GASTRIC ARTERY

ACCESSORY RIGHT HEPATIC ARTERY FROM SUPERIOR MESENTERIC ARTERY

ACCESSORY LEFT HEPATIC ARTERY FROM LEFT GASTRIC ARTERY

ACCESSORY LEFT HEPATIC ARTERY FROM RIGHT HEPATIC ARTERY

RIGHT HEPATIC ARTERY CROSSING ANTERIOR TO COMMON HEPATIC DUCT INSTEAD OF POSTERIOR

F. Netter, M.D. ©

or it anastomoses with a posterior branch of a common inferior pancreaticoduodenal, the latter receiving both the anterior and posterior arcades (60 per cent).

The main branches, arising from the retroduodenal and from the arcade it forms, comprise (1) several descending branches (two to three) to the first part of the duodenum, one of which, in about half of the cases, is the supraduodenal; (2) duodenal branches (five to ten, vasa recta) to the posterior surfaces of the descending, transverse and ascending duodenum; (3) small pancreatic branches that are far less numerous and are shorter than those of the anterior arcade; (4) ascending branches (one or more) to the supraduodenal portion of the common bile duct, which they supply; (5) a cystic artery (entire or its superficial branch) which, in about 4 per cent of cases, stems from the first part of the retroduodenal or at its site of origin from the gastroduodenal.

In the majority of instances, the anterior and posterior pancreaticoduodenal arcades have a variant anatomic structure, in the sense that the arcades may be double, triple or even quadruple, wholly or in part. When multiple arcades are present, it is the outer arcade near the duodenum that usually supplies the latter with its branches, whereas the inner arcades supply only pancreatic branches and ultimately become united with the celiac, dorsal pancreatic and other regional arteries.

With every duodenal resection three important vascular arrangements must be borne in mind:

(1) The entire blood supply of the duodenum and head of the pancreas may be completely dissociated from the superior mesenteric. This occurs when an aberrant right hepatic from the superior mesenteric, coursing behind the head of the pancreas, gives

(Continued on page 61)

(Continued from page 60)

off one or two inferior pancreaticoduodenals to receive the anterior or posterior or both pancreaticoduodenal arcades.

(2) The anterior or posterior pancreaticoduodenal arcade, or both, often ends via one or more inferior pancreaticoduodenals derived from the left side of the superior mesenteric or from its first, second or third jejunal branch, a fact to be explored in every gastrojejunostomy, lest the blood supply of the duodenum be impaired and rendered insufficient for viability of that section of the gut.

(3) In resections of the duodenum, extreme care should be taken to maintain an adequate blood supply to the anterior and posterior surfaces of the stumps. The duodenal rami (vasa recta) from the pancreaticoduodenal arcades are end arteries (Shapiro and Robillard), and, if these are evulsed or ligated in their entirety, the suture lines through the ischemic parts, which become necrotic, may break, with resultant "blowout" of the duodenal stump; such an event has repeatedly been fatal, excessive devascularization of the stump being the direct cause of the fatal issue.

SECTION III—PLATE 13

COLLATERAL CIRCULATION OF UPPER ABDOMINAL ORGANS

No other region in the body presents more diversified collateral pathways of blood supply than are found in the supracolonic organs (stomach, duodenum, pancreas, spleen, liver and gallbladder), there being at least twenty-six possible collateral routes to the liver alone (Michels). Because of the multiplicity of its blood vessels and the large amount and loose arrangement of its connective tissue, the great omentum is exceptionally well adapted as a terrain of compensatory circulation, especially for the liver and spleen, when either the hepatic or splenic artery is occluded. Via interlocking arteries, the stomach may receive its blood supply from six primary and six secondary sources (see page 56); the pancreas from the hepatic, splenic and superior mesenteric; the liver from three primary sources — celiac, superior mesenteric and left gastric and, secondarily, from communications with at least twenty-three other arterial pathways. In view of the relational anatomy of the splenic artery, it is quite obvious that most of the collateral pathways to the upper abdominal organs can be initiated via this vessel and its branches and completed through communications established by the gastroduodenal and superior mesenteric.

The most important collateral pathways in the upper abdominal organs are:

1. Arcus arteriosus ventriculi inferior. This infragastric omental pathway is made by the right and left gastro-epiploics as they anastomose along the greater curvature of the stomach. The arc gives off

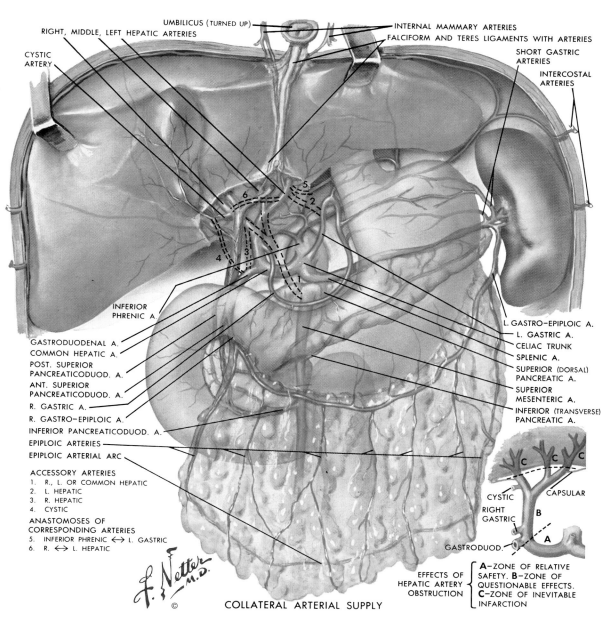

COLLATERAL ARTERIAL SUPPLY

ascending gastric and descending epiploic (omental) arteries.

2. Arcus arteriosus ventriculi superior. This supragastric pathway with branches to both surfaces of the stomach is made by the right and left gastrics anastomosing along the lesser curvature. Branches of the right gastric may unite with branches from the gastroduodenal, supraduodenal (see page 57), retroduodenal (see page 58), superior pancreaticoduodenal or right gastro-epiploic. Branches of the left gastric may anastomose with the short gastrics from the splenic terminals, left gastro-epiploic or with branches from the recurrent cardio-esophageal branch of the left inferior phrenic or with those of an accessory left hepatic, derived from the left gastric.

3. Arcus epiploicus magnus. This epiploic (omental) pathway is situated in the posterior layer of the great omentum below the transverse colon. Its right limb is made by the right epiploic from the right gastro-epiploic; its left limb by the left epiploic from the left gastro-epiploic. Arteries involved in this collateral route include hepatic, gastroduodenal, right gastro-epiploic, right epiploic, left epiploic, left gastro-epiploic and inferior terminal of the splenic.

4. Circulus transpancreaticus longus. This important collateral pathway is effected by the transverse pancreatic artery coursing along the inferior surface of the pancreas (see page 59). Via the dorsal pancreatic, of which it is the main left branch, it may communicate with the first part of the splenic, hepatic, celiac or superior mesenteric, depending on which artery gives

rise to the dorsal pancreatic. At the tail end of the pancreas, it communicates with the splenic terminals via the large pancreatic and caudal pancreatic, and at the head of the pancreas with the gastroduodenal, superior pancreaticoduodenal or right gastro-epiploic.

5. Circulus hepatogastricus. This is a derivative of the primitive, embryonic arched anastomosis between the left gastric and the left hepatic. In the adult the arc may persist in its entirety; the upper half may give rise to an accessory left gastric, the lower half to an "accessory" left hepatic from the left gastric (25 per cent).

6. Circulus hepatolienalis. Here an aberrant right hepatic or the entire hepatic, arising from the superior mesenteric, may communicate with the splenic via a branch of the dorsal pancreatic or gastroduodenal or via the transverse pancreatic and caudal pancreatic.

7. Circulus celiacomesentericus. Through the inferior pancreaticoduodenal, blood may be routed through the anterior and posterior pancreaticoduodenal arcades to enter the gastroduodenal, from which, via the right and left gastro-epiploics, it reaches the splenic, or, via the common hepatic, it reaches the celiac.

8. Circulus gastrolienophrenicus. It may be effected (a) via a communication between the short gastrics from the splenic terminals and the recurrent cardio-esophageal branches of the left inferior phrenic or (b) via a communication between the latter and the cardio-esophageal branches given off by the left gastric, its aberrant left hepatic branch or an accessory left gastric from the left hepatic.

VENOUS DRAINAGE OF STOMACH AND DUODENUM

The venous blood from the stomach and duodenum, along with that from the pancreas and spleen and that of the remaining portion of the intestinal tract (except anal canal), is conveyed to the liver by the *portal vein* (*P.*). The portal vein resembles a tree, in that its roots (capillaries) ramify in the intestinal tract, whereas its branches (sinusoids, capillaries) arborize in the liver. Typically, the portal vein is formed by the rectangular union of the superior mesenteric vein (*S.M.*) with the splenic vein, behind the neck of the pancreas. Its tributaries show many variations (Douglass, Baggenstoss and Hollinshead), which are extremely important in operative procedures (see CIBA COLLECTION, Vol. 3/III, page 73). The *inferior mesenteric vein* (*I.M.*) opens most commonly into the splenic (38 per cent) but, in many instances, drains into the junction point of the superior mesenteric and splenic (32 per cent) or into the superior mesenteric itself (29 per cent). Occasionally, it bifurcates, opening into both veins. From its point of formation to its division at the porta hepatis into a right and a left branch, the portal vein measures from 8 to 10 cm. in length and from 8 to 14 mm. in width (Michels).

The *coronary* (left gastric) *vein* (*C.*) accompanies the left gastric artery and runs from right to left along the lesser curvature of the stomach, at the cardioesophageal end of which it receives esophageal branches. It may empty into the junction point of the *superior mesenteric* (*S.M.*) and *splenic* (*S.*) (58 per cent), *portal vein* (24 per cent) or *splenic* (16 per cent). The pyloric (*right gastric*) (*R.G.*) vein accompanies the right gastric artery from left to right, receives veinlets from both surfaces of the upper part of the stomach and, usually, opens directly into the lower part of the portal vein (75 per cent). Frequently, it enters the *superior mesenteric* (22 per cent) and, occasionally, the *right gastro-epiploic* (*R.G-E.*) or inferior pancreaticoduodenal veins. In some instances it has a common termination with the coronary or is not identifiable. The *left gastro-epiploic* receives branches from the lower anterior and posterior surfaces of the stomach, great omentum and pancreas,

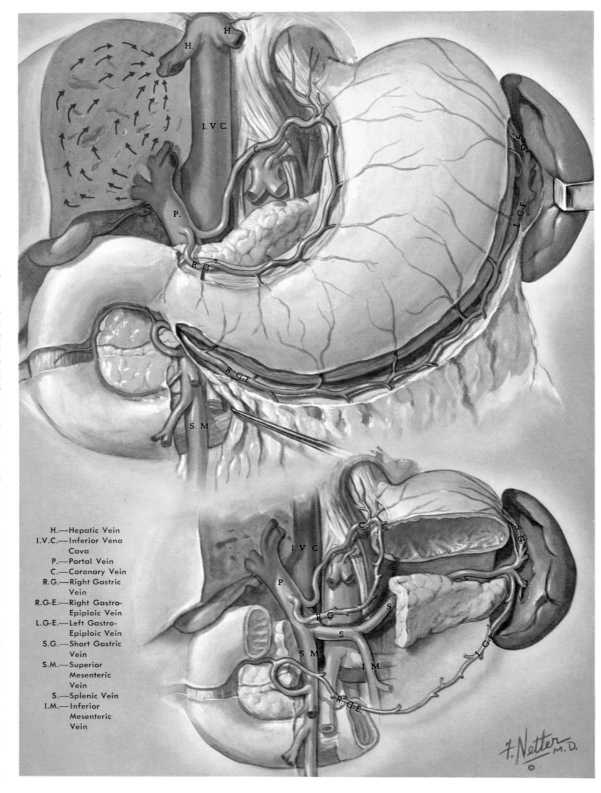

H.—Hepatic Vein
I.V.C.—Inferior Vena Cava
P.—Portal Vein
C.—Coronary Vein
R.G.—Right Gastric Vein
R.G-E.—Right Gastro-Epiploic Vein
L.G-E.—Left Gastro-Epiploic Vein
S.G.—Short Gastric Vein
S.M.—Superior Mesenteric Vein
S.—Splenic Vein
I.M.—Inferior Mesenteric Vein

opening, usually, into the distal part of the splenic trunk and, less frequently, into the inferior splenic terminal or one of its branches (3 to 6). *Short gastric veins* (*S.G.*), arising from the fundic and cardioesophageal end of the stomach, join the splenic terminals or the splenic branches of the left gastroepiploic, or they enter the spleen directly. The *right gastro-epiploic vein* (*R.G-E.*) courses along the greater curvature of the stomach, where it receives branches from its anterior and posterior surfaces and from the great omentum. Usually, it terminates in the superior mesenteric (83 per cent), just before that vessel joins the portal vein. Occasionally, it enters the first part of the splenic or portal vein (2 per cent).

The pancreaticoduodenal veins run with the anterior and posterior arterial pancreaticoduodenal arcades (see page 60) and fuse into a single vein that usually joins the superior mesenteric, a bit below the

right gastro-epiploic. Frequently, the posterior arcade empties directly into the portal vein. The cystic vein, formed by a superficial and deep tributary from the gallbladder, may enter the portal vein, its right branch (see CIBA COLLECTION, Vol. 3/III, page 19) or the liver directly. The majority of pancreatic venous branches, arising from the body and tail of the pancreas, join the splenic along its course, while others terminate in the upper part of the superior or inferior mesenteric or left gastro-epiploic vein. The left inferior phrenic vein receives a tributary from the cardioesophageal region of the stomach and, usually, enters the suprarenal but, in some instances, joins the renal vein.

Since all larger vessels of the portal system are devoid of valves, collateral venous circulation in portal obstruction is readily effected via communications with the caval system.

LYMPHATIC DRAINAGE OF STOMACH

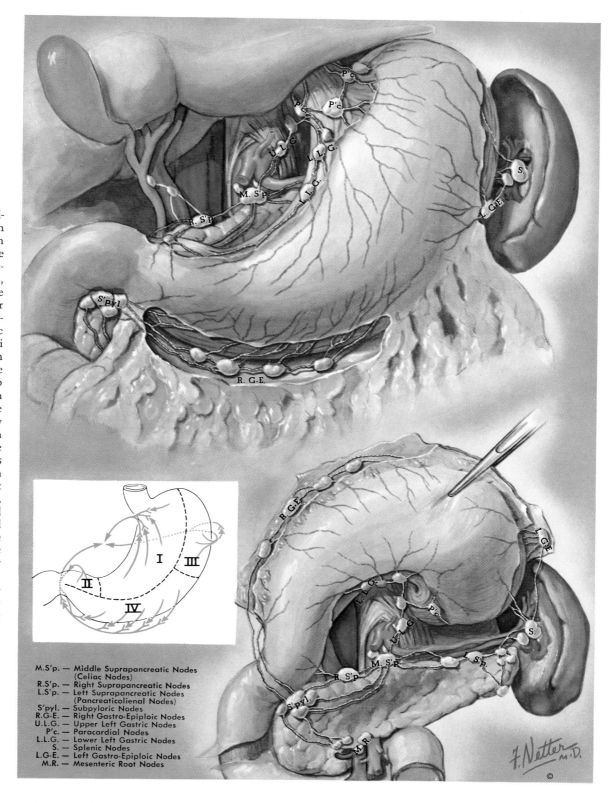

M.S'p. — Middle Suprapancreatic Nodes
(Celiac Nodes)
R.S'p. — Right Suprapancreatic Nodes
L.S'p. — Left Suprapancreatic Nodes
(Pancreaticolienal Nodes)
S'pyl. — Subpyloric Nodes
R.G-E. — Right Gastro-Epiploic Nodes
U.L.G. — Upper Left Gastric Nodes
P'c. — Paracardial Nodes
L.L.G. — Lower Left Gastric Nodes
S. — Splenic Nodes
L.G-E. — Left Gastro-Epiploic Nodes
M.R. — Mesenteric Root Nodes

The lymph from the gastric wall collects in the lymphatic vessels, which form a dense subperitoneal plexus on the anterior and posterior surfaces of the stomach. The lymph flows in the direction of the greater and lesser curvatures, where the first regional lymph nodes are situated. On the upper half of the lesser curvature, i.e., the portion near the cardia, are situated the *lower left gastric* (L.L.G.) *nodes* (lymphonodi gastrici superiores), which are connected with the *paracardial nodes* surrounding the cardia. Above the pylorus is a small group of suprapyloric nodes (not labeled). On the greater curvature, following the trunk of the right gastro-epiploic artery and distributed in a chainlike fashion within the gastrocolic ligament, are the *right gastro-epiploic* (R.G-E.) *nodes* (lymphonodi gastrici inferiores). From these nodes the lymph flows to the right toward the *subpyloric* (S'pyl.) *nodes*, which are situated in front of the head of the pancreas below the pylorus and the first part of the duodenum. There are a few smaller *left gastro-epiploic* (L.G-E.) *nodes* in the part of the greater curvature nearest to the spleen.

For purposes of simplification, a distinction can be made between four different drainage areas into which the gastric lymph flows, although, in point of fact, these areas cannot be so clearly separated. The lymph from the upper left anterior and posterior walls of the stomach (Region I in the diagram) drains through the lower left gastric and paracardial nodes. From here, the lymphatics follow the left gastric artery and the coronary vein toward the vascular bed of the celiac artery. Included in this system are the *upper left gastric* (U.L.G.) *nodes*, which lie on the left crus of the diaphragm. The lower left gastric nodes, the paracardial nodes and the upper left gastric nodes are known collectively as the "left gastric nodes". The pyloric segment of the stomach, in the region of the lesser curvature (Region II), discharges its lymph into the *right suprapancreatic* (R.S'p.) *nodes*, partly directly and partly indirectly, via the small suprapyloric nodes. The lymph from the region of the fundus facing the greater curvature, i.e., adjacent to the spleen, flows along lymphatic vessels running within the gastrosplenic ligament. Some of these lymphatics lead directly to the *left suprapancreatic* (L.S'p.) (pancreaticolienal) *nodes,* and others indirectly via the small *left gastro-epiploic* (L.G-E.) *nodes* and via the splenic nodes lying within the hilus of the spleen. Lymph from the dis-

tal portion of the corpus facing the greater curvature and from the pyloric region (Region IV) collects in the right gastro-epiploic nodes. From here, the lymph flows to the subpyloric nodes, which lie in front of the head of the pancreas, partly behind and partly below the pylorus. Leading to these nodes are also a few lymphatics from that part of the greater curvature which is immediately adjacent to the pylorus. From the subpyloric nodes, which are also connected with the superior mesenteric nodes by way of prepancreatic lymphatics, the lymph flows to the right suprapancreatic nodes through lymphatics situated behind the pylorus and duodenal bulb.

From the upper left gastric nodes (Region I), from the right suprapancreatic nodes (Regions II and IV) and from the left suprapancreatic nodes (pancreaticolienal nodes) (Region III), the lymph stream leads to the celiac (*middle suprapancreatic,* M.S'p.) nodes,

which are situated above the pancreas and around the celiac artery and its branches. From the celiac lymph nodes, the lymph flows through the gastro-intestinal lymphatic trunk to the thoracic duct, in the initial segment of which, i.e., at the point where it arises from the various trunks, there is generally a more or less pronounced expansion in the form of the cisterna chyli.

In the region where the thorax borders on the neck, the thoracic duct, before opening into the angle formed by the left subclavian and left jugular veins, receives inter alia the left subclavian lymphatic trunk. In cases of gastric tumor, palpable metastases may sometimes develop in the left supraclavicular nodes (also known as Virchow's or Troisier's nodes).

The lymphatics of the duodenum drain into the nodes which serve also the pancreas and are described on page 30 of CIBA COLLECTION, Vol. 3/III.

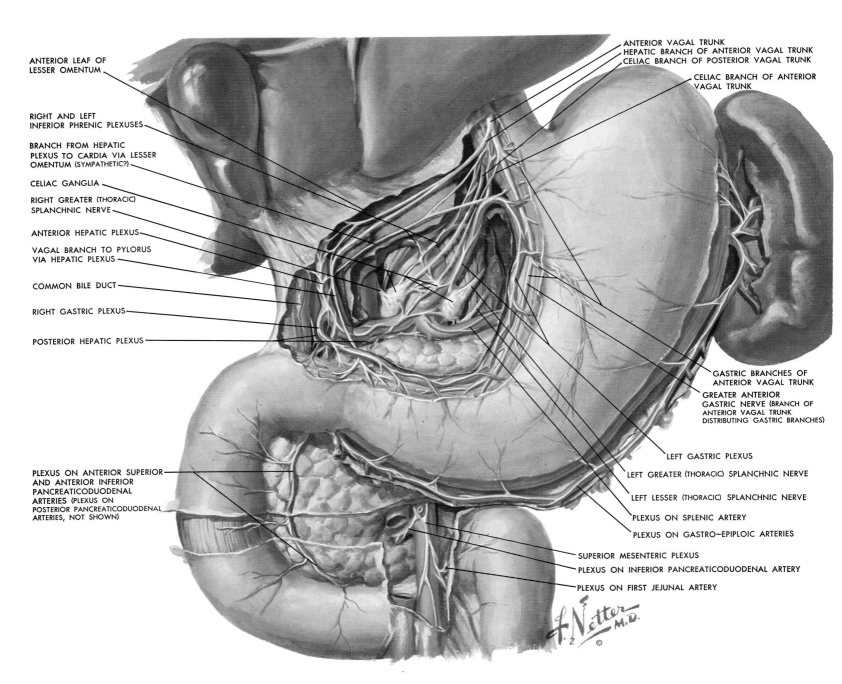

ANTERIOR LEAF OF
LESSER OMENTUM

RIGHT AND LEFT
INFERIOR PHRENIC PLEXUSES

BRANCH FROM HEPATIC
PLEXUS TO CARDIA VIA LESSER
OMENTUM (SYMPATHETIC?)

CELIAC GANGLIA

RIGHT GREATER (THORACIC)
SPLANCHNIC NERVE

ANTERIOR HEPATIC PLEXUS

VAGAL BRANCH TO PYLORUS
VIA HEPATIC PLEXUS

COMMON BILE DUCT

RIGHT GASTRIC PLEXUS

POSTERIOR HEPATIC PLEXUS

PLEXUS ON ANTERIOR SUPERIOR
AND ANTERIOR INFERIOR
PANCREATICODUODENAL
ARTERIES (PLEXUS ON
POSTERIOR PANCREATICODUODENAL
ARTERIES, NOT SHOWN)

ANTERIOR VAGAL TRUNK
HEPATIC BRANCH OF ANTERIOR VAGAL TRUNK
CELIAC BRANCH OF POSTERIOR VAGAL TRUNK

CELIAC BRANCH OF ANTERIOR
VAGAL TRUNK

GASTRIC BRANCHES OF
ANTERIOR VAGAL TRUNK

GREATER ANTERIOR
GASTRIC NERVE (BRANCH OF
ANTERIOR VAGAL TRUNK
DISTRIBUTING GASTRIC BRANCHES)

LEFT GASTRIC PLEXUS

LEFT GREATER (THORACIC) SPLANCHNIC NERVE

LEFT LESSER (THORACIC) SPLANCHNIC NERVE

PLEXUS ON SPLENIC ARTERY

PLEXUS ON GASTRO–EPIPLOIC ARTERIES

SUPERIOR MESENTERIC PLEXUS

PLEXUS ON INFERIOR PANCREATICODUODENAL ARTERY

PLEXUS ON FIRST JEJUNAL ARTERY

f. Netter M.D.

SECTION III—PLATES 16 AND 17

INNERVATION OF STOMACH AND DUODENUM

The stomach and duodenum are innervated by sympathetic and parasympathetic nerves which contain efferent and afferent fibers.

The SYMPATHETIC SUPPLY emerges in the anterior spinal nerve roots as preganglionic fibers, which are axons of lateral cornual cells located at about the sixth to the ninth or tenth thoracic segments. They are carried from the spinal nerves in rami communicantes which pass to the adjacent parts of the sympathetic ganglionated trunks and then in the thoracic splanchnic nerves to the *celiac plexus* and ganglia. Some of them form synapses in the sympathetic trunk ganglia, but the majority form synapses with cells in the celiac and superior mesenteric ganglia. The axons of these cells, the postganglionic fibers, are conveyed to the stomach and duodenum in the nerve plexuses alongside the various branches of the celiac and superior mesenteric arteries. These arterial plexuses are composed mainly of sympathetic fibers, but they contain some parasympathetic

fibers which reach the celiac plexus through the celiac branches of the vagal trunks. The afferent impulses are carried in fibers which pursue the reverse route of the one just described, but they do not form synapses in the sympathetic trunks; their cytons are located in the posterior spinal root ganglia and enter the cord via the posterior spinal nerve roots.

The *celiac plexus* is the largest of the autonomic plexuses and surrounds the celiac arterial trunk and the root of the superior mesenteric artery. It consists of right and left halves, each containing one larger *celiac ganglion,* a smaller *aorticorenal ganglion* and a superior mesenteric ganglion which is often unpaired. These and other still smaller ganglia are united by numerous nervous interconnections to form the plexus. It receives sympathetic contributions through the greater (superior), lesser (middle) and least (inferior) thoracic splanchnic nerves and through filaments from the first lumbar ganglia of the sympathetic trunks, whereas its parasympathetic roots are derived from the celiac division of the *posterior vagal trunk* and smaller celiac branches from the *anterior vagal trunk.*

The plexus sends direct filaments to some adjacent viscera, but most of its branches accompany the arteries from the upper part of the

abdominal aorta. Numerous filaments from the celiac plexus unite to form open-meshed nerve *plexuses* around the celiac trunk and the *left gastric, hepatic* and *splenic arteries.* Subsidiary plexuses from the hepatic arterial plexus are continued along the right gastric and gastroduodenal arteries and from the latter along the *right gastro-epiploic* and *anterior* and *posterior superior pancreaticoduodenal arteries.* The splenic arterial plexus sends offshoots along the short gastric and left gastro-epiploic arteries.

The *superior mesenteric plexus* is the largest derivative of the celiac plexus and contains the superior mesenteric ganglion or ganglia. The main superior mesenteric plexus divides into secondary plexuses, which surround and accompany the inferior pancreaticoduodenal, jejunal and other branches of the artery.

The *left gastric plexus* consists of one to four nervelets connected by oblique filaments which accompany the artery and supply twigs to the cardiac end of the stomach, communicating with offshoots from the left phrenic plexus. Other filaments follow the artery along the lesser curvature between the layers of the lesser omentum to supply adjacent parts of the stomach. They communicate profusely with the *right gastric*

(Continued on page 65)

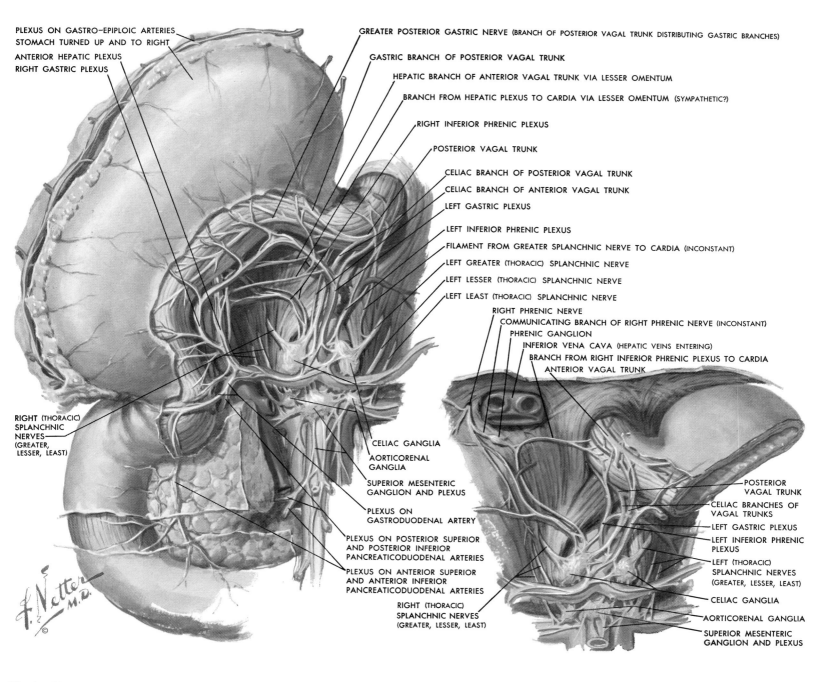

(*Continued from page 64*)

plexus and with gastric branches of the vagus.

The *hepatic plexus* also contains both sympathetic and parasympathetic efferent and afferent fibers and gives off subsidiary plexuses along all its branches. These, following the right gastric artery, supply the pyloric region, and the gastroduodenal plexus accompanies the artery between the first part of the duodenum and the head of the pancreas, supplying fibers to both structures and to the adjacent parts of the common bile duct. When the artery divides into its anterior superior pancreaticoduodenal and right gastroepiploic branches, the nerves also subdivide and are distributed to the second part of the duodenum, the terminations of the common bile and pancreatic ducts, the head of the pancreas and the parts of the stomach. The part of the hepatic plexus lying in the free margin of the lesser omentum gives off one or more (hepatogastric) *branches which pass to the left* between the layers of the lesser omentum to the cardiac end and lesser curvature of the stomach; they unite with and reinforce the left gastric plexus. The *splenic plexus* gives off subsidiary nerve plexuses around its pancreatic, short gastric and left gastro-epiploic branches, and these supply the structures indicated by their names. A filament

may curve upward to supply the fundus of the stomach.

The *phrenic plexuses* assist in supplying the cardiac end of the stomach. A *filament from the right plexus* sometimes turns to the left, postero-inferior to the *vena caval hiatus* in the diaphragm, and passes to the region of the cardiac orifice, whereas the left phrenic plexus supplies a constant twig to the cardiac orifice. A delicate branch from the left phrenic nerve (not illustrated) supplies the cardia.

The PARASYMPATHETIC SUPPLY for the stomach and duodenum arises in the dorsal vagal nucleus in the floor of the fourth ventricle, and the afferent fibers end in the same nucleus, which is a mixture of visceral efferent and afferent cells. The fibers are conveyed to and from the abdomen through the vagus nerves, esophageal plexus and vagal trunks. The vagal trunks give off *gastric,* pyloric, *hepatic* and *celiac branches.* The *anterior vagal trunk* gives off gastric branches which run downward along the lesser curvature, supplying the anterior surface of the stomach almost as far as the pylorus. Frequently, one branch, the *greater anterior gastric nerve,* is larger than the others. The various gastric branches can be traced for some distance beneath the serous coat before they sink into the muscle

coats, and, although they communicate with neighboring gastric nerves, a true anterior gastric plexus in the accepted sense of the term does not usually exist. The pyloric branches (not illustrated) arise from the anterior vagal trunk or from the greater anterior gastric nerve and run to the right between the layers of the lesser omentum before turning downward through or close to the hepatic plexus to reach the pyloric antrum, pylorus and proximal part of the duodenum. Small celiac branches run alongside the left gastric artery to the celiac plexus, often uniting with corresponding branches of the posterior vagal trunk.

The *posterior vagal trunk* gives off gastric branches which radiate to the posterior surface of the stomach, supplying it from the fundus to the pyloric antrum. One branch, the *greater posterior gastric nerve,* is usually larger than the others. As on the anterior aspect, these branches communicate with adjacent gastric nerves, although no true posterior gastric plexus exists. The celiac branch is large and reaches the celiac plexus alongside the left gastric artery. Vagal fibers from this celiac branch are distributed to the pylorus, duodenum, pancreas, etc., through the vascular plexuses derived from the celiac plexus.

Section IV

FUNCTIONAL AND DIAGNOSTIC ASPECTS OF THE UPPER DIGESTIVE TRACT

by

FRANK H. NETTER, M.D.

in collaboration with

WILLIAM H. BACHRACH, M.D., Ph.D.
Plates 1-5, 8-22, 24-29

MAX L. SOM, M.D., F.A.C.S.
Plate 23

BERNARD S. WOLF, M.D.
Plates 6 and 7

HUNGER AND APPETITE

The digestive processes are initiated by the ingestion of food in response to need (hunger) or desire (appetite). Hunger has been defined as "the complex of sensations evoked by depletion of body nutrient stores" (Grossman). Of these sensations the most common is a discomfort localized to the epigastrium and perceived as emptiness, gnawing, tension or pangs. The epigastric sensation was at one time considered (Carlson) to be an indispensable element in hunger; but the fact that hunger is experienced by individuals whose stomach has been removed or denervated is evidence that contractions of the empty stomach (*hunger contractions*) cannot be an essential component of the hunger phenomenon. Hunger engenders a desire for food (appetite), which leads to appetitive behavior, manifested in the unconditioned state, as in the newborn or anencephalic infant or decerebrate animal, by feeding reflexes, and in the conditioned or learned state by food-seeking and food-taking activities of varying complexity. Appetitive behavior is suppressed by the sensation of fullness or satiety brought on by adequate repletion with foodstuff.

The nervous regulation for all activities involved in obtaining and ingesting food has been thought, since Pavlov's investigations (1911), to be "centered" in *cell groups in the cerebral hemispheres* and at lower levels in the brain. According to one theory (Carlson), contractions of the empty or nearly empty stomach, activated by inherent automatism, give rise to impulses which pass up the *vagi* to the *nucleus solitarius*, thence to the *hypothalamus* and, finally, to the cerebral cortex. Some of the hunger reflexes are considered to be mediated in the medulla. More recently, the presence of two centers in the diencephalon — one in the lateral hypothalamic area concerned with the facilitation of feeding reflexes, the other a *medial hypothalamic inhibitory area* — has been established (Brobeck; see also CIBA COLLECTION, Vol. 1, Supplement, page 161). From these "appetite" and "satiety" centers, fibers have been assumed to descend and act upon the neurons of the pons, medulla and spinal cord, which govern the muscles concerned in appetitive behavior as well as the motility and secretion of the digestive organs. Such theory assumes that, when food is eaten, certain changes occur which suppress the activity of the

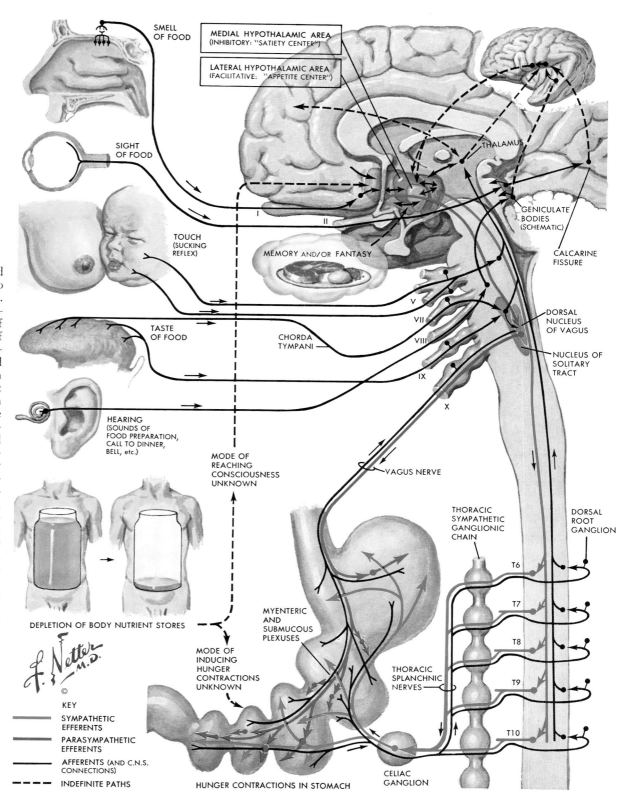

SMELL OF FOOD

MEDIAL HYPOTHALAMIC AREA
(INHIBITORY: "SATIETY CENTER")

LATERAL HYPOTHALAMIC AREA
(FACILITATIVE: "APPETITE CENTER")

SIGHT OF FOOD

THALAMUS

TOUCH (SUCKING REFLEX)

MEMORY AND/OR FANTASY

GENICULATE BODIES (SCHEMATIC)

CALCARINE FISSURE

TASTE OF FOOD

CHORDA TYMPANI

DORSAL NUCLEUS OF VAGUS

NUCLEUS OF SOLITARY TRACT

HEARING (SOUNDS OF FOOD PREPARATION, CALL TO DINNER, BELL, etc.)

MODE OF REACHING CONSCIOUSNESS UNKNOWN

VAGUS NERVE

THORACIC SYMPATHETIC GANGLIONIC CHAIN

DORSAL ROOT GANGLION

DEPLETION OF BODY NUTRIENT STORES

MODE OF INDUCING HUNGER CONTRACTIONS UNKNOWN

MYENTERIC AND SUBMUCOUS PLEXUSES

THORACIC SPLANCHNIC NERVES

T6

T7

T8

T9

T10

f. Netter M.D.

KEY

— SYMPATHETIC EFFERENTS

— PARASYMPATHETIC EFFERENTS

— AFFERENTS (AND C.N.S. CONNECTIONS)

--- INDEFINITE PATHS

HUNGER CONTRACTIONS IN STOMACH

CELIAC GANGLION

lateral hypothalamus, thus decreasing appetite while stimulating the medial portion, thus promoting satiety. The searching for, the examination, and the ingestion or rejection of food involve other nervous reflex mechanisms, of which those provoked by *visual, olfactory and auditory stimuli* must be mediated via cortical connections to the hypothalamus (see CIBA COLLECTION, Vol. 1, page 161). *Tactile, gustatory and enteroceptive stimuli* could act through infracortical pathways.

Since food-taking behavior is not abolished by denervation of the gastro-intestinal tract, it is evident that "the composition of the blood is a stimulus for the food center" (Carlson). Efforts to identify specific metabolic or chemical changes which govern the intervals of food taking and the amount of food eaten have resulted in hypotheses such as the glucostatic-lipostatic theory (J. Mayer, 1955). According to this

theory the short-term or meal-to-meal regulation of food intake is concerned with the acute energy requirements and depends upon the operation of glucoreceptors sensitive to the rate of glucose utilization, as reflected in the arteriovenous glucose difference. It is further hypothesized that the long-term regulation of food intake, directed at stabilizing body weight, is accomplished by a lipostatic mechanism which controls the daily mobilization of a quantity of fat proportional to the total fat content of the body. It is presumed that these glucostatic and lipostatic mechanisms influence hunger and appetite via the hypothalamus. The ultimate validity of such theories will depend on the results of investigations stimulated by them. Presently not enough evidence is available to decide precisely what blood or tissue changes, or other factors, are responsible for the seeking and taking of food.

DISTURBANCES OF HUNGER AND APPETITE

Deviations from the normal pattern of food-taking may theoretically be based on disturbances of (1) the central nervous regulatory mechanism, (2) the hunger contractions of the stomach or (3) the hypothetical peripheral receptors. Clinically, the most important problem is anorexia, which may be viewed as a condition in which the depletion of body nutrients fails to evoke the sensations which normally lead to appetitive behavior. In pathologic and experimental *febrile states,* as well as in some infectious illnesses with little or no fever, gastric tonus and contractions are inhibited. Whether this occurs in connection with anorexia in *gastro-intestinal diseases,* such as hepatitis and colitis, is unknown. The fact that a profound anorexia is one of the earliest symptoms in viral hepatitis and that in the severest cases encephalopathy may occur permits the speculation that the virus may affect the appetite centers in the brain. On teleologic grounds any inflammatory disease of the digestive organs would be expected to depress appetite as a protective measure. In acute pancreatitis it is deemed clinically astute to abet this tendency, not only withholding everything by mouth but actually aspirating the stomach. In acute hepatitis, on the other hand, clinical judgment holds that the anorexia has no good biologic purpose and is to be thwarted by forced feeding.

Anorexia nervosa, a loss of appetite amounting to a disgust or distaste for food in the absence of any somatic provocation, is an extreme example of the effect of emotion on the intake of food. The mechanism here is entirely neural, involving the cortical and probably the hypothalamic centers. The anorexia in *nutritional, metabolic, fluid and electrolyte deficiencies,* while poorly understood, usually responds to correction of the underlying condition. The depressing effect on the appetite of *excessive smoking* may be explained by inhibition of gastric hunger contractions, impairment of taste sensations, distraction from hunger sensations to those associated with smoking and a possible central effect of nicotine or other tobacco-combustion products.

Drugs, particularly *amphetamine* and its derivatives, have been employed to impair the appetite deliberately in the

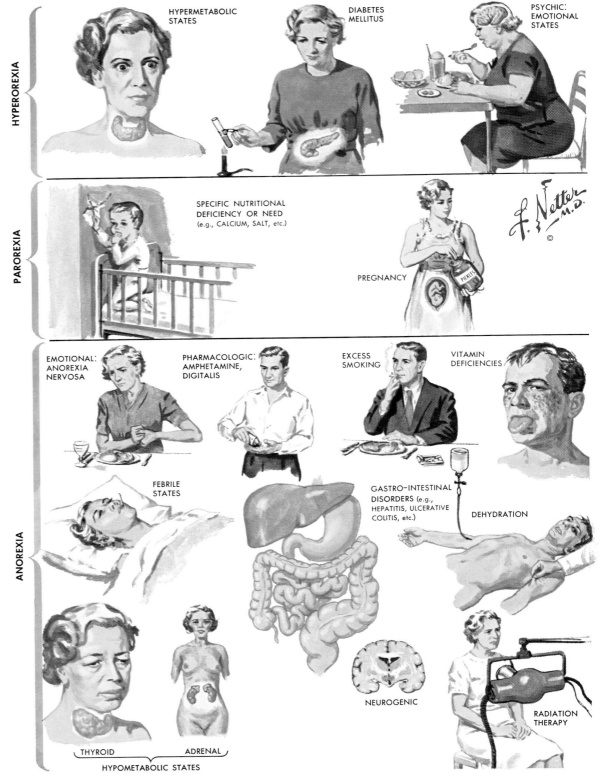

management of obesity. Evidence bearing on the mechanism of their action has been obtained recently (Brobeck) by recording increased electrical activity from the medial hypothalamic area after amphetamine administration. Amara, or "bitters", have been alleged to have appetite-stimulating properties, but no convincing evidence is available that they do so.

Hyperorexia, or food intake in excess of body requirements, has become a pressing medical problem in view of the increasing incidence of obesity. The fact that fat people cannot suppress their desire to eat, in spite of being disgusted and ashamed of their body form, has been advanced in some quarters as evidence that the causes are primarily emotional. The solution of this problem will have to come from the discovery and control of the physiologic mechanism by which the hunger sensation of these people is mediated. Extreme hunger after prolonged starvation

drives normal individuals to the very limits of antisocial behavior—even to cannibalism; thus, one could understand that some drive of unknown origin in an obese patient makes it an ordeal to refrain from eating. The hyperorexia of *diabetes* and *hyperthyroidism* does not result in obesity, because the body nutrient stores are depleted by concomitant nutritional wastage or energy expenditure. On the other hand, pancreatic islet cell tumor with hyperinsulinemia often results in hyperorexia with weight gain.

Parorexia, meaning an abnormal desire for certain substances, like the salt craving in uncontrolled Addison's disease or the drive for chalk in calcium deficiency states, clearly has its origin in blood and tissues, but the mechanism of this phenomenon is not known. The desire in early pregnancy for sour foodstuffs or comestibles normally not desired has also not yet been explained.

SALIVARY SECRETION

Stimulation of areas in the *premotor region of the cortex cerebri* (in the vicinity of the masticatory center) and in the *hypothalamus* evokes salivation. No information is available as to nervous connections between these two areas or between the hypothalamus and the superior and inferior *salivary nuclei* in the medulla. The nervous pathways from these nuclei and the sympathetic and parasympathetic innervation of the salivary glands have been described on page 31.

During the resting or recovery phase, when no secretory stimuli are acting, granules of mucinogen, the precursor of mucin, are formed in the mucous cells, and granules of zymogen, the precursor of ptyalin, in the serous or demilune cells (see also page 14). Extrusion of these substances, together with other components (see below), into the lumen of the alveoli and into the ducts is activated entirely by impulses reaching the cells over the nervous pathways; no hormonal regulation of salivary secretion has been demonstrated. The *parasympathetic nerves* supply the mucin-secreting and the intralobular duct cells, while the *sympathetics* govern the serous cells and the myo-epithelial or *"basket" cells,* which lie between the basal membrane and the secretory cells and are presumed to account for the contractile action which permits a gush of saliva. The quantity and composition of saliva are adapted to the nature of the agent which stimulates, chemically or mechanically, the nerve endings (V and IX) of the oral mucosa (unconditioned reflex). Thus, edible substances generally produce a viscid saliva, rich in mucin and enzyme. Inedible substances, *e.g.,* sand, evoke a watery secretion. Acid material stimulates saliva with buffering (high protein content) and diluting properties. Milk, in contrast to other fluids, evokes a copious flow of saliva, rich in organic material — a fact which has been thought (Pavlov) to help the digestion of the coagulum by the gastric juice. These unconditioned reflex responses do not depend on any learning process and have been elicited experimentally in decerebrated animals. The conditioned reflexes, on the other hand, are manifested by the flow of saliva in association with the thought or sight of food and with events the individual has learned to relate to

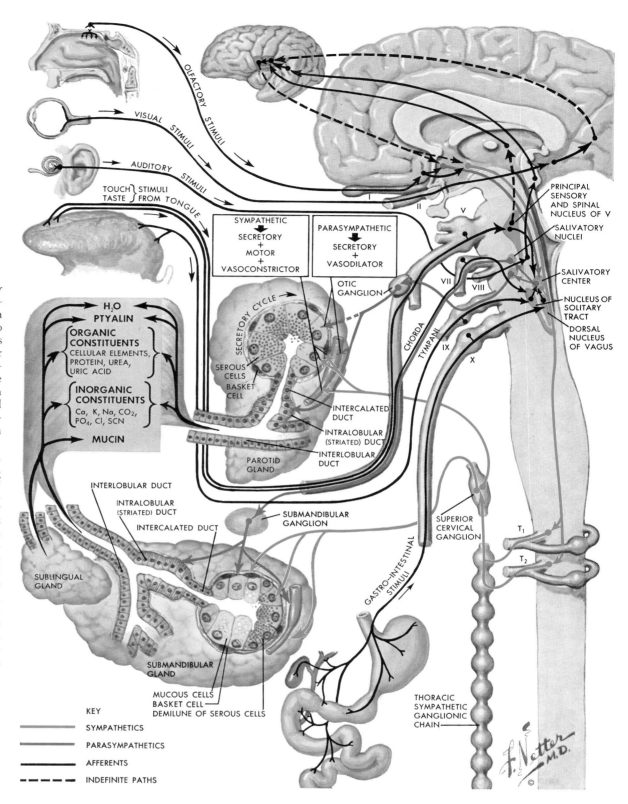

food, such as the sound of a tuning fork in Pavlov's famous experiment with dogs.

The total amount of saliva secreted per day is estimated at 1000 to 1500 ml. The specific gravity varies from 1003 to 1008 and the pH from 6.2 to 7.6. Resting saliva is usually acid; freely flowing, usually alkaline. The viscosity varies with the type of stimulus and the rate of flow. The *parotid gland* forms a watery fluid containing protein, salts and ptyalin but no mucus. The *sublingual gland* is predominantly mucous, while the *submandibular* is intermediate, though predominantly serous in man. Saliva is hypotonic, and its osmotic pressure increases as flow rate increases. The only salivary enzyme, *ptyalin,* is produced by the parotid and submandibular glands and converts cooked starch into dextrins and maltose at a pH range of 4.5 to 9 (optimum 6.5). Ptyalin is inactivated at pH below 4.5 and destroyed by heating to

65° C. Other *organic constituents* include cellular elements from the buccal mucosa and the glands, urea, uric acid and traces of urease. The *inorganic constituents* consist of the anions Cl⁻, PO₄⁻ and HCO₃⁻ and the cations Ca, Na and K. The ratio of the last two in the saliva mirrors their presence in the blood serum. Present in the saliva is also a small amount of thiocyanate, which is assumed to act as a coenzyme, since it can activate ptyalin in the absence of NaCl. The saliva of smokers is relatively rich in KCNS.

Saliva has a cleansing action which plays a significant rôle in oral hygiene, but the salivary glands have also a still more important function inasmuch as they present an essential regulative factor for the water balance. The glands stop secreting saliva whenever the body fluid content falls to a low level, and this leads to a dryness of the oral mucosa and, therewith, arouses the sensation of thirst.

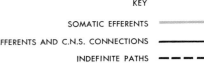

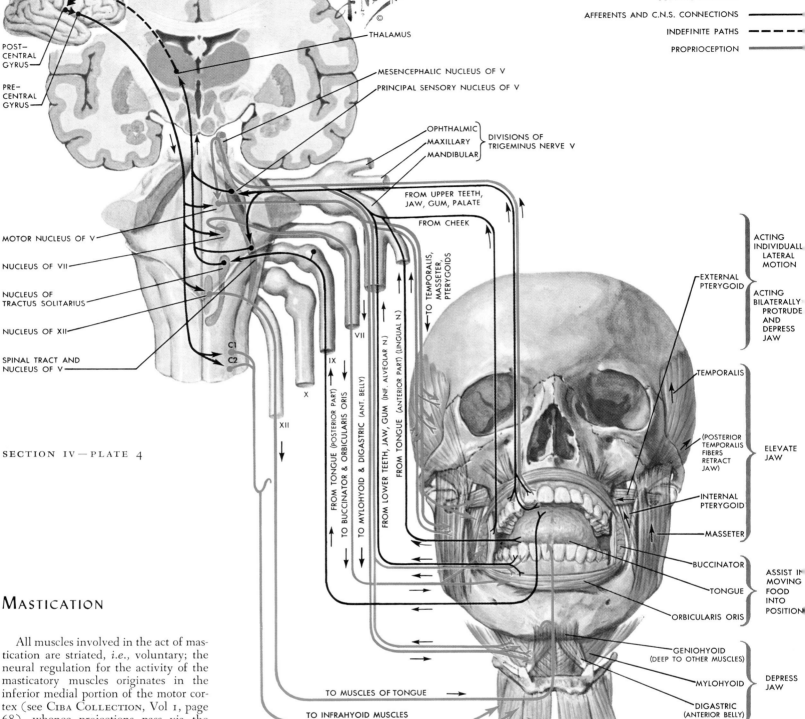

KEY

SOMATIC EFFERENTS	
AFFERENTS AND C.N.S. CONNECTIONS	
INDEFINITE PATHS	
PROPRIOCEPTION	

POST–CENTRAL GYRUS

PRE–CENTRAL GYRUS

THALAMUS

MESENCEPHALIC NUCLEUS OF V

PRINCIPAL SENSORY NUCLEUS OF V

OPHTHALMIC
MAXILLARY
MANDIBULAR

DIVISIONS OF TRIGEMINUS NERVE V

FROM UPPER TEETH, JAW, GUM, PALATE

FROM CHEEK

MOTOR NUCLEUS OF V

NUCLEUS OF VII

NUCLEUS OF TRACTUS SOLITARIUS

NUCLEUS OF XII

SPINAL TRACT AND NUCLEUS OF V

C1
C2

TO TEMPORALIS, MASSETER, PTERYGOIDS

VII

IX

X

XII

FROM TONGUE (POSTERIOR PART)

TO BUCCINATOR & ORBICULARIS ORIS

TO MYLOHYOID & DIGASTRIC (ANT. BELLY)

FROM LOWER TEETH, JAW, GUM (INF. ALVEOLAR N.)

FROM TONGUE (ANTERIOR PART) (LINGUAL N.)

ACTING INDIVIDUALLY LATERAL MOTION

ACTING BILATERALLY PROTRUDE AND DEPRESS JAW

EXTERNAL PTERYGOID

TEMPORALIS

(POSTERIOR TEMPORALIS FIBERS RETRACT JAW)

ELEVATE JAW

INTERNAL PTERYGOID

MASSETER

BUCCINATOR

TONGUE

ORBICULARIS ORIS

ASSIST IN MOVING FOOD INTO POSITION

GENIOHYOID (DEEP TO OTHER MUSCLES)

MYLOHYOID

DIGASTRIC (ANTERIOR BELLY)

DEPRESS JAW

TO MUSCLES OF TONGUE

TO INFRAHYOID MUSCLES (FIX HYOID BONE)

SECTION IV — PLATE 4

MASTICATION

All muscles involved in the act of mastication are striated, *i.e.,* voluntary; the neural regulation for the activity of the masticatory muscles originates in the inferior medial portion of the motor cortex (see CIBA COLLECTION, Vol 1, page 68), whence projections pass via the pyramidal tract to the pons to co-ordinate the motor nuclei of the nerves supplying the muscles of mastication (see page 29). The complex movements of these muscles are centrally integrated, and co-ordination is aided by the impulses carrying sensation from the teeth and mucosal surface of the mouth, as well as proprioceptive sensibility of the muscles themselves. From the tooth sockets, proprioceptive pathways lead to the principal mesencephalic sensory nucleus (the only sensory root that has its cells of origin within the central nervous system) and thence to the motor nucleus (see CIBA COLLECTION, Vol. 1, pages 47 and 59), effecting control of the masticatory pressure and preventing the breaking of teeth.

Mastication begins with the cutting of the food (if necessary) by the incisor teeth and continues by bringing food in position between the grinding surfaces of the molars and premolars, in which act the tongue and the muscles of the cheek are involved. This done, the necessary muscular forces come into action to accomplish the grinding. The mandible is alternately elevated (masseter, temporal, internal pterygoid muscles) and depressed (digastric, mylohyoid, geniohyoid), moved forward (external pterygoid) and backward (lower fibers of temporal), and from side to side (external pterygoid and elevators of the opposite side). The strength with which this grinding is performed may be appreciated by the fact that the molars have been shown to exert a biting force as high as 270 lb. (For the muscles involved in these movements and their innervation, see pages 8, 9 and 22.)

The primary purpose of mastication is to facilitate deglutition by reducing the size of the food particles and lubricating them with saliva. How much chewing is required to accomplish this depends on the type of food, the amount taken into the mouth at one time, the strength of the bite, the intensity of hunger, etc. Ordinarily, by the time food is swallowed, most of it has been reduced to particles less than 2 mm. in diameter. The largest particles usually do not exceed 12 mm. The nerve endings in the mouth sense the size of the particles which form the bolus and determine when the latter is ready to be swallowed. The efficiency of this function is such that rarely does a bolus become lodged in the normal esophagus.

Mere facilitation of swallowing is, however, not the only result of mastication. Thorough chewing also aids digestion. The prolonged contact of tasty food with the oral mucosa increases the psychic secre-

(Continued on page 73)

MASTICATION

(Continued from page 72)

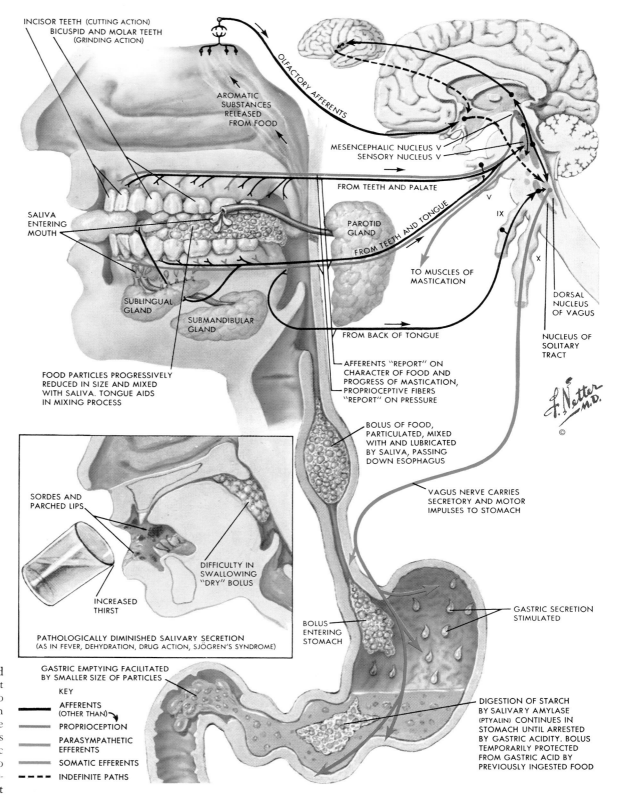

INCISOR TEETH (CUTTING ACTION)
BICUSPID AND MOLAR TEETH (GRINDING ACTION)

AROMATIC SUBSTANCES RELEASED FROM FOOD

OLFACTORY AFFERENTS

MESENCEPHALIC NUCLEUS V
SENSORY NUCLEUS V

FROM TEETH AND PALATE

SALIVA ENTERING MOUTH

PAROTID GLAND

FROM TEETH AND TONGUE

V

IX

X

TO MUSCLES OF MASTICATION

DORSAL NUCLEUS OF VAGUS

NUCLEUS OF SOLITARY TRACT

SUBLINGUAL GLAND

SUBMANDIBULAR GLAND

FROM BACK OF TONGUE

FOOD PARTICLES PROGRESSIVELY REDUCED IN SIZE AND MIXED WITH SALIVA. TONGUE AIDS IN MIXING PROCESS

AFFERENTS "REPORT" ON CHARACTER OF FOOD AND PROGRESS OF MASTICATION, PROPRIOCEPTIVE FIBERS "REPORT" ON PRESSURE

BOLUS OF FOOD, PARTICULATED, MIXED WITH AND LUBRICATED BY SALIVA, PASSING DOWN ESOPHAGUS

VAGUS NERVE CARRIES SECRETORY AND MOTOR IMPULSES TO STOMACH

SORDES AND PARCHED LIPS

DIFFICULTY IN SWALLOWING "DRY" BOLUS

INCREASED THIRST

BOLUS ENTERING STOMACH

GASTRIC SECRETION STIMULATED

PATHOLOGICALLY DIMINISHED SALIVARY SECRETION
(AS IN FEVER, DEHYDRATION, DRUG ACTION, SJÖGREN'S SYNDROME)

GASTRIC EMPTYING FACILITATED BY SMALLER SIZE OF PARTICLES

KEY

— AFFERENTS (OTHER THAN) ↘

— PROPRIOCEPTION

— PARASYMPATHETIC EFFERENTS

— SOMATIC EFFERENTS

- - - INDEFINITE PATHS

DIGESTION OF STARCH BY SALIVARY AMYLASE (PTYALIN) CONTINUES IN STOMACH UNTIL ARRESTED BY GASTRIC ACIDITY. BOLUS TEMPORARILY PROTECTED FROM GASTRIC ACID BY PREVIOUSLY INGESTED FOOD

F. Netter M.D.

tion of gastric juice (see page 82) and prepares the stomach for a more efficient action on the material it is going to receive. The greater the reduction in particulate size, the greater is the surface of ingested food, and the more readily is it exposed to both salivary and gastric enzymes. Reduction of particle size also facilitates gastric evacuation. It has, furthermore, been suggested (Cannon) that a more effective peristalsis is engendered by a "psychic tonus" — paralleling the psychic secretion — of the stomach, which results from adequate chewing of agreeable food. The significance of these effects may be appreciated from the fact that a patient, on whom a gastrostomy has been performed for esophageal obstruction, does better nutritionally if he chews the food before introducing it into the stomach.

An important aspect of thorough mastication relates to the salivary secretion (see page 71), which it stimulates. Besides the diluting and lubricating effects of the saliva, its solvent action improves the taste and thereby further enhances the psychic secretion of the stomach. A copious flow permits more

complete digestion of starches in the stomach before the bolus is penetrated by the gastric acid, which inactivates ptyalin. With diminished salivary secretion, termed xerostomia or aptyalism, as occurs in dehydration, fever, Mikulicz's disease and Sjögren's syndrome (the two latter now thought to be rheumatic diseases of the salivary glands), all these effects are lost, and mastication is rendered extremely difficult. Certain agents, such as quinine, sympatholytics and, particularly, anticholinergic drugs, inhibit salivary secretion and may therewith produce undesirable effects on the digestion. The opposite disturbance, namely, excessive salivary secretion, called ptyalism or sialorrhea, may result from a local irritation (jagged edges of teeth, poorly fitting dentures, dissimilar metals in fillings, lesions such as canker sores or stomatitis) or as a reflex of visceral disease. When extreme, the loss of the secreted fluid may lead

to dehydration. Sialorrhea of a degree not clinically manifest has been observed in association with gastric hypersecretion in ulcer patients.

The most common disturbance of mastication probably is that resulting from the absence of teeth. Edentulous individuals attempting to eat food which requires effective chewing may swallow particles large enough to tax the triturating action of the stomach. The same holds true for ill-fitting dentures. Thus, faulty mastication should be seriously considered as a cause of indigestion in an edentulous patient. Loss of function of the buccinator and orbicularis oris muscles, as occurs in central or peripheral paralysis of the facial nerve, usually results in the pocketing of food between the teeth and the adjacent lips and cheek, and thereby interferes with mastication on the affected side. Inability to chew food thoroughly may be one of the early signs of myasthenia gravis.

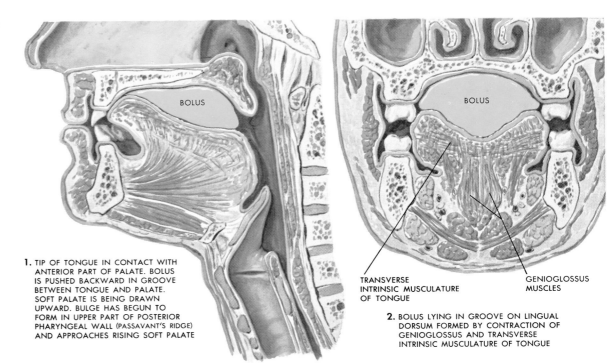

1. TIP OF TONGUE IN CONTACT WITH ANTERIOR PART OF PALATE. BOLUS IS PUSHED BACKWARD IN GROOVE BETWEEN TONGUE AND PALATE. SOFT PALATE IS BEING DRAWN UPWARD. BULGE HAS BEGUN TO FORM IN UPPER PART OF POSTERIOR PHARYNGEAL WALL (PASSAVANT'S RIDGE) AND APPROACHES RISING SOFT PALATE

2. BOLUS LYING IN GROOVE ON LINGUAL DORSUM FORMED BY CONTRACTION OF GENIOGLOSSUS AND TRANSVERSE INTRINSIC MUSCULATURE OF TONGUE

TRANSVERSE INTRINSIC MUSCULATURE OF TONGUE

GENIOGLOSSUS MUSCLES

DEGLUTITION

6. SOFT PALATE HAS BEEN PULLED DOWN AND APPROXIMATED TO ROOT OF TONGUE BY CONTRACTION OF PHARYNGOPALATINE MUSCLES (POSTERIOR PILLARS), AND BY PRESSURE OF DESCENDING "STRIPPING WAVE". OROPHARYNGEAL CAVITY CLOSED BY CONTRACTION OF UPPER PHARYNGEAL CONSTRICTORS. CRICOPHARYNGEUS MUSCLE IS RELAXING TO PERMIT ENTRY OF BOLUS INTO ESOPHAGUS. TRICKLE OF FOOD ENTERS ALSO LARYNGEAL ADITUS BUT IS PREVENTED FROM GOING FARTHER BY CLOSURE OF VENTRICULAR FOLDS

SOFT PALATE

ROOT OF TONGUE

VALLECULA

EPIGLOTTIS TURNED DOWN (SECTIONED)

THYROID CARTILAGE

ARYEPIGLOTTIC FOLD

VENTRICULAR FOLD

VENTRICLE OF LARYNX

VOCAL FOLD

CRICOID CARTILAGE

RESIDUUM OF BOLUS

7. LARYNGEAL VESTIBULE IS CLOSED BY APPROXIMATION OF ARYEPIGLOTTIC AND VENTRICULAR FOLDS, PREVENTING ENTRY OF FOOD INTO LARYNX (CORONAL SECTION: A–P VIEW)

Although deglutition is a continuous process, it is traditional to divide it into three stages: (1) oral, (2) pharyngeal and (3) esophageal. The original deductions as to the course of events during these stages have recently become susceptible to accurate observation in man as the result of the development of techniques for cineradiography and intraluminal pressure recordings. The essential physiologic requirements for deglutition consist of: (1) preparation of a bolus of suitable size and consistency; (2) prevention of dispersal of this bolus during the various phases of swallowing; (3) creation of differential pressures which will propel the bolus in a forward direction; (4) prevention of the entrance of food or fluid into the nasopharynx and larynx; (5) rapid passage of a bolus through the pharynx in order to shorten the time during which respiration is suspended; (6) prevention of gastric reflux into the esophagus during the period of free communication between both organs; (7) provision for wiping of residual material from (final clearance of) the tract.

During the oral phase, which follows mastication (see pages 72 and 73), the bolus is gathered in a groove on the dorsum of the free portion of the tongue and thrown backward by the tongue, while the soft palate, fauces and posterior wall of the oropharynx are approximated to close the opening into the nasopharynx. Contraction of the soft palate and a posterior movement of the tongue displace the bolus into the oropharynx, where a stripping peristaltic wave is created which progressively propels the bolus distally. Though most easily observed on the posterior aspect of

the oropharynx, the peristaltic wave is actually of concentric nature. With the entrance of material into the oropharynx, the hyoid bone and the larynx are abruptly elevated. The upward movement, combined with a forward motion and a tilting posteriorly of the larynx, creates a pulling force and increases the anteroposterior diameter of the laryngopharynx, producing a zone of relatively negative pressure which abruptly "sucks" the bolus into the laryngopharynx. Air leaving the respiratory tract at this time would oppose this sucking effect, but contraction of the intrinsic laryngeal muscles, shortening and widening the aryepiglottic folds and true and false bands, produces an airtight, soft stopper for the subglottic region, thus closing the air conduit. It is likely that the laryngeal ventricles are also obliterated during this

phase. An approximation of the thyroid cartilage to the hyoid bone, displacing the intervening pre-epiglottic fat pad backward, results in a downward and backward move of the epiglottis. The depression of the epiglottis, however, does not completely close the laryngeal aditus, and small particles of the bolus may insert themselves a short distance into the opening. It is characteristic for a liquid bolus to be split by the epiglottis and to travel on each side of the larynx through the piriform recesses, to rejoin each other behind the cricoid cartilage.

The distal travel of the stripping wave, which rapidly follows the bolus, is not delayed at the level of the cricopharyngeal muscle, because this region relaxes prior to the entrance of the bolus into the hypophar-

(Continued on page 75)

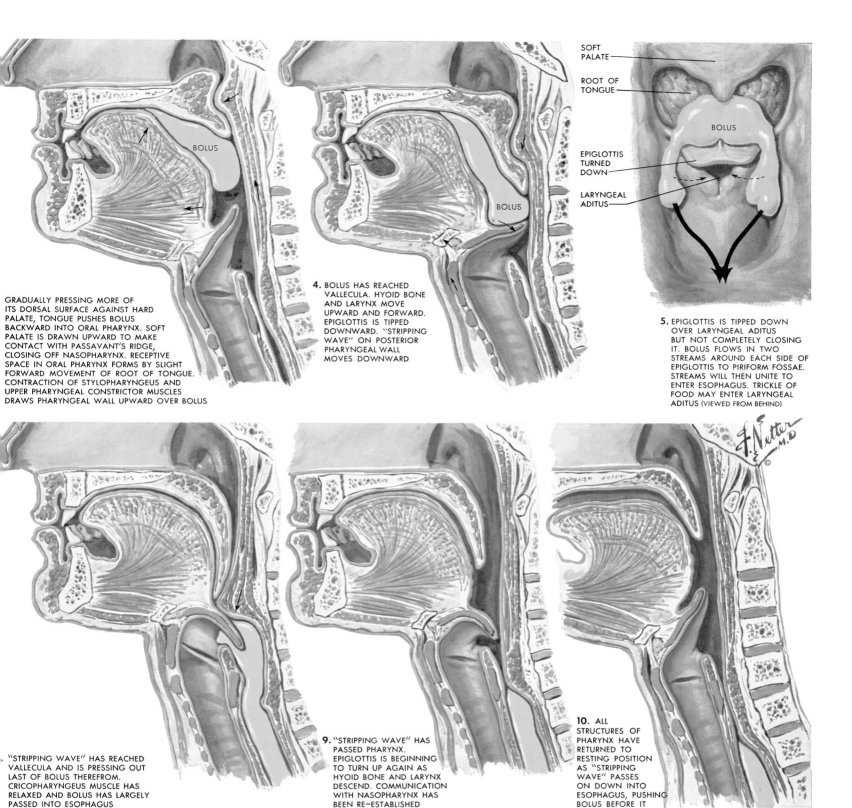

GRADUALLY PRESSING MORE OF ITS DORSAL SURFACE AGAINST HARD PALATE, TONGUE PUSHES BOLUS BACKWARD INTO ORAL PHARYNX. SOFT PALATE IS DRAWN UPWARD TO MAKE CONTACT WITH PASSAVANT'S RIDGE, CLOSING OFF NASOPHARYNX. RECEPTIVE SPACE IN ORAL PHARYNX FORMS BY SLIGHT FORWARD MOVEMENT OF ROOT OF TONGUE. CONTRACTION OF STYLOPHARYNGEUS AND UPPER PHARYNGEAL CONSTRICTOR MUSCLES DRAWS PHARYNGEAL WALL UPWARD OVER BOLUS

4. BOLUS HAS REACHED VALLECULA. HYOID BONE AND LARYNX MOVE UPWARD AND FORWARD. EPIGLOTTIS IS TIPPED DOWNWARD. "STRIPPING WAVE" ON POSTERIOR PHARYNGEAL WALL MOVES DOWNWARD

SOFT PALATE

ROOT OF TONGUE

BOLUS

EPIGLOTTIS TURNED DOWN

LARYNGEAL ADITUS

5. EPIGLOTTIS IS TIPPED DOWN OVER LARYNGEAL ADITUS BUT NOT COMPLETELY CLOSING IT. BOLUS FLOWS IN TWO STREAMS AROUND EACH SIDE OF EPIGLOTTIS TO PIRIFORM FOSSAE. STREAMS WILL THEN UNITE TO ENTER ESOPHAGUS. TRICKLE OF FOOD MAY ENTER LARYNGEAL ADITUS (VIEWED FROM BEHIND)

"STRIPPING WAVE" HAS REACHED VALLECULA AND IS PRESSING OUT LAST OF BOLUS THEREFROM. CRICOPHARYNGEUS MUSCLE HAS RELAXED AND BOLUS HAS LARGELY PASSED INTO ESOPHAGUS

9. "STRIPPING WAVE" HAS PASSED PHARYNX. EPIGLOTTIS IS BEGINNING TO TURN UP AGAIN AS HYOID BONE AND LARYNX DESCEND. COMMUNICATION WITH NASOPHARYNX HAS BEEN RE-ESTABLISHED

10. ALL STRUCTURES OF PHARYNX HAVE RETURNED TO RESTING POSITION AS "STRIPPING WAVE" PASSES ON DOWN INTO ESOPHAGUS, PUSHING BOLUS BEFORE IT

(*Continued from page 74*)

ynx. Relaxation and contraction of the crico-pharyngeus and the intrinsic laryngeal muscula-ture are so co-ordinated that air is directed into the respiratory passages during breathing and fluid into the esophagus during deglutition. Once the peristaltic wave has traversed the crico-pharyngeus, marking the end of the pharyn-geal phase of swallowing, this muscle remains contracted, closing the esophagus superiorly; the hyoid bone, larynx and epiglottis return to their original positions, and air re-enters the air channels.

The peristaltic wave starting in the orophar-ynx continues without interruption into the body of the esophagus at the rate of 2 to 3 cm. per sec-

ond. It is now generally agreed that the terminal portion of the esophagus, from 1 or 2 cm. above the diaphragm to its junction with the stomach, referred to as the gastro-esophageal vestibule or "high-pressure zone", plays a significant rôle in the swallowing mechanism. In the resting state, the pressure within this region is higher than in the remainder or body of the esophagus. With the onset of swallowing, the vestibule appears to relax, by reflex mechanisms, to a limited degree, but it does not relax completely until the pres-sure immediately proximal to it is great enough not only to allow thorough evacuation of the ves-tibule, when it opens, but also to inhibit reflux of the stomach's content into the esophagus. The function of the vestibule, thus, is that of a physi-

ologic valve. The portion of the esophagus imme-diately proximal to the vestibule, termed the ampulla,* serves as a collecting area, within which the pressure is built up by the efforts of the peristaltic wave to progress distally, and in which the bolus is temporarily delayed.

The stripping peristaltic wave in the body of the esophagus, which creates a transient peak or climactic pressure wave immediately behind the bolus, stops in front of the vestibule. After

---

*This functional "ampulla of the esophagus", recognized on intraluminal pressure studies, appears to correspond with the anatomical description (Lerche) but cannot be said to be identical with current roentgen usage of the term "phrenic ampulla".

(*Continued on page 76*)

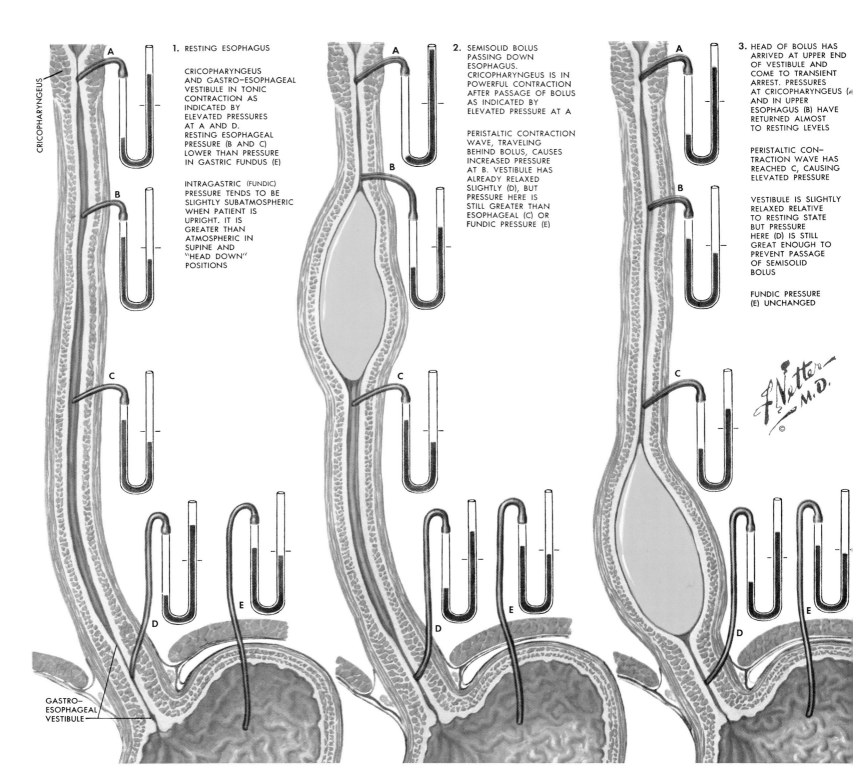

CRICOPHARYNGEUS

1. RESTING ESOPHAGUS

CRICOPHARYNGEUS AND GASTRO-ESOPHAGEAL VESTIBULE IN TONIC CONTRACTION AS INDICATED BY ELEVATED PRESSURES AT A AND D. RESTING ESOPHAGEAL PRESSURE (B AND C) LOWER THAN PRESSURE IN GASTRIC FUNDUS (E)

INTRAGASTRIC (FUNDIC) PRESSURE TENDS TO BE SLIGHTLY SUBATMOSPHERIC WHEN PATIENT IS UPRIGHT. IT IS GREATER THAN ATMOSPHERIC IN SUPINE AND "HEAD DOWN" POSITIONS

2. SEMISOLID BOLUS PASSING DOWN ESOPHAGUS. CRICOPHARYNGEUS IS IN POWERFUL CONTRACTION AFTER PASSAGE OF BOLUS AS INDICATED BY ELEVATED PRESSURE AT A

PERISTALTIC CONTRACTION WAVE, TRAVELING BEHIND BOLUS, CAUSES INCREASED PRESSURE AT B. VESTIBULE HAS ALREADY RELAXED SLIGHTLY (D), BUT PRESSURE HERE IS STILL GREATER THAN ESOPHAGEAL (C) OR FUNDIC PRESSURE (E)

3. HEAD OF BOLUS HAS ARRIVED AT UPPER END OF VESTIBULE AND HAS COME TO TRANSIENT ARREST. PRESSURES AT CRICOPHARYNGEUS (A) AND IN UPPER ESOPHAGUS (B) HAVE RETURNED ALMOST TO RESTING LEVELS

PERISTALTIC CONTRACTION WAVE HAS REACHED C, CAUSING ELEVATED PRESSURE

VESTIBULE IS SLIGHTLY RELAXED RELATIVE TO RESTING STATE BUT PRESSURE HERE (D) IS STILL GREAT ENOUGH TO PREVENT PASSAGE OF SEMISOLID BOLUS

FUNDIC PRESSURE (E) UNCHANGED

GASTRO-ESOPHAGEAL VESTIBULE

(Continued from page 75)

the bolus has entered the stomach, the pressure in the vestibular region increases for a considerable period of time before returning to the resting level.

Complete prevention of dispersal of the bolus frequently fails, and small amounts of material may remain in the esophagus, particularly if the bolus is thick in consistency or if swallowing is performed in the recumbent position. As a result of the persistent distention, or simultaneously with the swallowing of a small amount of saliva, a "secondary" peristaltic wave originates at about the level of the arch of the aorta and strips residual material distally in a fashion similar to the primary peristaltic wave. In both instances a small amount of material, usually mixed with air, may remain just above the hiatus in a small saclike collection, which, after a short interval,

empties into the stomach by a concentric type of contraction.

Retrograde peristalsis has not been observed in the esophagus. "Tertiary" waves are often seen, particularly in elderly individuals and in patients with hiatal hernias. They consist of nonperistaltic, repeated, ringlike contractions at multiple levels in the distal half of the esophagus, usually during stages of incomplete distention. If "tertiary" waves are marked or occur prematurely, functional disturbances, described as "diffuse spasm of the esophagus", may result.

In the description given above, sphincteric activity has been attributed to the entire vestibular area, which measures about 3 cm. in length, rather than to isolated muscle bands at either its proximal or its distal margins. Such specialized bands have been described by some authors as "the inferior esophageal sphincter" at the prox-

imal margin of the vestibule and the "cardiac sphincter" at its distal margin, the esophagogastric junction. From a physiologic point of view, however, isolated sphincteric activity at these sites seems to be of little significance under normal circumstances.

The activity of the vestibule during deglutition suggests that reflux of gastric contents into the esophagus is prevented by contraction of this area. To some extent this is true, since it can be demonstrated in some patients with sliding hiatal hernias that, in the Trendelenburg position, a barium-fluid mixture will fill the hernial sac but will not enter the esophagus. If, however, intraabdominal pressure is increased further, barium can be made to flow freely into the esophagus. The maximum "barrier" pressure which the vestibule can create is about 20 cm. of water.

(Continued on page 77)

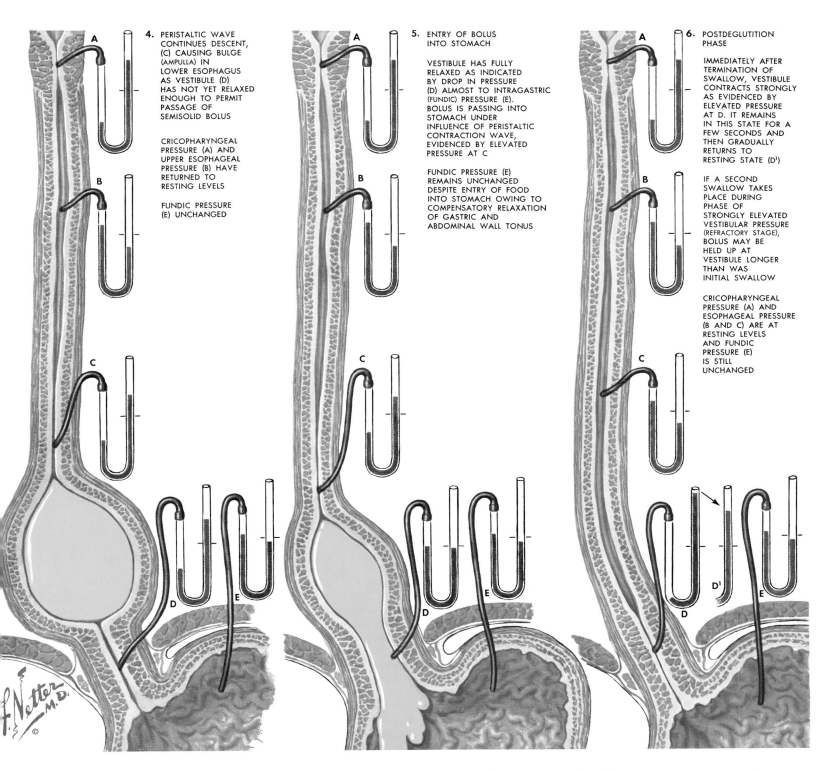

(Continued from page 76)

Under normal circumstances, *i.e.*, with the esophagogastric junction below the hiatus, intra-abdominal pressure must be increased to about 20 cm. of water before gastric contents can be forced into the esophagus. Thus, an additional mechanism operating normally must be assumed, which is more important than vestibular contraction. The nature of this mechanism is not entirely clear, but it appears to be valvular and related to the acute-angled entry of the esophagus into the side of the stomach at a considerable distance below the fundus of the stomach. While this acute-angled entry is partly attributable to the configuration of the intrinsic muscle bundles at the "cardiac incisura", it is likely that the maintenance of this relationship is dependent on the presence of a normal hiatus. The "hiatus" is, in reality, a short, funnel-shaped channel (see page 39) with its thick left margin occupying the cardiac incisura. Valvular action, as a result of redundant mucosa at the cardia, has been observed in animals and may possibly play a rôle in man.

Additional evidence that the diaphragm plays a rôle in the closing mechanism is provided by the fact that swallowing is impossible in deep inspiration. If one observes fluoroscopically the region of the hiatus while an individual continuously swallows a fluid-barium mixture, the barium column is seen to be cut off at the level of the hiatus during deep inspiration. This has been referred to as the "pinchcock" action of the diaphragm. During this interval the peristaltic wave in the body of the esophagus continues to travel distally. As a result, barium trapped in the esophagus collects above the hiatus in a pear-shaped configuration to which the term "phrenic ampulla" has been applied. The nature of this

"pinchcock" action remains a matter of controversy. It is possible that, in deep inspiration, the crura of the diaphragm constrict the hiatus to a size so small as to close completely the lumen of the esophagus. Attempts to demonstrate this during the course of operative exposure have not been successful. Another possible explanation is that, simultaneously with inspiration, a reflex contraction of the vestibule occurs. "Pinchcock" action is, however, also observed at the hiatus in patients with sliding types of hiatal hernia in whom the vestibule is located well above the diaphragm, and, moreover, pressure studies do not demonstrate reflex contraction of the vestibule with inspiration. It would seem, therefore, that the mechanism, which must be postulated at the level of the hiatus to explain prevention of reflux, also plays a rôle in "pinchcock" action.

NEUROREGULATION
OF DEGLUTITION

V TO TENSOR VELI PALATINI MUSCLE

X (XI) TO LEVATOR VELI PALATINI MUSCLE

PHARYNGEAL PLEXUS

V FROM SOFT PALATE

V FROM TONGUE (LINGUAL NERVE)

V TO MYLOHYOID & ANT. BELLY OF DIGASTRIC

IX FROM SOFT PALATE, FAUCES, PHARYNX

IX TO STYLOPHARYNGEUS

X {FROM PHARYNX, LARYNX, UPPER ESOPHAGUS
{FROM LOWER ESOPHAGUS & G.I. TRACT

X {TO MUSCLES OF PHARYNX, LARYNX, UPPER ESOPHA·
{TO MUSCLE OF LOWER ESOPHAGUS & G.I. TRACT

XII TO MUSCLES OF TONGUE & GENIOHYOID

ANSA HYPOGLOSSI TO INFRAHYOID MUSCLES
SYMPATHETIC EFFERENTS

AFFERENTS

SYMPATHETIC EFFERENTS

AFFERENTS

(MYLOHYOID NERVE)

RECURRENT LARYNGEAL NERVE

SYMPATHETIC EFFERENTS
THORACIC GREATER SPLANCHNIC NERVE

AFFERENTS

SOFT PALATE (SLIGHT)

PHARYNGEAL WALL

ANTERIOR PILLAR

TONSIL

POSTERIOR PILLAR

POSTERIOR PART OF TONGUE

AREAS FROM WHICH DEGLUTITION
REFLEX MAY BE EXCITED (STIPPLED)

CELIAC GANGLION

A cortical area which, on electrical stimulation, evokes swallowing movements has been located in the inferior portion of the *precentral gyrus* just as it turns under into the insula. Efferent connections are presumably made via the hypothalamus with the medulla, where a deglutition center has been identified in close relationship with the ala cinerea and the *nuclei of the X nerve*. The medullary deglutition center co-ordinates the activities of the structures concerned in the act of swallowing.

Sensory impulses reaching this center via afferent fibers from the mucosa of the *mouth (soft palate, tongue), fauces, pharynx and esophagus* initiate the reflex regulation of the muscle groups controlling respiration, the position of the larynx and the movement of the bolus into and down the esophagus (see pages 74-77).

The voluntary component of the deglutitory act terminates when the bolus comes into contact with certain sensitive areas, principally the faucial surfaces and the posterior pharyngeal wall. From this point, swallowing becomes an involuntary process. *Afferents* from the sensitive zone pass *via the V, IX and X nerves* to their respective nuclei, whence association fibers make connections with the adjacent deglutition center. Under the co-ordination of this center, impulses pass

outward in flawlessly timed sequence via the V, X and XII nerves to the levator muscles of the soft palate, via the X nerve to the constrictor muscles of the pharynx, via the cervical and thoracic spinal nerves to the diaphragm and intercostal muscles, via the V and XII nerves to the extrinsic muscles of the larynx, and via the X nerve to the intrinsic muscles of the larynx and the musculature of the esophagus. The bolus is carried down the esophagus by a sequential series of discharges over the vagus nerves. It has been demonstrated in experimental animals that in addition to the recurrent laryngeal nerve, the cervical esophagus receives an additional efferent supply from either a pharyngo-esophageal nerve arising just proximal to the nodose ganglion or from an esophageal

branch of the external laryngeal branch of the superior laryngeal. A number of clinical observations suggest that a double innervation exists also in human beings, but it has not been demonstrated by physiologic methods. On teleologic grounds a margin of safety for the cervical esophagus in the form of an extra nerve supply is understandable, since deglutition is impossible if the cervical esophagus, in contrast to the thoracic portion, is deprived of its extrinsic nervous control.

The musculature at successive levels of the esophagus contracts in response to the impulses coming down from the medullary center, and, by a sequential series of such discharges, the bolus is moved smoothly along the esophagus. Contraction of the more proxi-

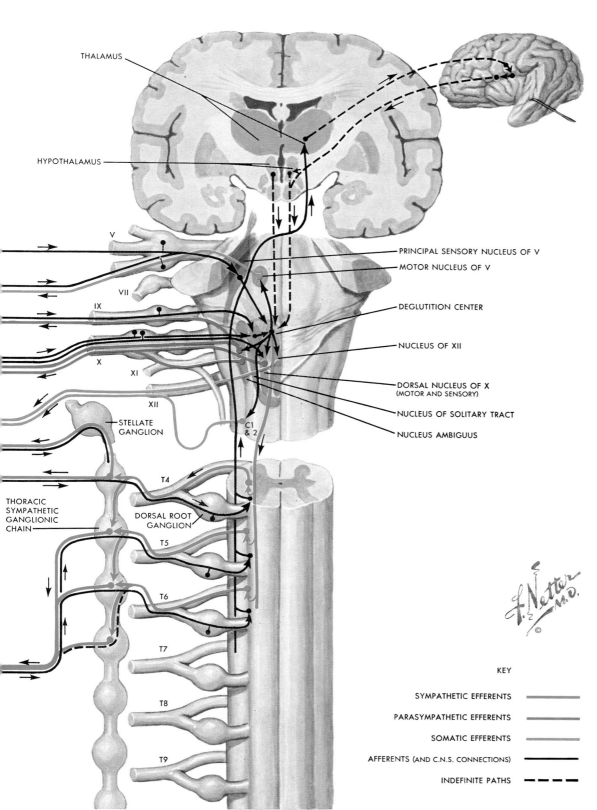

THALAMUS

HYPOTHALAMUS

V

VII

IX

X

XI

XII

STELLATE GANGLION

THORACIC SYMPATHETIC GANGLIONIC CHAIN

DORSAL ROOT GANGLION

T4

T5

T6

T7

T8

T9

PRINCIPAL SENSORY NUCLEUS OF V

MOTOR NUCLEUS OF V

DEGLUTITION CENTER

NUCLEUS OF XII

DORSAL NUCLEUS OF X (MOTOR AND SENSORY)

NUCLEUS OF SOLITARY TRACT

NUCLEUS AMBIGUUS

C1 & 2

KEY

SYMPATHETIC EFFERENTS	
PARASYMPATHETIC EFFERENTS	
SOMATIC EFFERENTS	
AFFERENTS (AND C.N.S. CONNECTIONS)	
INDEFINITE PATHS	— — —

mal segments of the esophagus inhibit the more distal segments (Hwang), but the nervous mechanism of this inhibitory effect has not been elucidated. The peristaltic waves continue over the esophagus if the reflexes are initiated by stimulation of the pharynx, even when the esophagus has been severed somewhere at its upper two thirds, provided the vagal innervation of the tube has remained intact. If, however, the vagus nerve has been cut or if its esophageal branches or plexus have been separated from the trunk, no peristalsis can be elicited. A series of discharges along the esophageal tube may be set in motion by afferent impulses reaching the deglutition center from moderate distention of the cervical esophagus; thus, a peristaltic wave initiated within the

upper esophagus will sweep down the entire tube as effectively as that originating from a conventional pharyngeal swallowing movement. Increased distention of the cervical esophagus, simulating the pressure of a bolus lodged there, causes reflex swallowing. In the more distal portion (lower third) the progression of a bolus does not require the participation of the extrinsic or vagal reflex arc, since the musculature may function effectively under the control of the intrinsic nervous apparatus (see page 46). Thus, if the extrinsic innervation of the esophagus is interrupted, the bolus does not move normally through the esophagus until it reaches the level of the local nerve networks; on the other hand, if the intrinsic innervation does not function in an orderly fashion

as, for example, is presumed to occur in certain types of cardiospasm (see pages 98 and 145), a swallowing wave passes normally along the portion with preserved extrinsic nerve supply, then becomes inco-ordinated in the diseased distal part.

Stimuli arising from esophageal distention, chemical irritation, spasm or temperature variations are conveyed by visceral afferent nerves passing in the upper five or six thoracic sympathetic roots to the thalamus, thence presumably to reach consciousness in the inferior portion of the postcentral gyrus, where they are interpreted as sensations of pressure, burning, "gas", dull aching or pain in the tissues innervated by the somatic nerves from the corresponding spinal levels. Thus, pain from esophageal disease may be referred to the middle or either side of the chest, to the sides of the neck, to the jaws, the teeth or the ears. The similarity to referred pain of cardiac origin often poses a problem in the differential diagnosis of cardiac and esophageal disease. Distention, hypertonus or obstruction of the distal esophagus may give rise to a reflex contraction of the superior esophageal sphincter, with a resulting sensation of a "lump" at the level of the suprasternal notch and difficulty in swallowing.

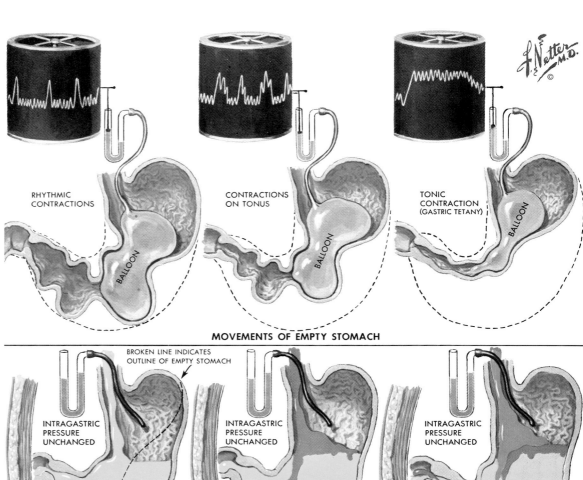

RHYTHMIC CONTRACTIONS

CONTRACTIONS ON TONUS

TONIC CONTRACTION (GASTRIC TETANY)

MOVEMENTS OF EMPTY STOMACH

MOTILITY OF STOMACH, EMPTY STOMACH, FILLING OF STOMACH, EMPTYING OF STOMACH AND DUODENAL MOTOR ACTIVITY

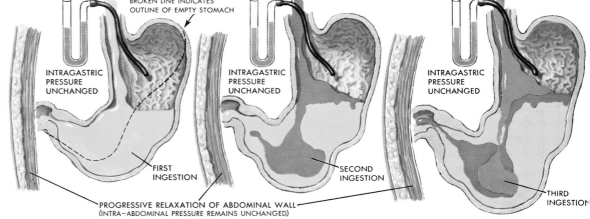

BROKEN LINE INDICATES OUTLINE OF EMPTY STOMACH

INTRAGASTRIC PRESSURE UNCHANGED

INTRAGASTRIC PRESSURE UNCHANGED

INTRAGASTRIC PRESSURE UNCHANGED

FIRST INGESTION

SECOND INGESTION

THIRD INGESTION

PROGRESSIVE RELAXATION OF ABDOMINAL WALL (INTRA-ABDOMINAL PRESSURE REMAINS UNCHANGED)

GASTRIC FILLING

The internal pressure of the empty stomach, as recorded by appropriate techniques (*e.g.,* balloon introduced into stomach, connected with manometer recording on a kymograph), changes periodically and with sufficient consistency to suggest distinct types of contractions. The interdigestive or "hunger" periods frequently begin with mild, rhythmic pressure waves occurring at a rate of three per minute, a pattern designated as *tonus rhythm* (Carlson), indicating that it represents regular changes in the tonus or state of gastromuscular tension. After a variable period of time, higher pressure elevations are recorded, which appear as spikes of about 30 seconds' duration occurring at progressively closer intervals. These waves, termed Type I contractions, are assumed to represent *peristaltic contractions* originating at or proximal to the incisure and passing down to the pylorus. As the activity of the empty stomach becomes more vigorous, the contraction waves succeed each other at such a rate that new pressure waves are superimposed upon previous ones (Type II contractions). In occasional individuals, especially after periods of prolonged fasting, the gastric motility increases and exhibits a Type III contraction, also termed *"gastric tetanus"*, which is characterized by rapid passage of peristaltic waves along a stomach in a state of sustained tonus.

The cause of this motor activity of the empty stomach is not known, but, since it is present (though less vigorous) in the denervated stomach, it is assumed that the intrinsic nerves could serve as an autonomous pacemaker. The possibility

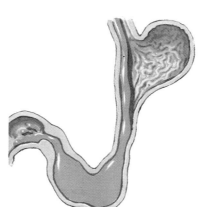

FLUID ENTERING EMPTY STOMACH

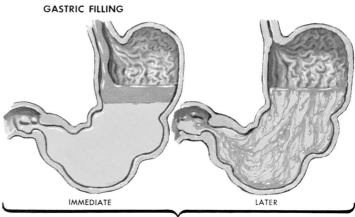

IMMEDIATE

LATER

FLUID ENTERING DIGESTING STOMACH

of a humoral factor must be considered, because an autotransplanted fundic pouch contracts almost synchronously with the main stomach in experimental animals.

The "hunger" contractions of the empty stomach terminate when food is ingested. The cardiac and fundic regions relax in advance of the first swallowed bolus, and more so with successive increments of food entering the stomach. This relaxation of the gastric musculature (see page 53), manifesting its ability to elongate without change in tension, enables the stomach to enlarge to a volume adequate for a full meal, *i.e.,* to serve as a reservoir. Together with the slackening of the abdominal muscles, which occurs as the stomach fills, this "receptive relaxation" accounts also in great measure for the *constancy of the intragastric pressure* while a meal is being eaten. Food entering the stomach passes down to the most

dependent part. Successive portions of ingesta occupy the more central part of the mass, so that a sort of crude layering of the gastric content ensues. *Fluids* taken *when food is in the stomach* temporarily float on top but soon gravitate down to the distal portion, whence they are promptly evacuated.

Peristalsis commences usually within a matter of minutes after food reaches the stomach, at first in the pyloric portion, which, owing to the greater thickness of its musculature, has the strongest triturating power. The contractions, as seen fluoroscopically in the presence of an opaque medium, originate as *shallow indentations in the region of the incisura angularis* and deepen as they move toward the pylorus. After 5 to 10 minutes the contractions start at higher levels on the stomach and become progressively more vigorous. The pylorus, during this phase, opens only

(*Continued on page 81*)

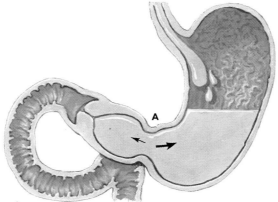

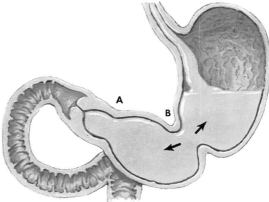

1. STOMACH IS FILLING. A MILD PERISTALTIC WAVE (A) HAS STARTED IN ANTRUM AND IS PASSING TOWARD PYLORUS. GASTRIC CONTENTS ARE CHURNED AND LARGELY PUSHED BACK INTO BODY OF STOMACH

2. WAVE (A) FADING OUT AS PYLORUS FAILS TO OPEN. A STRONGER WAVE (B) IS ORIGINATING AT INCISURE AND IS AGAIN SQUEEZING GASTRIC CONTENTS IN BOTH DIRECTIONS

MOTILITY OF STOMACH, EMPTY STOMACH, FILLING OF STOMACH, EMPTYING OF STOMACH AND DUODENAL MOTOR ACTIVITY

(Continued from page 80)

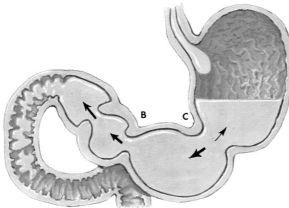

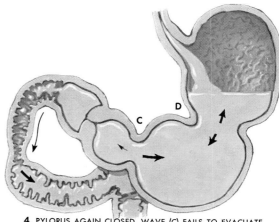

3. PYLORUS OPENS AS WAVE (B) APPROACHES IT. DUODENAL BULB IS FILLED AND SOME CONTENTS PASS INTO SECOND PORTION OF DUODENUM. WAVE (C) STARTING JUST ABOVE INCISURE

4. PYLORUS AGAIN CLOSED. WAVE (C) FAILS TO EVACUATE CONTENTS. WAVE (D) STARTING HIGHER ON BODY OF STOMACH. DUODENAL BULB MAY CONTRACT OR MAY REMAIN FILLED, AS PERISTALTIC WAVE ORIGINATING JUST BEYOND IT EMPTIES SECOND PORTION

incompletely and intermittently as the waves advance toward it. Most of the material reaching the pyloric portion is forced back into the fundus, this process continuing until part of the content has been reduced to a fluid or semifluid consistency suitable for the small intestine. The evacuation is regulated, once the gastric content has the correct consistency, by the influence of the chyme in the upper intestine, where any adverse mechanical (too rapid distention) or physicochemical (osmotic, pH) impact gives rise to intrinsic or extrinsic nervous reflexes, which modify the tone of the pyloric sphincter as well as the motor activity of the pyloric region. "The tonus of the pyloric sphincter in gastric emptying is chiefly determined by stimuli affecting the stomach muscle as a whole. Hence, its tonus changes are in the same direction and not opposed to the tone changes of the remainder of the pars pylorica. It serves as a constant resistance to the passage of chyme and blocks the exit of solid particles. By maintaining a narrow orifice it 'filters' the gastric contents. By contracting when the duodenum contracts, it limits regurgitation" (Thomas).

Ordinarily, gastric emptying proceeds smoothly while well-masticated food, free of gross irritants, is exposed to the digestive effect of the gastric secretion (see page 84). Mechanical interference is minimized by the consistency to which the gastric chyme is reduced by the triturating effect of the gastric movements and the solubilizing effect of the secretory products.

"Receptive relaxation" of the first part of the duodenum permits the gastric

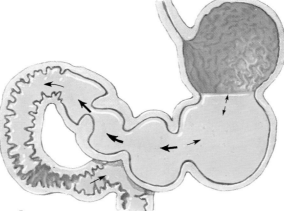

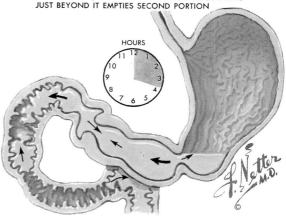

5. PERISTALTIC WAVES ARE NOW ORIGINATING HIGHER ON BODY OF STOMACH. GASTRIC CONTENTS ARE EVACUATED INTERMITTENTLY. CONTENTS OF DUODENAL BULB AREA PUSHED PASSIVELY INTO SECOND PORTION AS MORE GASTRIC CONTENTS EMERGE

6. 3 TO 4 HOURS LATER STOMACH ALMOST EMPTY. SMALL PERISTALTIC WAVE EMPTYING DUODENAL BULB WITH SOME REFLUX INTO STOMACH. REVERSE AND ANTEGRADE PERISTALSIS PRESENT IN DUODENUM

content to be admitted without excessive distention. Physicochemical irritation by the gastric acidity is counteracted by the diluting and neutralizing actions of the secretion of Brunner's glands and of the bile and pancreatic juice. The relaxation of the bulb persists during a series of gastric contractions, allowing the material to be pushed through it and into the second duodenal portion (see page 50), where peristaltic waves develop. *Antral and duodenal contractions* seem to be fairly well synchronized (Wheelon and Thomas), apparently by intrinsic nervous reflexes, so that a continuous flow of chyme results. Though intrinsic mechanisms come into play by chemical stimuli or by distention of the duodenal wall, no "substantial experimental evidence" is available "to support the concept of regulation of the gastric emptying by a sphincteric action of the pylorus" (Thomas). The older theory that a certain acid concentration in the

intestine would regulate the activity of the pyloric sphincter, plausible as it seemed, had to be abandoned in the light of numerous newer experimental observations, which point to the fact that gastric emptying rests upon the stimuli that increase and decrease the tone and peristalsis of the stomach and that the rôle of the sphincter is to control the volume of evacuated chyme and to prevent regurgitation of the duodenal content.

At the height of gastric propulsive activity, two peristaltic waves — occasionally three or four — may follow one another at intervals of from 5 to 15 seconds. This activity may continue without interruption or may be interspersed with periods of relative rest until the stomach is empty. Even before the gastric content has been completely evacuated, the motility characteristic of the "hunger period" (see above) may begin to develop.

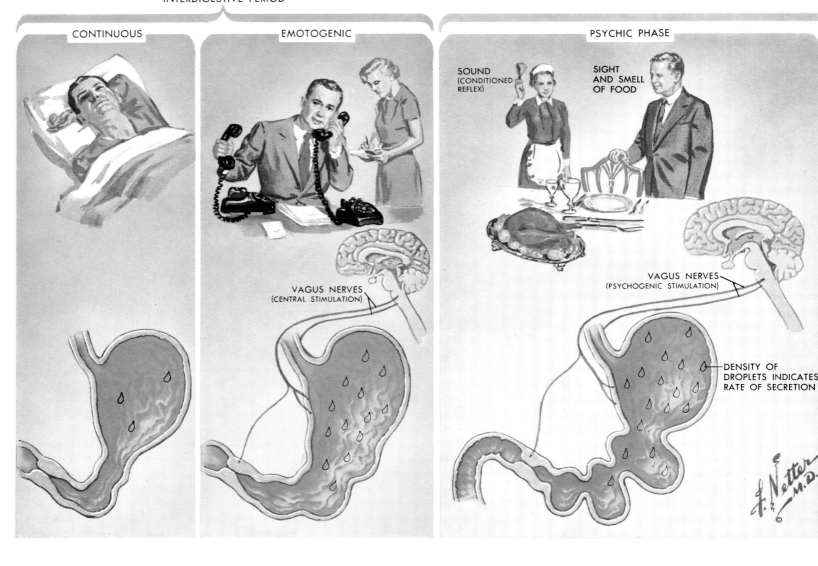

CONTINUOUS

EMOTOGENIC

PSYCHIC PHASE

SOUND (CONDITIONED REFLEX)

SIGHT AND SMELL OF FOOD

VAGUS NERVES (CENTRAL STIMULATION)

VAGUS NERVES (PSYCHOGENIC STIMULATION)

DENSITY OF DROPLETS INDICATES RATE OF SECRETION

SECTION IV—PLATE II

MECHANISMS OF GASTRIC SECRETION

Just as the empty or fasting stomach manifests periods of motility, so does it secrete intermittently. The secretion of gastric juice, when food is absent from the stomach and intestine and in the absence of any sight or thought of food, is referred to as the *"interdigestive period"* of secretion. Included in this category are the *"continuous"* secretion — somewhat of a misnomer, since the secretion is actually intermittent — and the *"emotogenic"* secretion.

The continuous secretion is that which occurs in the absence of all known stimuli; it has been observed in variable amounts throughout a 40-day fast, and it is present after vagotomy. The mechanism of this secretion is unknown. It has been variously attributed to alterations in blood flow to the gastric glands, to digestion of cellular detritus, to the intermittent release of small amounts of gastric secretory hormone and to the mechanical expression of the glands by the con-

tractions which occur during fasting periods.

The *emotogenic secretion* is that which has been reported to occur in emotional states such as anger, resentment and hostility. Most theories of the psychodynamics of this secretion explain it as being associated in the unconscious mind with the concept of food; if this should prove to be correct, the emotogenic secretion would not properly be classified in the interdigestive period.

A neurohormonal pathway for gastric secretion in the interdigestive period has been postulated (Gray *et al.*), involving the hypothalamus, the pituitary and the adrenal cortex. Reports of experimental verification of this mechanism have not been confirmed.

The *"digestive period"* of secretion is that secretion which is related to food. It consists of three phases. The first, or cephalic, phase includes the secretory response to all stimuli acting in the region of the head. These may be

unconditioned (unlearned) reflexes, such as the secretion to sham feeding in a decorticate animal, or conditioned (learned) reflexes, as exemplified by the secretory effect of the thought, odor, sight or taste of food. The conditioned, or "psychic", secretion (Pavlov) is the principal component of the cephalic phase; the copious flow of gastric juice which occurs when appetizing food is masticated amounts to almost half the volume output of the gastric glands during the digestive period and is rich in all components of the gastric secretion; its presence contributes to both the effective initiation and the subsequent efficiency of gastric digestion. The cephalic phase is abolished by section of the vagi; thus, it is entirely neurogenic.

The second, or *gastric, phase* is so named because the stimuli concerned act in the stomach. The effective stimuli are of two types — mechanical and chemical. The only adequate

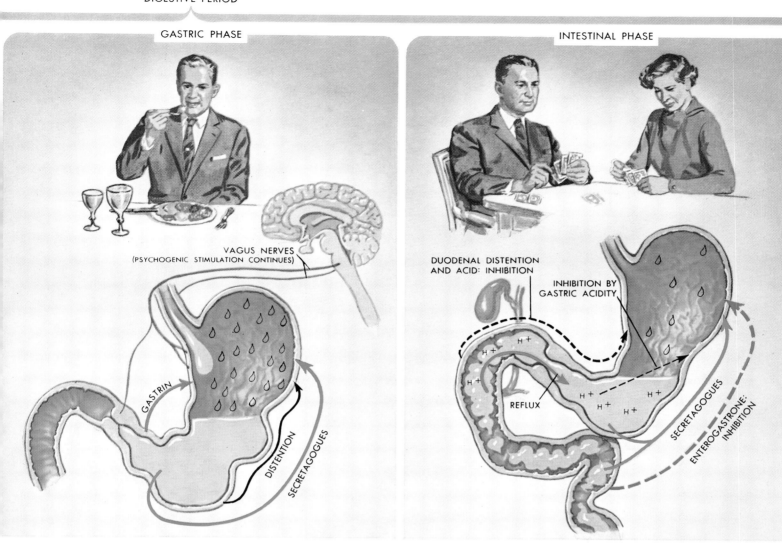

mechanical stimulus is distention; this is demonstrated in the experimental situation by the inflation of a balloon in the stomach and is provided in the normal digestive process by the distending effect of the meal. Thus, the mere presence of an ordinary stomach tube or other foreign object does not excite the gastric glands. It has been shown (Hunt and Macdonald) that up to a certain point the intensity of the mechanical stimulation is proportional to the size of the meal. Chemical stimulation of secretion is ascribed to substances called *secretagogues* which are naturally present in certain foods or are released therefrom in the process of digestion. Both the mechanical and chemical stimuli evoke gastric secretion principally by contact with the mucosa of the pyloric portion to release a hormone, *gastrin,* which acts on the secretory elements of the fundus. The chemical identity of the secretagogues and of the secretory hormone from the

pyloric mucosa has not been established. The possibility that the release of histamine or a histaminelike substance is involved in the chemical phase is not entirely excluded.

The high gastric secretagogue potency of such foods as meat, particularly liver and fish, and of their extractives, *e.g.,* bouillon, is the basis for their exclusion from the diet in the acute phase of peptic ulcer.

An appreciable secretion of gastric juice occurs as a result of stimulation originating in the small intestine; this constitutes the third, or *intestinal, phase* of the digestive period. The only effective agency in this phase is the action of secretagogues; the precise mechanism of this effect is not known, but it is apparently a humoral one.

By the time a significant amount of the gastric content has been delivered into the intestine, regulatory mechanisms are already in operation to terminate the digestive period of gastric secre-

tion. The filling of the stomach and the beginning of absorption of the products of intestinal digestion bring on satiety and, with it, the cessation of eating and the withdrawal of the stimuli for psychic secretion. The attainment within the stomach of an acidity of pH 1.5 or less acts upon the antral mucosa to inhibit the release of gastrin or, conceivably, to cause the production of a secreto-inhibitory hormone from the antrum; together with the progression of gastric emptying, this results in the withdrawal of the hormonal, humoral and mechanical stimuli of the gastric phase. These effects are abetted by the active inhibitory influences of the chyme in the upper intestine, including hormonal (release of gastric inhibitory agent, enterogastrone), mechanical (distention), chemical (acidity) and physical (osmolarity); mechanical and physiochemical factors exert their inhibitory action by vagal (perhaps also by intrinsic) nervous reflexes.

DIGESTIVE ACTIVITY OF STOMACH

Almost all of the available evidence points to the parietal cell (see page 52) as the source of the *HCl of the gastric secretion.* The exact site within (or adjacent to) the cell where the acid is liberated has not been agreed upon. Nor have the physicochemical processes involved been elucidated.

The concentration of the acid, as it leaves the parietal cell, is in the neighborhood of 0.160 N; more common expressions for the same value are 160 mEq./l., or 160 clinical units or degrees of acidity. This theoretical maximal concentration of HCl is never actually attained, because the observed acidity at any given time depends upon the relative proportions of parietal and nonparietal secretions. In general, the more rapid the rate of secretion, the higher the acidity.

Aside from the normal physiologic mechanisms (see pages 82 and 83), a number of systemic and local factors affect the secretion of acid. The stimulating effect of the oral administration of sodium bicarbonate, popularly called "acid rebound", is probably the result of a combination of factors, including a direct stimulating action on the gastric mucosa, annulment of the antral acid-inhibitory influence and acceleration of gastric emptying.

The *alkaline tide,* or decrease in urinary acidity which may occur after a meal, is generally attributed to an increased alkalinity of the blood resulting from the secretion of HCl. The occurrence of an alkaline tide is not predictable, being influenced by (1) the relative rate of formation of HCl and alkaline digestive secretions, mainly pancreatic with its high content of NaHCO₃, (2) the rate of absorption of HCl from the gut, (3) neutralizing capacity of the food, (4) respiratory adjustments after the meal and (5) diuretic effect of the meal.

Pepsin, the principal enzyme of gastric juice, is preformed and stored in the chief cells as pepsinogen. At pH below 6, *pepsinogen* is converted to pepsin, a reaction which then proceeds autocatalytically; *i.e.,* the free pepsin activates the continued transformation of pepsinogen to pepsin. Pepsin exerts its proteolytic activity by attacking peptid linkages containing the amino groups of the aromatic amino acids, with the liberation principally of intermediate protein moieties and very few polypeptids and amino acids. An accessory digestive function of pepsin is the *clotting of milk,* which serves to improve the utilization of this food by preventing its too rapid passage through the alimentary tract and by rendering it more susceptible to enzymatic hydrolysis. Anything which mobilizes vagal impulses to the stomach serves as a powerful stimulus for pepsin secretion; thus, a gastric juice rich in pepsin content is evoked by sham feeding, by hypo-

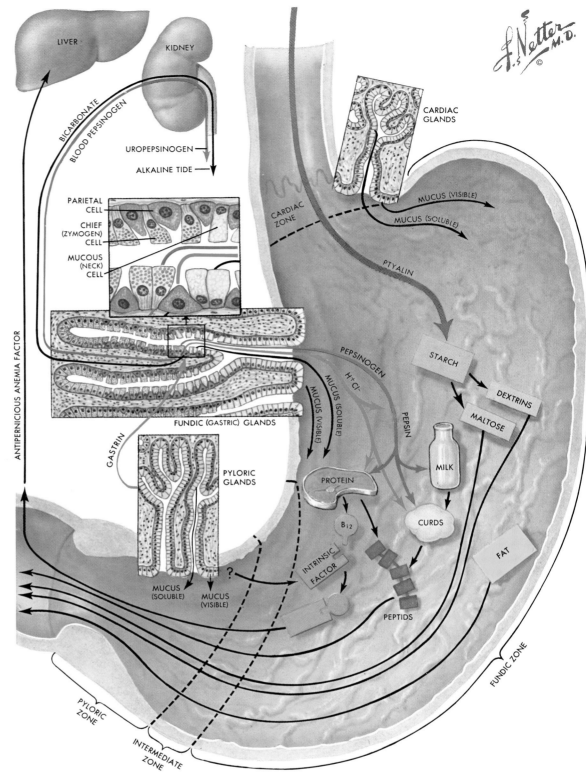

glycemia (which stimulates the vagal centers) or by direct electrical stimulation of the vagus nerves.

The pepsinogen of the gastric chief cells, besides being secreted externally into the lumen of the stomach, is to some extent secreted internally into the blood stream and appears in the urine as uropepsinogen, which provides the basis for attempts to use *uropepsinogen* determinations as an index of the peptic secretory activity of the stomach (see also page 101).

The mucoid component of gastric juice consists of at least two distinct mucoproteins. One of these substances, the so-called *"visible mucus",* has a gelatinous consistency and, in the presence of HCl, forms a white coagulum; the evidence indicates that it is secreted by the surface epithelium. The other, usually referred to as the *soluble* or dissolved *mucus,* appears to be a product of the neck chief cells and the mucoid cells of the pyloric and cardiac glands.

The secretion of soluble mucus is activated primarily by vagal impulses, while the secretion of visible mucus occurs principally in response to direct chemical and mechanical irritation of the surface epithelium. By virtue of its adherent properties and its resistance to penetration by pepsin, the mucous secretion protects the mucosa of the stomach against damage by various acid irritating agents, including its own acid-pepsin.

A normal constituent of the gastric juice, but characteristically deficient or absent in patients with pernicious anemia, is the *"intrinsic factor",* the chemical nature of which is unknown. It interacts with cobalamine (vitamin B₁₂) to prepare it for absorption in the intestine.

The gastric juice, furthermore, contains the proteolytic enzyme, cathepsin (of undetermined significance and unknown cellular origin), a weak lipase, urea, amino acids, histamine and a number of inorganic ions (Na⁺, K⁺, Ca⁺⁺, Mg⁺⁺, Cl⁻, HCO₃⁻, SO₄⁼ and phosphates).

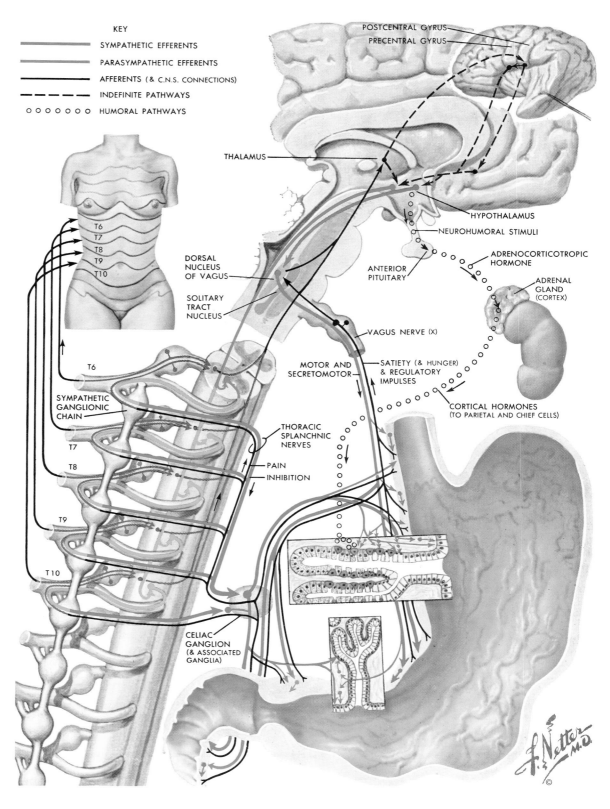

KEY
━━━	SYMPATHETIC EFFERENTS
━━━	PARASYMPATHETIC EFFERENTS
———	AFFERENTS (& C.N.S. CONNECTIONS)
– – –	INDEFINITE PATHWAYS
∘∘∘∘∘∘	HUMORAL PATHWAYS

Neuroregulation of Gastric Activity

Such evidence as is available places the cortical area that influences gastric motility and secretion in the *posterior orbital gyrus* and the *adjacent anterior cingulate gyrus.* Connections are made, via the medial *thalamic nuclei,* with the *hypothalamus,* whence fibers descend in the dorsal longitudinal fasciculus, at least as far as the *dorsal nucleus of the vagus.* Impulses from the anterior hypothalamic region act, it is assumed, on *cranial parasympathetic nuclei in the brain stem,* while the *posterior hypothalamus* probably makes connections with the *neurons of the lateral horns* of gray matter in the thoracolumbar segments of the spinal cord.

The innervation of the stomach and duodenum, including the course of the vagus and sympathetic nerves, has been described on pages 64 and 65. The vagi, the principal innervation to the stomach, exert augmentative and inhibitory effects on both motility and secretion. Gastric tonus, motility and secretory activity are permanently reduced when the vagi are sectioned, whereas section of the splanchnic nerve does not essentially alter the functions of the stomach. By virtue of the autonomy exercised by the intramural plexus and nerves, the stomach is able to function adequately after complete extrinsic denervation, *i.e.,* after bilateral vagotomy and splanchnicotomy.

The *afferent fibers,* which take their course with the vagi and sympathetic nerves, mediate the visceral sensations, some of which, such as nausea and hunger, have been taken up elsewhere (see pages 69, 90 and 91, respectively). Pain sensations are carried by afferent fibers accompanying the sympathetic

nerves. In contrast to the somatic sensory nerves, the visceral afferents or their receptors are relatively insensitive to stimuli such as cutting or burning. The effective stimulus for visceral pain is tension transmitted to the nerve endings by strong muscular contraction, by distention or by inflammation. Normal peristaltic movements of the stomach do not ordinarily give rise to any sensation, but forceful contractions may be perceived as a feeling of gnawing and tension or as actual pain in the abdomen, particularly in the presence of an inflammatory or ulcerative process. In addition to the discomfort which the individual locates in the involved viscus, pain may be felt which is subjectively interpreted as arising in the abdominal or thoracic wall. The *areas* to which this *"referred pain"* is ascribed depend upon the distribution of the afferent fibers and their course. Pain from the stomach is conveyed mainly in the afferents

which run in the *sympathetic nerves of the fifth to the tenth thoracic segments,* but the pathways may also extend as low as the twelfth. The impulses reach the spinal cord by way of the white communicating rami and the dorsal root ganglia. Within the cord the impulses are "transferred" to the neurons of the somatic sensory nerves, with the result that pain originating in the stomach may be referred to any of the somatic structures receiving their sensory supply from the fifth to the twelfth thoracic segments. Many of the details of visceral and "referred" pain remain to be clarified. Several theories and concepts still await unification and experimental confirmation.

In the interpretation of visceral pain, the phenomenon of "habit reference" must be taken into account. This term denotes the referral of pain in any visceral disease to the same area in which the pain of a previous disease was felt.

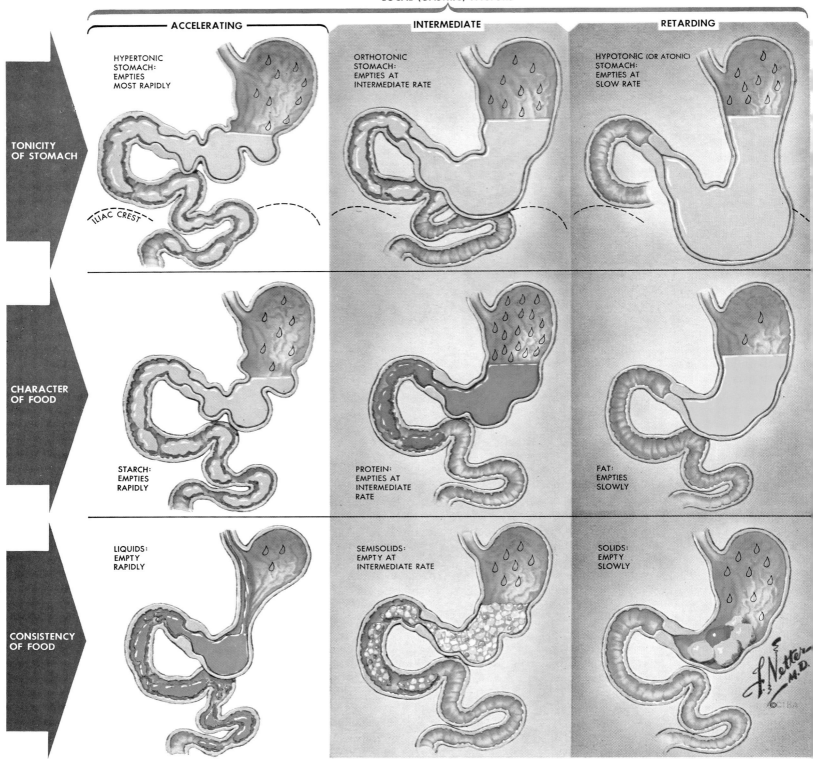

ACCELERATING

INTERMEDIATE

RETARDING

TONICITY OF STOMACH

HYPERTONIC STOMACH: EMPTIES MOST RAPIDLY

ORTHOTONIC STOMACH: EMPTIES AT INTERMEDIATE RATE

HYPOTONIC (OR ATONIC) STOMACH: EMPTIES AT SLOW RATE

ILIAC CREST

CHARACTER OF FOOD

STARCH: EMPTIES RAPIDLY

PROTEIN: EMPTIES AT INTERMEDIATE RATE

FAT: EMPTIES SLOWLY

CONSISTENCY OF FOOD

LIQUIDS: EMPTY RAPIDLY

SEMISOLIDS: EMPTY AT INTERMEDIATE RATE

SOLIDS: EMPTY SLOWLY

SECTION IV—PLATE 14

FACTORS INFLUENCING GASTRIC ACTIVITY

Motor and secretory activities of the stomach are modified, usually simultaneously and in the same direction, by a number of factors, chief among which are the following:

1. TONUS OF THE STOMACH. The *hypertonic,* or steer-horn, stomach (see page 49) tends to be hypermotile and to empty relatively rapidly as contrasted with the *hypotonic,* or fishhook, type. Also, individuals with a hypertonic stomach tend toward secretion of more HCl and, as

a corollary, to accelerated secretion and diminished intragastric stasis, and thereby also to peptic ulcers of the duodenum, whereas it is in those with *orthotonic* and, particularly, hypotonic stomachs, that gastric ulcers are more likely to be found. A residue of barium in the stomach 4 or 5 hours after an upper gastro-intestinal X-ray examination must be interpreted with due consideration for the fact that the organ's inherent tonicity is a factor in its emptying rate.

2. CHARACTER OF THE FOOD. A meal which is sufficiently *high in fat* to yield an intragastric fat content in excess of about 10 per cent empties much more slowly and stimulates considerably less acid secretion than does a meal *predominantly of protein.* The inhibitory effect of fat on gastric secretion is not a local one but a result of enterogastrone formation after fat has

entered the upper intestine. The interval half-milk-half-cream feeding to ulcer patients does not necessarily accomplish the motor and secretory inhibiting action which the fat content of the mixture implies. With whole milk having a maximum of 4 per cent butter fat, and cream usually 18 per cent, the resulting 11 per cent fat concentration is high enough to initiate the formation of enterogastrone only if the "half-and-half" reaches the intestine undiluted. This is not likely to happen unless the stomach is empty and the mixture is discharged from the stomach before an appreciable secretion of gastric juice occurs. The enterogastric inhibitory action of fat is much more effectively achieved by the ingestion of 15 to 30 ml. of a vegetable oil before meals.

A meal exclusively or *mainly of starch* tends

(Continued on page 87)

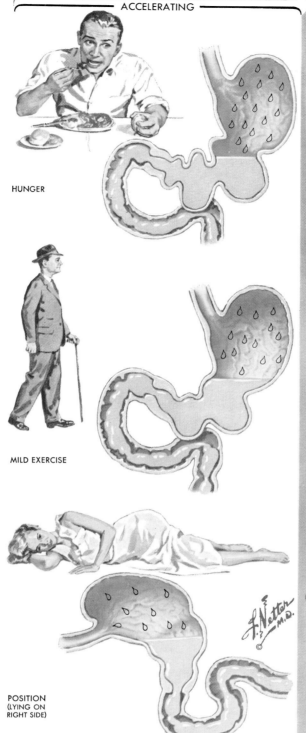

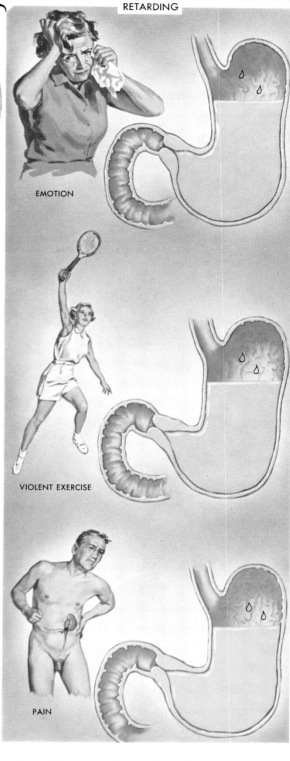

Factors Influencing Gastric Activity

(*Continued from page 86*)

to empty more rapidly, though stimulating less secretion, than does a protein meal. Thus, other factors being equal, a person may expect to be hungry sooner after a breakfast of fruit juice, cereal, toast and tea than after one of bacon, eggs and milk. The amount of total secretion and of acid content is highest with the ingestion of proteins. However, the relationship of quantity and rate of secretion and its acid or pepsin concentration is subject to great individual variations as well as variations in a single individual under different conditions.

3. Consistency of the Food. *Liquids,* whether ingested separately or with solid food, leave the stomach more rapidly than do *semisolids* or *solids*. This does not apply to liquids such as milk, from which solid material is precipitated on contact with gastric juice. In the case of any foods requiring mastication, the consistency of the material reaching the stomach should normally be semisolid, thereby facilitating gastric secretion, digestion and evacuation. Important exceptions to the general rule that liquids are weak stimulants of gastric secretion are (1) the broth of meat or fish, by virtue of their high secretagogue content and (2) coffee, which derives its secretory potency from its content both of caffeine and of the secretagogues formed in the roasting process.

4. Hunger. A meal eaten at a time of intense hunger tends to be evacuated more rapidly than is normally the case, apparently in consequence of the heightened gastric tonus. Since hunger results from the depletion of body nutrient stores (see page 69), it is understandable on teleologic grounds that in the hunger state the body should have some mechanism for hastening the delivery of ingested nutrients into the intestine.

5. Exercise. Mild exercise, particularly just after eating, shortens the emptying time of the meal. With strenuous exercise, gastric contractions are temporarily inhibited, then augmented, so that final emptying is not significantly delayed. Secretory activity does not appear to be materially influenced by exercise.

6. Position. In certain individuals, gastric emptying is facilitated when the position of the body is such that the pylorus and duodenum are in a dependent position, *i.e.,* with the individual lying on the right side. In the supine position, particularly in infants and in adults with a cascade stomach, the gastric content pools in the dependent fundic portion, and emptying is delayed. No evidence is available that secretion is affected by position.

7. Emotion. The retarding effect of emotional states on gastric motility and secretion has been well documented by clinical and experimental observa-

tions. More recently, evidence has been submitted (Wolf and Wolff) to indicate that the influence of emotions on gastric activity may be augmentative or inhibitory, depending on whether the emotional experience is of an aggressive (hostility, resentment) or depressive (sorrow, fear) type, respectively. One point of view (Margolin *et al.*) holds that it is not the manifest or conscious emotion which determines whether the stomach will be stimulated or inhibited, but rather the unconscious or symbolic content of the emotional state, and that, further, certain emotions may be accompanied by a dissociation in the response among the various components of the gastric secretions.

8. Pain. Severe or sustained pain in any part of the body, *e.g.,* kidney- or gallbladder stone, migraine, sciatic neuritis, etc., inhibits gastric motility and evacuation by nervous reflex pathways.

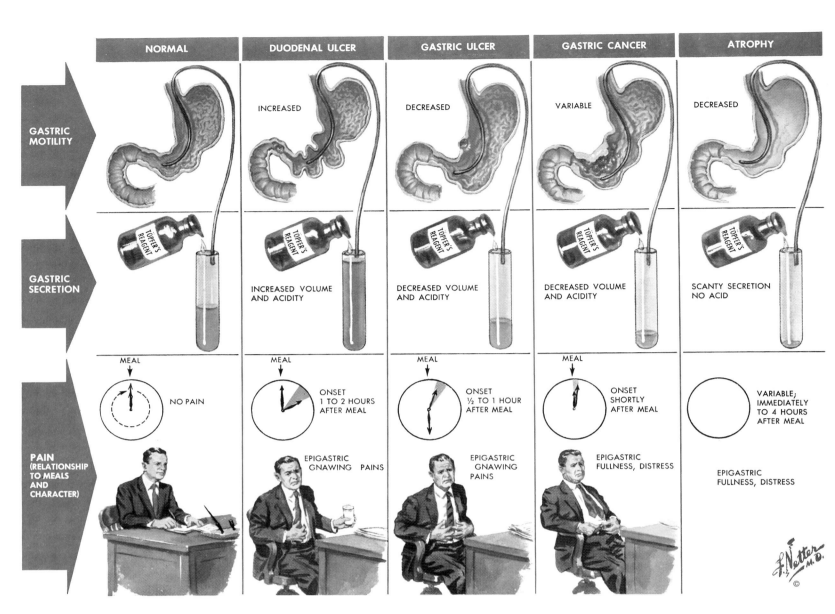

NORMAL	DUODENAL ULCER	GASTRIC ULCER	GASTRIC CANCER	ATROPHY

GASTRIC MOTILITY — INCREASED (Duodenal Ulcer); DECREASED (Gastric Ulcer); VARIABLE (Gastric Cancer); DECREASED (Atrophy)

GASTRIC SECRETION — TÖPFER'S REAGENT; INCREASED VOLUME AND ACIDITY (Duodenal Ulcer); DECREASED VOLUME AND ACIDITY (Gastric Ulcer); DECREASED VOLUME AND ACIDITY (Gastric Cancer); SCANTY SECRETION NO ACID (Atrophy)

PAIN (RELATIONSHIP TO MEALS AND CHARACTER) — MEAL; NO PAIN (Normal); ONSET 1 TO 2 HOURS AFTER MEAL, EPIGASTRIC GNAWING PAINS (Duodenal Ulcer); ONSET ½ TO 1 HOUR AFTER MEAL, EPIGASTRIC GNAWING PAINS (Gastric Ulcer); ONSET SHORTLY AFTER MEAL, EPIGASTRIC FULLNESS, DISTRESS (Gastric Cancer); VARIABLE; IMMEDIATELY TO 4 HOURS AFTER MEAL, EPIGASTRIC FULLNESS, DISTRESS (Atrophy)

FUNCTIONAL CHANGES IN GASTRIC DISEASES

Normally, gastric secretion and motility vary considerably from one individual to another and in the same individual from time to time. In the stomachs of subjects in whom no disease of the upper gastro-intestinal tract can be demonstrated, the emptying time of a standard meal may vary over 100 per cent from the average, and the concentration of HCl secreted in the basal state or in response to the standard stimuli ranges from 0 to 100 mEq./l. or more.

A tendency to gastric hypertonicity and hypermotility is observed in many *duodenal ulcer* patients. Initial emptying of a meal may be delayed for a considerable time because of reflex antral spasm incited from the ulcerated duodenal cap; after the pressure by the active contractions of the stomach overcomes the pyloro-antral resistance, evacuation proceeds so rapidly that the final emptying time may be considerably shortened. The most important motility change occurs when the ulcer area becomes so inflamed and edematous, or so scarred, that the gastric outlet is obstructed (see pages 89 and 174). After a preliminary period of hypermotility the stomach becomes atonic, a condition immediately recognized roentgenologically with the first swallow of barium. The stomach, in cases of duodenal

ulcer, tends to secrete excessively as regards both *volume and concentration of acid,* so that the average output of acid in duodenal ulcer patients greatly exceeds the average of all other categories, including the normal.*

Almost all patients secreting 6 mEq. or more per hour under basal conditions will be found in the duodenal ulcer category. The hourly basal acid output of 8 mEq. or higher, found in about 10 per cent of duodenal ulcer patients, is so rarely attained in any other circumstances as to be diagnostic of this disease.

It is not certain whether a hypersecretion exists before the ulcer starts to develop, but it does persist after the ulcer heals, and the neutralizing capacity of the duodenal bulb area is more readily exhausted in duodenal ulcer patients than in normals.

The pain in duodenal ulcer is most often described as a gnawing or intense hunger sensation, coming on characteristically from 1 to 2 hours after a meal.

The pathophysiologic phenomena caused by a *gastric ulcer* depend on the site of the ulcer in the stomach. The closer the ulcer is to the pylorus, the more the manifestations resemble those of duodenal ulcer. In peptic ulcer of the lesser curvature at or proximal to the incisure, gastric motility is not notably altered from the normal, except for some local hypertonicity of the musculature at, and frequently opposite, the ulcer site. When the gastric emptying is delayed in a case of ulcer of the body of the stomach, the presence of a coexisting duodenal ulcer should be sus-

pected. In fact, it has been postulated (Dragstedt) that the gastric stasis resulting from chronic pyloric narrowing by a duodenal ulcer is in many instances the etiologic factor for a gastric ulcer.

The pain of gastric ulcer tends to occur relatively soon after eating, because the gastric content is in immediate contact with the lesion; for the same reason, smoothness and blandness of the diet are much more important in gastric than in duodenal ulcer, although evidence has been submitted to the effect that the blandness of the diet is not of overriding importance in either.

Gastric carcinoma is not characterized by any general motility pattern, except for the obvious changes to be expected in an area of infiltration into muscle or where the tumor produces obstruction (see pages 180, 182 and 185).

In *atrophy of the gastric mucosa* (schematically indicated in the picture by a flattened mucosal surface [see also page 164], although the thinning of the mucosa by loss of the normal glandular arrangement does not necessarily result in obliteration of the rugal folds), the reduction in glandular elements results in a greatly diminished secretion containing no HCl even with maximal stimulation, *e.g.,* by an augmented histamine test. If motility is affected at all, it is in the direction of a decrease.

---

*The only known exception is the rare disease described by Ellison and Zollinger, which is characterized by peptic ulceration in the upper intestine distal to the duodenal bulb, multiple endocrinopathies and secretion of such enormous quantities of HCl as to require total gastrectomy to abolish the ulcerative process.

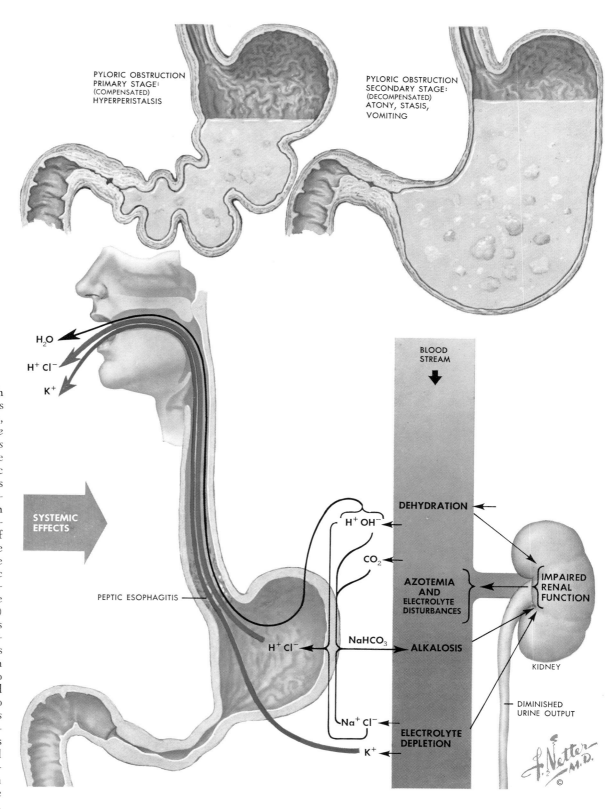

PYLORIC OBSTRUCTION
PRIMARY STAGE:
(COMPENSATED)
HYPERPERISTALSIS

PYLORIC OBSTRUCTION
SECONDARY STAGE:
(DECOMPENSATED)
ATONY, STASIS,
VOMITING

PYLORIC OBSTRUCTION, EFFECTS OF VOMITING

When the outlet of the stomach becomes narrowed to the point of serious interference with gastric emptying (see, e.g., page 174), the *gastric musculature responds at first with increased peristalsis* in an effort to build up sufficient pressure to overcome the resistance at its pyloric end. At this stage the patient experiences a sensation of "burning" in the epigastrium or left hypochondrium. With persisting obstruction and further stagnation of the stomach content, both of ingested food and of gastric secretion, the *stomach begins to dilate;* the musculature becomes atonic, and very little peristaltic activity is present. The patient now complains of fullness, vomiting (in the late afternoon, evening or during the night) of undigested food eaten many hours earlier, and foul eructation. If the obstruction is unrelieved, vomiting becomes more frequent and more copious. With so little gastric content now passing into the intestine because of the profound gastric atony, the patient is powerless to keep up with the *fluid and electrolytes lost* in the vomitus; dehydration, hypochloremia, hypokalemia and alkalosis supervene. These, in turn, affect renal function, with the consequent development of oliguria, azotemia and retention of other electrolytes. Clinically, the patient is weak, anorexic and drowsy. Unless measures are instituted to correct the metabolic disorder and relieve the obstruction, the condition progresses to irreversible tissue damage and a fatal outcome.

Pyloric obstruction is, of course, not the only cause of vomiting (see pages 90 and 91); the diagnosis may be suspected by reason of the preceding history, the pattern of the emesis and the appearance of the vomitus. In duodenal ulcer, which is the most common cause of pyloric obstruction, the patient usually gives a history of ulcer symptoms. The vomiting is at first intermittent, perhaps 2 or 3 days apart, and the vomitus often contains recognizable particles of food eaten the previous day. The quantity of fluid

and ions lost by vomiting is largely dependent upon the degree of gastric dilatation and, thereby, upon the length of time during which the pyloric obstruction develops and remains incomplete; in other words, upon the time between the *primary stage,* in which the obstruction is "compensated" (see also page 174) by increased peristalsis, and the *secondary stage,* in which the stomach becomes atonic.

As with any excessive vomiting from whatever cause, the *patient loses,* besides appreciable amounts of *fluids, hydrogen ions, chloride ions and potassium.* Since the gastric juice is poor in sodium, usually no sodium deficiency occurs, and while sodium remains in the blood, bicarbonate ion substitutes for the chloride ion. The loss of potassium is attributable to the fact that the parietal cell secretes significant amounts of this ion.

Vomiting does not ordinarily occur in uncompli-

cated ulcer disease, except when the ulcer is located in the pyloric canal, but many ulcer patients empty the stomach by means of vomiting to obtain relief from the pain.

Management of the consequences of repeated or excessive vomiting consists of fluid and electrolyte replacement, evacuation of the stomach with an Ewald tube, followed by continuous gastric aspiration with a Levin tube for from 48 to 72 hours. If the obstruction itself is not relieved thereby, surgery is necessary to re-establish gastro-intestinal passage, but it should not be undertaken before the fluid and electrolyte balance has been restored.

A clinical and physiologic disturbance closely resembling that of pyloric obstruction may result from excessive ingestion of a soluble alkali and a rich source of calcium, e.g., milk; this is called the milk-alkali or Burnett syndrome.

NAUSEA AND VOMITING

Nausea is a disagreeable experience as difficult to define as it is distressing to experience. It is variously described as a sick feeling, a tightness in the throat, a sinking sensation or a feeling of imminent vomiting. It generally precedes vomiting, a notable exception being in brain tumors. Also, nausea may occur, continuously or in waves, without vomiting, especially if the stomach is empty. Salivation, pallor, tachycardia, faintness, weakness and dizziness are frequent concomitants.

The biologic purpose of nausea appears to be the prevention of food intake, and of vomiting the expulsion of food or other substances already ingested, in circumstances where their presence in the upper gastro-intestinal tract is unfavorable to the functioning of the organism. For instance, the loss of gastric tonus and peristalsis, which occurs in motion sickness, may make it expedient for the gastric content to be gotten rid of in that condition. Since nausea and vomiting may result from disturbances in practically any part of the body, the teleologic significance of these symptoms is not always apparent; indeed, in certain situations they appear to be contrary to the welfare of the individual.

Nausea and vomiting may be precipitated by emotional disturbances; by intracranial vasomotor and pressure changes; by unpleasant olfactory, visceral or gustatory stimuli; by functional or anatomic alterations in the thoracic and abdominal viscera, including the urogenital tract; by intense pain in somatic parts; by exogenous or endogenous toxins; by drugs (notably the opiates); and by stimulation of the vestibular apparatus (most commonly by motion). Impulses from all of these sources reach the central nervous system via the corresponding sensory nerves. Just how these impulses are channeled into the stream of consciousness cannot be stated with certainty, but it is possible that the medullary emetic elements make ascending connections with some cortical area concerned in the perception of nausea, and that these connections are activated before the impulses stimulating the emetic mechanism have reached the vomiting threshold.

The central nervous control of vomiting has for many years been ascribed to a vomiting center in the medulla,

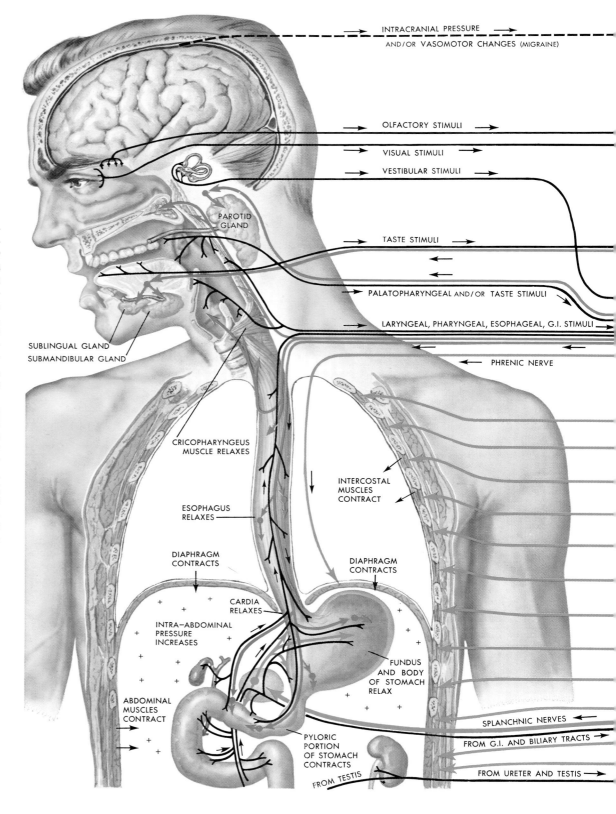

INTRACRANIAL PRESSURE AND/OR VASOMOTOR CHANGES (MIGRAINE)

OLFACTORY STIMULI

VISUAL STIMULI

VESTIBULAR STIMULI

PAROTID GLAND

TASTE STIMULI

PALATOPHARYNGEAL AND/OR TASTE STIMULI

LARYNGEAL, PHARYNGEAL, ESOPHAGEAL, G.I. STIMULI

SUBLINGUAL GLAND
SUBMANDIBULAR GLAND

PHRENIC NERVE

CRICOPHARYNGEUS MUSCLE RELAXES

INTERCOSTAL MUSCLES CONTRACT

ESOPHAGUS RELAXES

DIAPHRAGM CONTRACTS

DIAPHRAGM CONTRACTS

CARDIA RELAXES

INTRA–ABDOMINAL PRESSURE INCREASES

FUNDUS AND BODY OF STOMACH RELAX

ABDOMINAL MUSCLES CONTRACT

SPLANCHNIC NERVES

FROM G.I. AND BILIARY TRACTS

PYLORIC PORTION OF STOMACH CONTRACTS

FROM URETER AND TESTIS

FROM TESTIS

but only recently have the structural and functional details of this mechanism been clarified. The central control of vomiting is vested in two areas: one, called the *vomiting center,* is located *in the lateral reticular formation,* in the midst of the cell groups governing such related activities as salivation and respiration. The other, called the *chemoreceptor trigger zone,* is in a narrow strip along the floor of the fourth ventricle in close proximity to the vomiting center. The functions of the two areas are distinct, though not independent. The vomiting center is activated by impulses from the gastro-intestinal tract and other peripheral structures. The chemoreceptor trigger zone is stimulated by circulating toxic agents and by impulses from the cerebellum; influences of this zone on the vomiting center produce the resulting emetic action. Thus, ablation

of the chemoreceptor zone abolishes the emetic response to apomorphine, a centrally acting emetic, and to intravenously injected copper sulfate, which acts in the same way, but not to orally administered copper sulfate, because the latter exerts a peripheral action via the autonomic nerves to the vomiting center. Ablation of the vomiting center, on the other hand, abolishes the emetic response to apomorphine and to injected copper sulfate, because vomiting does not occur when the vomiting center is destroyed.

In the light of this newer concept of the nervous mechanisms, vomiting may be analyzed as follows: Impulses set up by irritation in any somatic or visceral parts or in any of the sense organs pass, by way of their respective sensory nerves, to reach the medulla, where they activate the vomiting center; toxic agents, whether

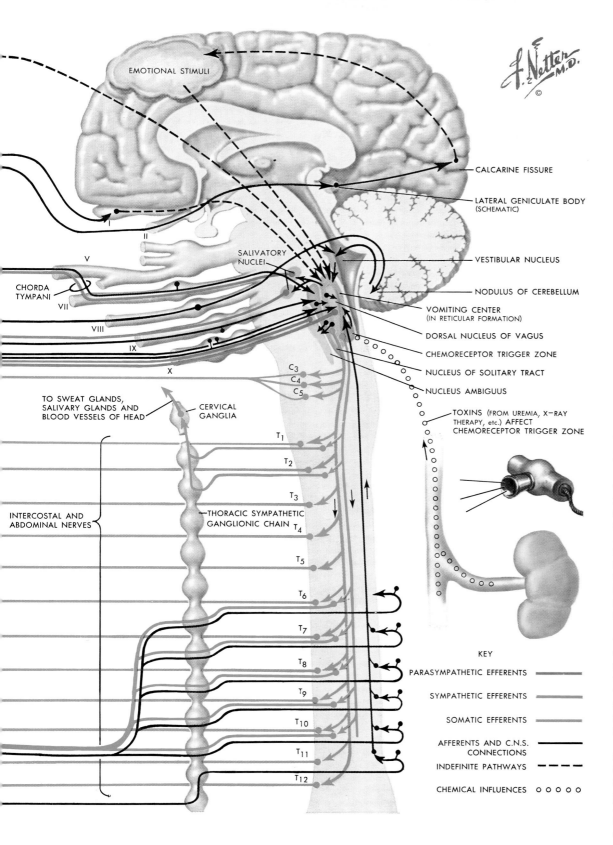

EMOTIONAL STIMULI

CALCARINE FISSURE

LATERAL GENICULATE BODY (SCHEMATIC)

VESTIBULAR NUCLEUS

NODULUS OF CEREBELLUM

VOMITING CENTER (IN RETICULAR FORMATION)

DORSAL NUCLEUS OF VAGUS

CHEMORECEPTOR TRIGGER ZONE

NUCLEUS OF SOLITARY TRACT

NUCLEUS AMBIGUUS

SALIVATORY NUCLEI

CHORDA TYMPANI

I
II
V
VII
VIII
IX
X

C_3
C_4
C_5

TO SWEAT GLANDS, SALIVARY GLANDS AND BLOOD VESSELS OF HEAD

CERVICAL GANGLIA

TOXINS (FROM UREMIA, X−RAY THERAPY, etc.) AFFECT CHEMORECEPTOR TRIGGER ZONE

INTERCOSTAL AND ABDOMINAL NERVES

THORACIC SYMPATHETIC GANGLIONIC CHAIN

T_1
T_2
T_3
T_4
T_5
T_6
T_7
T_8
T_9
T_{10}
T_{11}
T_{12}

KEY

PARASYMPATHETIC EFFERENTS ————

SYMPATHETIC EFFERENTS ————

SOMATIC EFFERENTS ————

AFFERENTS AND C.N.S. CONNECTIONS ————

INDEFINITE PATHWAYS - - - -

CHEMICAL INFLUENCES o o o o o

introduced into the body or accumulated endogenously, act upon the chemosensitive trigger zone, whence impulses reach and activate the nearby vomiting center. Before the vomiting threshold is exceeded, impulses passing up to the cortex give rise to the sensation of nausea. The vomiting center co-ordinates the discharge of impulses from adjacent neural components to the various structures which participate in the act of vomiting. *Salivation,* which almost invariably precedes the actual ejection of the vomitus, is stimulated by impulses from the salivary nuclei. Contraction of the *intercostal muscles* and of the *diaphragm* produces a sharp inspiratory movement and *increased intra-abdominal pressure,* an effect which is abetted by *contraction of the abdominal muscles.* Closure of the glottis forestalls aspiration into the respiratory passages. The *pyloric portion of the*

stomach contracts; the body of the stomach, the *cardia,* the *esophagus* and the *cricopharyngeus muscle relax,* and the gastric contents are forced out through the mouth and, in a vigorous emesis, through the nose as well.

The nausea and vomiting, brought on by motion, result from stimulation of the *vestibular organs* by movements of the head, neck and eye muscles, and by traction on the abdominal organs. The type of motion necessary to precipitate motion sickness does not require a vertical component, as is evident from the fact that some individuals develop the symptoms merely from being rotated or from riding backward in a train. In such instances, attempts to resolve the visual disorientation by movements of the eyes and head may result in stimulation of the labyrinth, either directly or by the fall in gastric tonus which may

occur with eye movements of this type. That visual stimuli are not essential for the development of motion sickness is evident from the fact that even blind persons may be susceptible.

Rapid downward motion which comes to a sudden stop or is followed by upward motion causes the abdominal viscera to sag and pull on their attachments; this is the origin of the sinking feeling experienced at the end of a rapid descent in an elevator or in a sudden sharp drop in a plane. The sensation does not occur if the subject stands on his head in the elevator, and it is reduced if he assumes a horizontal position when the plane is bouncing up and down, since the viscera cannot be displaced as far in the anteroposterior as in the craniocaudal direction. Nausea and retching may be induced in a patient under spinal anesthesia by downward traction on the exposed stomach. Impulses set up by these visceral stimuli pass in the autonomic nerves, chiefly the vagi, to the vomiting center. Yet the vestibular mechanism is in some way concerned in the effect, since motion sickness does not occur in the absence of the vestibular organs.

Impulses mediating nausea and vomiting by vestibular stimulation originate principally in the utricular maculae of the labyrinth, pass by way of the VIII cranial nerve to the vestibular nuclei, to the uvula and *nodulus of the cerebellum,* to the chemoreceptor trigger zone and, finally, to the vomiting center.

Nausea, besides being an unpleasant symptom which is sometimes difficult to relieve, becomes a serious clinical problem if it is sufficiently prolonged to interfere with nutrition. Primary nausea, *i.e.,* nausea occurring in the postabsorptive state, occasionally accompanies eye strain, myocardial infarction, azotemia and visceral neoplastic disease, but it is usually of psychologic origin.

Protracted vomiting is detrimental not only from the nutritional standpoint but also because of electrolyte depletion (see page 89) and the possible development of tears in the gastro-esophageal mucosa which may bleed (Mallory-Weiss syndrome), and of esophagitis. If vomiting does not respond to the administration of anti-emetic drugs, nasogastric suction should be instituted; correction of a gastric hypotonus may prove to be the factor which brings the condition under control.

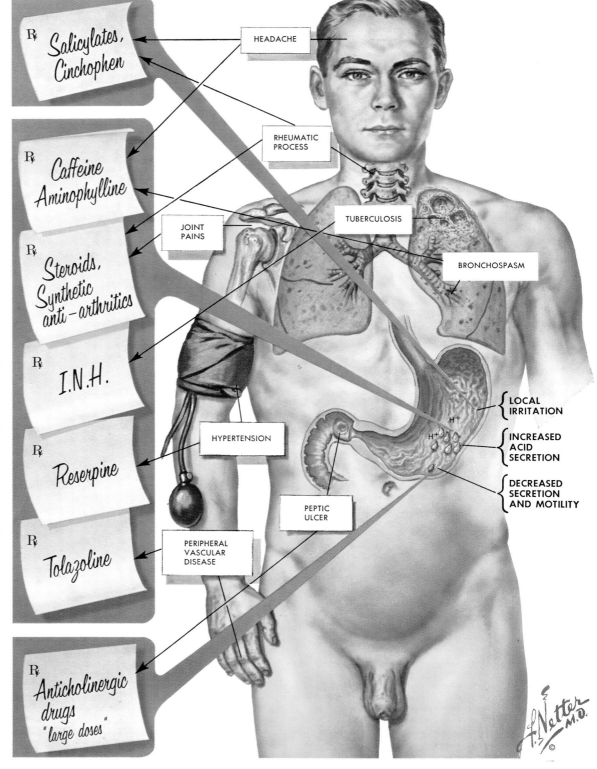

EFFECTS OF DRUGS ON GASTRIC FUNCTION

A number of the pharmacologic agents most widely employed in medical therapy may adversely affect the upper gastro-intestinal tract. Therefore, every patient with symptoms referable to the esophagus, stomach or duodenum should be questioned carefully regarding the recent use of drugs.

1. *Salicylates.* All antirheumatic drugs are potential gastric irritants; salicylates, whether alone or in combination with other analgesics, antacids, opiates or steroids, head the list of offenders. The inflammatory reaction produced by salicylates in the stomach of susceptible individuals engenders consequences varying from mild dyspepsia to massive hemorrhage.

2. *Cinchophen,* now less frequently prescribed, has been shown experimentally to be an ulcerogenic agent. Similar effects on the gastric mucosa have been observed with certain synthetic antiarthritic drugs, as, *e.g.*, phenylbutazone.

3. *Caffeine* (trimethylxanthine), a favorite component of headache remedies, is a gastric irritant and potent stimulant of gastric secretion in man. The caffeine test (see also page 101) for gastric secretion is based on the latter property. Individuals predisposed to peptic ulcer and patients with a peptic ulcer in remission have been shown to respond to caffeine with a higher average acidity than do nonulcer individuals.

Beverages containing caffeine, such as coffee and tea, have the same effect as has the pure xanthine preparation, and since a cup of coffee contains 100 to 150 mg. of caffeine, it is to be expected that the abusive use of coffee or its use by persons with a sensitive stomach may cause gastric hypersecretion and irritation. The quantity of caffeine in a cup of tea or coffee is about the same if the beverages are brewed to comparable concentration, but tea is often taken much weaker than coffee and, from that standpoint, is less objectionable.

4. *Aminophylline,* a water-soluble salt of theophylline, being a xanthine derivative, is chemically closely related to caffeine. Though used therapeutically for other purposes than is caffeine,

namely, essentially for the relief of bronchospasms, it has similar effects on the stomach.

5. The adrenal *steroids* and, consequently, the adrenocorticotropic hormone which stimulates their production or release, increase hydrochloric acid and pepsin secretion in man when administered over a period of days or weeks; this is thought to be one of the factors in the development of peptic ulcers in some patients receiving adrenocorticoids therapeutically (see also page 165).

6. Isonicotinic acid hydrazide (I.N.H.), used in the treatment of tuberculosis, and the related drug, iproniazid, stimulate gastric secretion when administered in large doses.

7. The antihypertensive and tranquilizing alkaloid, *reserpine,* produces gastric hyperemia and hypersecretion in doses of 0.5 mg. or more. In rare instances, gastroduodenal hemorrhage has followed

the use of this drug, necessitating its discontinuance.

8. *Tolazoline,* a powerful vasodilator, stimulates both acid and pepsin secretion and for this reason has been proposed as a test agent for secretory capacity. It may aggravate peptic ulcer pain.

9. *Anticholinergic drugs,* both the naturally occurring and the synthetic, are employed primarily for their effects on the stomach, particularly to reduce gastric motility and secretion in duodenal ulcer patients. The only phase of gastric secretion sufficiently inhibited by these drugs to be of value is the interdigestive or basal secretion, and even this accomplishment depends on the administration of large doses, *i.e.*, doses sufficient to produce perceptible xerostomia. Evidence indicates that anticholinergic drugs are most rationally administered at bedtime in maximum tolerated dosage and in conjunction with antacids for the control of the night secretion.

EFFECTS OF GASTRECTOMY

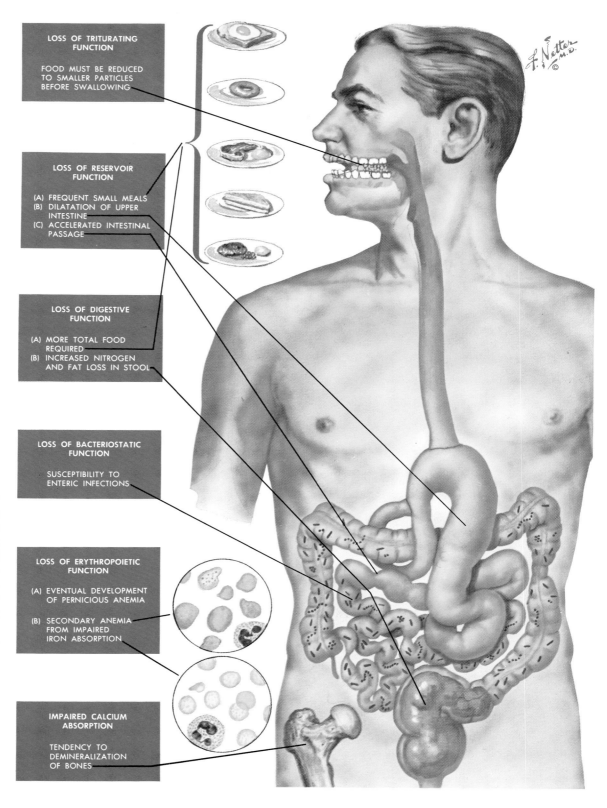

LOSS OF TRITURATING FUNCTION

FOOD MUST BE REDUCED TO SMALLER PARTICLES BEFORE SWALLOWING

LOSS OF RESERVOIR FUNCTION

(A) FREQUENT SMALL MEALS
(B) DILATATION OF UPPER INTESTINE
(C) ACCELERATED INTESTINAL PASSAGE

LOSS OF DIGESTIVE FUNCTION

(A) MORE TOTAL FOOD REQUIRED
(B) INCREASED NITROGEN AND FAT LOSS IN STOOL

LOSS OF BACTERIOSTATIC FUNCTION

SUSCEPTIBILITY TO ENTERIC INFECTIONS

LOSS OF ERYTHROPOIETIC FUNCTION

(A) EVENTUAL DEVELOPMENT OF PERNICIOUS ANEMIA

(B) SECONDARY ANEMIA FROM IMPAIRED IRON ABSORPTION

IMPAIRED CALCIUM ABSORPTION

TENDENCY TO DEMINERALIZATION OF BONES

The stomach, as has been proved by the numerous patients surviving after its surgical removal, is not an indispensable organ, but it is of sufficient importance to justify very careful consideration of the indications for partial or total gastrectomy (see page 186). In the management of patients who, for one reason or another, have undergone gastrectomy, it is well to keep in mind those gastric functions the loss of which may have serious consequences on the general health and well-being of the total organism.

Loss of the *reservoir function* deprives the patient of the capacity to hold a normal meal, necessitating the ingestion of frequent small feedings. A compensatory dilatation of the upper jejunum results, which, in some cases, eventually permits the resumption of normal eating habits. However, this does not replace the triturating action of the gastric musculature, and thorough mastication becomes correspondingly more important; also, it does not replace the mechanism of controlled gastric emptying geared to the readiness of the intestine to receive the chyme; therefore, intestinal passage is accelerated, with resulting impairment of intestinal digestion and almost invariable loss of weight. The well-nourished appearance of the gastrectomized individual presenting the frame for the schematic drawing, in which the essential points to be considered after gastrectomy are summarized, is definitely an exception to the rule.

Loss of the *digestive function* of the stomach in combination with the loss of the motor function, which controls the rate of discharge of fat into the intestine, eventuates in an increased fat and nitrogen loss in the stool, in compensation for which a greater total caloric intake is required.

The recovery of bacteria from much higher levels in the small bowel of the gastrectomized than in that of the eugastric patient is attributed to the loss of the *bacteriostatic functions* of the normal gastric secretion. This allows of a greater susceptibility to enteric infections and should alert the clinician to the possibility that an acute diarrhea in a gastrectomized patient may be the work of one representative of the Salmonella group.

Both the acid of the stomach and the controlled rate of gastric emptying favor the intestinal absorption of iron, and the absence of these functions predisposes to iron-deficiency anemia. Loss of another *erythropoietic function, i.e.,* of the intrinsic factor (see page 84), practically assures that every gastrectomized patient who lives long enough (about 5 years) will eventually develop pernicious anemia, unless the physician in charge administers some B12 at appropriate intervals after the operation.

Likewise, the impairment of the graded delivery of ingested calcium into the intestine and the absence of acid to bring it into soluble form interfere with *absorption of calcium;* hence, a tendency for the organism to draw on its endogenous calcium stores, with consequent demineralization of bones.

(For other manifestations after gastrectomy, see pages 188 and 189.)

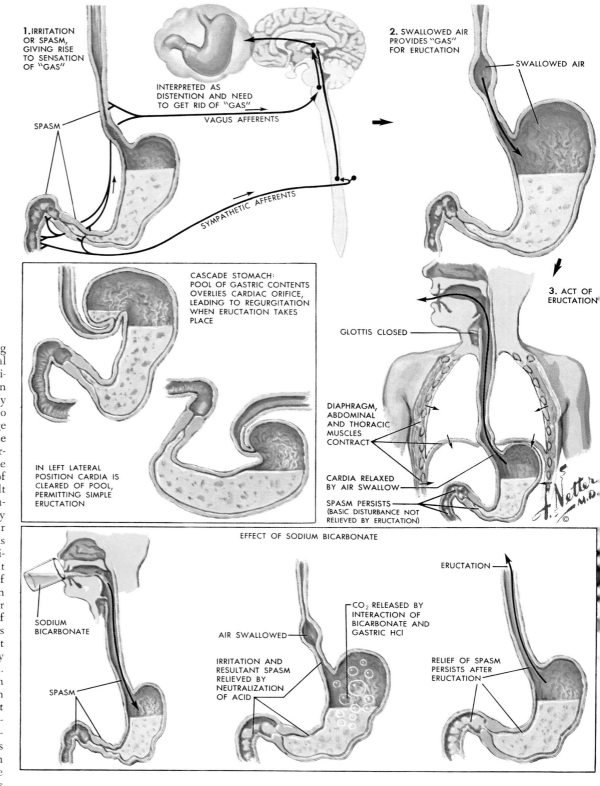

1. IRRITATION OR SPASM, GIVING RISE TO SENSATION OF "GAS"

INTERPRETED AS DISTENTION AND NEED TO GET RID OF "GAS"

VAGUS AFFERENTS

SPASM

SYMPATHETIC AFFERENTS

2. SWALLOWED AIR PROVIDES "GAS" FOR ERUCTATION

SWALLOWED AIR

3. ACT OF ERUCTATION

GLOTTIS CLOSED

DIAPHRAGM, ABDOMINAL AND THORACIC MUSCLES CONTRACT

CARDIA RELAXED BY AIR SWALLOW

SPASM PERSISTS (BASIC DISTURBANCE NOT RELIEVED BY ERUCTATION)

CASCADE STOMACH: POOL OF GASTRIC CONTENTS OVERLIES CARDIAC ORIFICE, LEADING TO REGURGITATION WHEN ERUCTATION TAKES PLACE

IN LEFT LATERAL POSITION CARDIA IS CLEARED OF POOL, PERMITTING SIMPLE ERUCTATION

EFFECT OF SODIUM BICARBONATE

SODIUM BICARBONATE

SPASM

AIR SWALLOWED

IRRITATION AND RESULTANT SPASM RELIEVED BY NEUTRALIZATION OF ACID

CO_2 RELEASED BY INTERACTION OF BICARBONATE AND GASTRIC HCl

ERUCTATION

RELIEF OF SPASM PERSISTS AFTER ERUCTATION

Aerophagia and Eructation

The release of air swallowed during a meal is a rather common and natural process in the normal individual, initiated voluntarily to relieve the sensation of fullness in the epigastric region. Early in life it is practiced by infants, who "burp" or are made to "burp" by change of position and are then able to resume the intake of the meal which was interrupted because the distention of the stomach by air created the feeling of satiety. Frequent eructation by adult individuals may become a habit, particularly on the part of those who eat hastily and, with each bite, swallow more air than is necessary. But this aerophagia as a nervous habit is an exceptional condition. Most instances of eructation result from motor disturbances in the form of a *segmental hypertonus or "spasm"* in the *esophagus, stomach, duodenum* or biliary tract. According to the theories of visceral pain, the adequate stimulus is pressure on the nerve endings in the gut wall; this pressure may be produced by intense contraction as well as distention. By conditioning or past experience, such impulses reaching the *brain* from an inflamed or contracted visceral segment are *interpreted* as representing a *distention* of the involved part; hence, the individual describes the sensation as a "gas pain" or a feeling of distention from which he would be relieved if he were to belch. Since it is not actually gaseous distention which is distressing him, he has nothing to eructate or bring up; he therefore swallows air, sometimes only into the esophagus but usually into the stomach, so that he will have something to belch. The process is usually repetitive, because the underlying motor disturbance remains unaltered. For example, a patient with "heartburn" or pyrosis may try to relieve the pressure by eructation, but the attempt is unsuccessful, because the source of the discomfort is not "gas" but an inflammation or a segmental contraction of the esophagus.

In the *act of belching,* the *glottis* is *closed* and the *diaphragmatic and thoracic muscles contract;* when the increased intra-abdominal pressure transmitted to

the stomach is sufficient to overcome the resistance of the cardia, the swallowed air is eructated. In the simple belching which follows a meal so large as to engender a feeling of fullness, the gas may be eructated at the instant the cardia is opened by a bolus of swallowed air.

In some individuals eructation is extremely difficult, because the *shape and position of the stomach* are such that the esophagus enters at a relatively acute angle; increased intragastric pressure then has the effect of shutting off the gastro-esophageal segment of expulsion. In these cases eructation may be facilitated by a change in position of the body, which temporarily changes the esophagogastric angle. The appropriate position is usually found by trial and error.

Some people, instead of swallowing air, are able to suck it in through a relaxed superior esophageal sphincter. This may occur, *e.g.,* in an emphysematous

patient who is "pulling" for air. Or it may be done deliberately, as in the case of some accomplished "belchers". The same principle is put to practical use in the development of "esophageal speech" in laryngectomized patients.

The aerophagic and the *bicarbonate consumer* do not differ basically unless the bicarbonate is taken to relieve the "gas" pains of a peptic ulcer. In this case the CO_2 generated in the stomach is eructated, and the patient gets real relief, which he does not get by belching swallowed air. The relief which follows the ingestion of soda must be explained not by decompression of a distended stomach by belching, but by neutralization of the acid which is irritating the ulcer and causing spasm of the duodenum and pylorus.

Obviously, the rational management of aerophagia and eructation depends upon correction of the underlying disturbance.

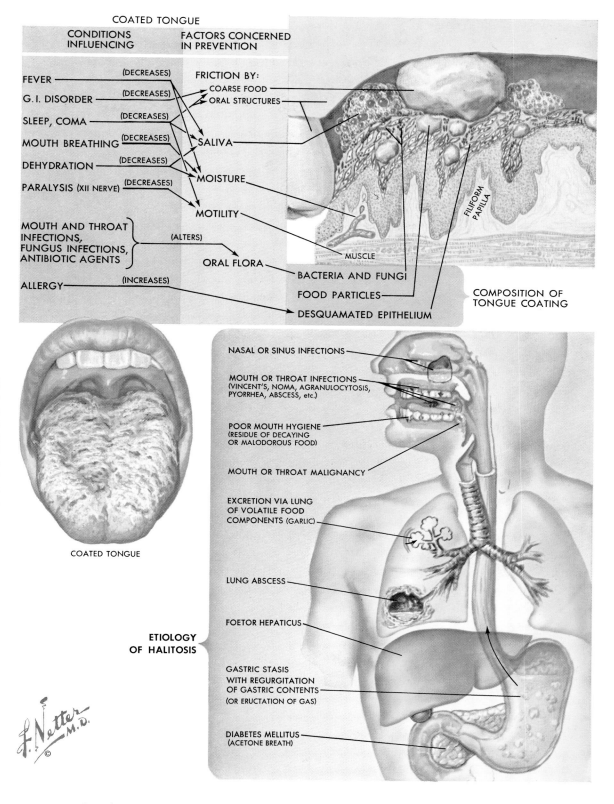

COATED TONGUE

CONDITIONS INFLUENCING		FACTORS CONCERNED IN PREVENTION
FEVER	(DECREASES)	FRICTION BY:
G.I. DISORDER	(DECREASES)	COARSE FOOD
		ORAL STRUCTURES
SLEEP, COMA	(DECREASES)	
MOUTH BREATHING	(DECREASES)	SALIVA
DEHYDRATION	(DECREASES)	MOISTURE
PARALYSIS (XII NERVE)	(DECREASES)	
		MOTILITY
MOUTH AND THROAT INFECTIONS, FUNGUS INFECTIONS, ANTIBIOTIC AGENTS	(ALTERS)	ORAL FLORA
ALLERGY	(INCREASES)	

FILIFORM PAPILLA

MUSCLE

BACTERIA AND FUNGI

FOOD PARTICLES

DESQUAMATED EPITHELIUM

COMPOSITION OF TONGUE COATING

COATED TONGUE

ETIOLOGY OF HALITOSIS

NASAL OR SINUS INFECTIONS

MOUTH OR THROAT INFECTIONS (VINCENT'S, NOMA, AGRANULOCYTOSIS, PYORRHEA, ABSCESS, etc.)

POOR MOUTH HYGIENE (RESIDUE OF DECAYING OR MALODOROUS FOOD)

MOUTH OR THROAT MALIGNANCY

EXCRETION VIA LUNG OF VOLATILE FOOD COMPONENTS (GARLIC)

LUNG ABSCESS

FOETOR HEPATICUS

GASTRIC STASIS WITH REGURGITATION OF GASTRIC CONTENTS (OR ERUCTATION OF GAS)

DIABETES MELLITUS (ACETONE BREATH)

COATED TONGUE AND HALITOSIS

Inspection of the tongue may not yield as much information as the older clinicians professed to derive therefrom, but it is true that certain disorders may be suspected from the appearance of the tongue. The tongue is kept clean and normally colored by the cleansing action of saliva, the mechanical action of mastication, the customary oral flora and adequate nutrition. Consequently, when salivary secretion is insufficient, when the dietary regimen eliminates chewing, when the bacterial flora is altered or when certain vitamins necessary for the preservation of the normal epithelium are deficient, the *tongue* may change its normal appearance. It may become coated, *i.e., food particles, sloughed epithelial cells, inflammatory exudates or fungous growths may be deposited on its surface,* in an individual on a diet for an ulcer or other gastro-intestinal disorder, or in a patient whose saliva is diminished by mouth breathing, dehydration or anticholinergic drugs, or in a comatose patient unable to eat, drink or rinse his mouth, or in one with impaired mobility of the tongue in consequence of a XII nerve paralysis, or in the presence of an exudative oral or pharyngeal inflammatory process, or on antibiotic therapy which destroys the normal flora and permits an overgrowth of fungi. In the latter case a hypertrophy of the papillae may, in the smoker especially, give the appearance of "black", or hairy, tongue (see page 112).

Sometimes in pernicious anemia, a varicolored appearance due to patchy loss of papillae may evolve, the so-called geographic tongue, but a geographic tongue (see page 113) does not make a diagnosis of pernicious anemia. In allergic reactions in the mouth, usually a manifestation of sensitivity to some ingested food, the tongue may swell, and epithelial elements may desquamate and coat the surface.

A complaint of unpleasant breath, frequently a figment of the patient's fancy, is voiced at times by people who have sensations of unpleasant taste and conclude that this must be a reflection of, or be reflected in, the odor of the breath. Often enough, however, *halitosis* is a real occurrence, brought to the attention of the victim by a spouse or other member of the family. Some of the more obvious causes may be discovered by a search for one of the following conditions: infection or neoplasm in the oro-nasopharyngeal structures, poor oral hygiene, bronchiectasis or lung abscess, cirrhosis of the liver with hepatic fetor, gastric stasis inducing aerophagia and eructation, or diabetes.

The odor of garlic remains on the breath for many hours, because garlic is absorbed into the portal circulation and passes through the liver into the general circulation. It has also been shown that volatile oils applied to the denuded or even intact skin surface are recognizable on the breath. On the basis of such observations, it has been suggested that the enzymatic processes in the intestine may, in certain individuals, liberate incompletely digested but absorbable substances of offensive odor. The fact that material not normally found in the upper gastro-intestinal tract may, when introduced rectally, be recovered from the stomach, gives credence to the possibility that retrograde passage of other, odoriferous substances may reach the mouth from the intestine. However, in a patient with pyloric obstruction, the breath is ordinarily offensive only at times of eructation. It has also been postulated that substances like fats, fatty acids or some abnormal end products of faulty digestion of fats may cause halitosis and that a trial of a low-fat diet is indicated to improve this condition. All too often the search for the cause of halitosis, though diligent enough, is unavailing, and one must have recourse to frequent mouth rinsings with antiseptic solutions flavored with pleasant-smelling ingredients.

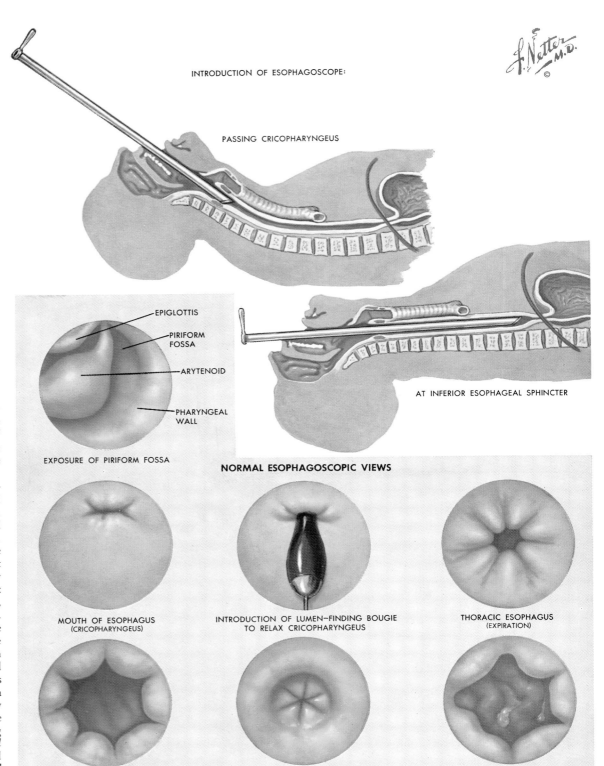

INTRODUCTION OF ESOPHAGOSCOPE:

PASSING CRICOPHARYNGEUS

AT INFERIOR ESOPHAGEAL SPHINCTER

EPIGLOTTIS

PIRIFORM FOSSA

ARYTENOID

PHARYNGEAL WALL

EXPOSURE OF PIRIFORM FOSSA

NORMAL ESOPHAGOSCOPIC VIEWS

MOUTH OF ESOPHAGUS (CRICOPHARYNGEUS)

INTRODUCTION OF LUMEN–FINDING BOUGIE TO RELAX CRICOPHARYNGEUS

THORACIC ESOPHAGUS (EXPIRATION)

THORACIC ESOPHAGUS (INSPIRATION)

INFERIOR ESOPHAGEAL SPHINCTER

GASTRO–ESOPHAGEAL JUNCTURE

Esophagoscopy

Endoscopic visualization of the esophagus is an essential procedure in the diagnosis and treatment of diseases of the gullet. Introduced primarily for the removal of foreign bodies, this technique has become much more inclusive.

Adequate sedation (Demerol®), atropine and local anesthesia of throat and hypopharynx precede the introduction of the instrument, which is performed with the patient in a recumbent position. His neck is flexed at the aperture of the thorax and is then slightly extended at the occipital region. The instrument may be brought into the mouth and pharynx from either side; the epiglottis is passed, and the arytenoid brought into view. Distending the piriform fossa by the lumen of the esophagoscope, the crevice in the anterior portion of the piriform fossa is visualized. Hugging the lateral wall of the piriform fossa, the scope is passed toward the midline, assuming a position behind the cricoid cartilage. By gentle elevation controlled by pressure from the thumb, with the hand resting upon the chin, the *cricopharyngeal sphincter* is brought into view and appears as a pitlike depression situated anteriorly at the lower level of the cricoid cartilage. Further gentle pressure permits overcoming the sphincteric action of the cricopharyngeus. If resistance is encountered, a small *bougie or lumen finder* may be used through the esophagoscope into the dimple which represents the contracted cricopharyngeal muscle. When this bougie has been passed beyond into the proximal esophagus, the esophagoscopic tube can be gently guided along the course of the bougie to enter the thoracic esophagus. The mucosa appears thrown into folds and is of a distinctive pinkish color. The lumen of the *thoracic esophagus* can be seen to dilate with each *inspiration* and to become smaller with *expiration*. The pulsation of the aortic arch at about 23 cm. from the upper incisor teeth may be recognizable. The head is now slightly lowered and tilted to the right, and the esophagoscope directed to the left and anteriorly, allowing the esophagoscopic tube to pass into the terminal esophagus. At a distance of 38 or 39 cm. from the upper incisor teeth, a puckering of the mucosa comes into view, which has the appearance of a rosette. At this point no further influence of the respiration on the lumen of the esophagus can be noticed. Instead, one encounters a tonic contracture of the musculature at this level, indicating the active mechanism of the *inferior esophageal sphincter* and the gastro-esophageal vestibule (see pages 76 and 77). When the mucosa of the rosette is touched, it promptly opens, and the tube slips into the abdominal portion of the esophagus and then, at a distance of 1½ cm. or slightly more distally, into the stomach proper. The *entrance of the esophagoscope into the stomach* is unmistakably heralded by the appearance of gastric juice in the tube and the recognition of gastric rugae which have a distinctly more reddish color.

Esophagoscopy as a diagnostic procedure should not be denied any patient except under the most unusual conditions. Difficulties in the introduction of the tube are encountered in cases of extreme kyphosis or lordosis of the cervical vertebra and in patients with dermatomyositis and difficulty in opening the mouth, in cases of aneurysm of the aorta, and in extremely old and debilitated patients. Although perforations (see page 151) inevitably occur in a very small percentage of cases, this accident is less apt to happen in the hands of the skilled endoscopist who is performing these procedures constantly. An essential part of the procedure rests with getting the confidence of the patient and having him relax during the introduction of the esophagoscope. Comforting encouragement and advice to relax are always helpful before the introduction of the tube.

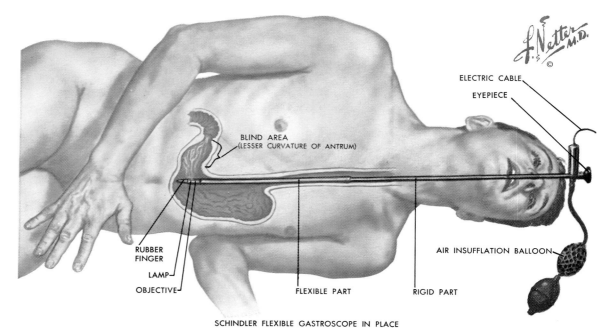

ELECTRIC CABLE
EYEPIECE
BLIND AREA
(LESSER CURVATURE OF ANTRUM)
AIR INSUFFLATION BALLOON
RUBBER FINGER
LAMP
OBJECTIVE
FLEXIBLE PART
RIGID PART

SCHINDLER FLEXIBLE GASTROSCOPE IN PLACE

GASTROSCOPY

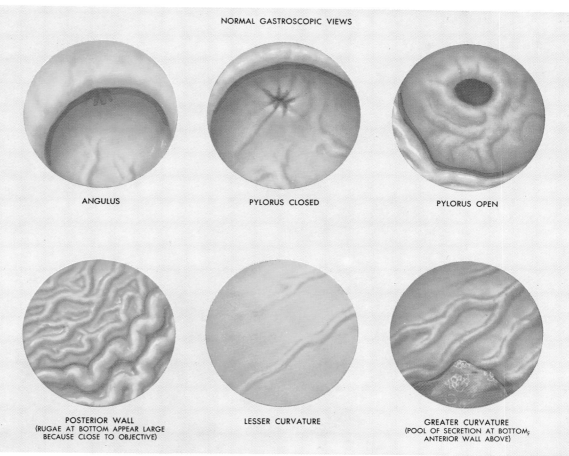

NORMAL GASTROSCOPIC VIEWS

ANGULUS

PYLORUS CLOSED

PYLORUS OPEN

POSTERIOR WALL
(RUGAE AT BOTTOM APPEAR LARGE BECAUSE CLOSE TO OBJECTIVE)

LESSER CURVATURE

GREATER CURVATURE
(POOL OF SECRETION AT BOTTOM; ANTERIOR WALL ABOVE)

Except for special investigative projects, gastroscopy should be restricted to those cases where the diagnosis is not clarified by the X-ray examination (e.g., unexplained bleeding, gastric ulcer and possible marginal ulcer). Any distortion of the outline of the stomach which the radiologist cannot confidently interpret should be brought to the attention of the gastroscopist for an opinion as to whether he might be able to contribute to the diagnosis. If the stomach is radiologically normal, a gastroscopic examination will rarely contribute to the management of the case. Gastritis, in most instances, is strictly a gastroscopic diagnosis, but the types of gastritis visualized only by the gastroscope have not yet attained sufficient clinical significance to remove them from the realm of a gastroscopic investigative problem.

Gastroscopy should not be attempted in the presence of aortic aneurysm, angina pectoris, esophageal obstruction or varices, any abnormality of the spinal or thoracic structures which prevents the esophagus from being brought into a straight line, or in any case of known or suspected corrosive or phlegmonous gastritis.

For the preparation of the patient, who should not have eaten during the previous 12 hours, any sequence or combination of drugs is acceptable which produces the maximum degree of sedation compatible with adequate co-operation by the patient. The pharynx is anesthetized with a 2 per cent Pontocaine® solution, which is gargled, sprayed or applied directly to the pharynx 10 minutes and again 5 minutes before the examination. Antifoam emulsion, 5 ml., may be used to abolish bubbles and foam.

A *rubber finger* attached to the *flexible part* of the instrument leads the latter through the esophagus and along the posterior gastric wall. The flexible part carries an objective which collects the rays reflected from the wall as illuminated by an *electric lamp* mounted inside the end of the flexing tube. The small picture, as produced by the objective, is transmitted through a lens system to the *eyepiece* (ocular) through which the gastroscopist receives a sharp picture owing to the arrangement of the lenses within the flexible tube. An electric cable running through the whole instrument is needed to provide the light source (lamp). To inflate the stomach with air, which is necessary for an adequate inspection, an insufflation balloon is connected with the tube system. Visualization is usually satisfactory for all parts of the organ, except for a few *blind areas* which include that portion of the posterior wall in immediate contact with the objective and the distal part of the lesser curvature.

Any sustained resistance to passage of the instrument is a signal to terminate the examination. A skillful gastroscopy is usually a brief one.

Any interpretation of intragastric appearances, as seen by the gastroscope, depends upon a familiarity with the normal pictures, some of which are illustrated.

DIAGNOSTIC AIDS IN ESOPHAGEAL AND GASTRIC DISORDERS

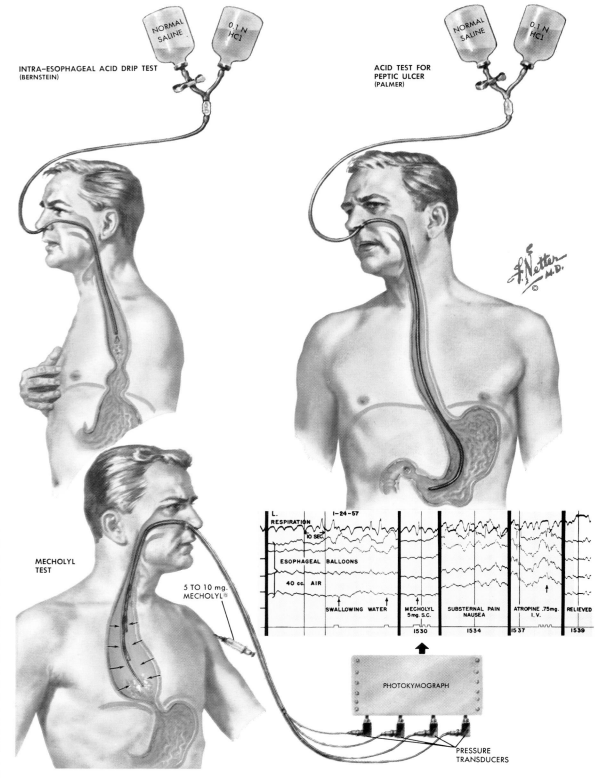

Though the X-ray findings of esophageal peristalsis in cardiospasm (see page 145) are usually quite characteristic, observation of the effect of a parasympathomimetic drug (Mecholyl) has proved valuable in ascertaining the diagnosis in cases that have remained doubtful. The *Mecholyl test* is based on the development of a diffuse contraction of the esophagus after administration of this acetylcholine derivative in the presence of cardiospasm (Kramer and Ingelfinger). Such hypersensitivity is explained by the fact that autonomically denervated organs are more responsive to a humoral neurotransmitter (Cannon and Rosenblueth) and is supported by the discovery of degenerated nerve cells in the intramural plexuses in patients with achalasia (Rake, Damioni) (see also page 46). The test may be performed under fluoroscopic observation with barium in the esophagus, or by kymographic recording with a pressure transmitting system. After the subcutaneous injection of 5 to 10 mg. Mecholyl, a diffuse, sustained contraction of the esophagus occurs, usually accompanied by substernal pain. These effects are characteristic of cardiospasm, the only known exception being the infrequent destruction of the intrinsic plexus by a carcinoma of the cardia infiltrating the wall of the esophagus.

The *intra-esophageal acid drip test* (Bernstein) is a useful diagnostic procedure in patients who complain of heartburn for which no anatomic basis can be found clinically, radiologically and endoscopically. In such cases the reproduction of the patient's symptoms by introduction of acid into the esophagus establishes the diagnosis of esophagitis. A thin polyethylene tube is introduced via the nostril to a distance of 25 cm., so that its tip is located in the midthoracic part of the esophagus. The tube is connected to a bottle of normal saline solution and a second bottle containing 0.1 N HCl. The saline solution is used first and permitted to drip into the esophageal lumen at a rate of 150 drops per minute. If the patient does not complain within 5 minutes, the acid solution is dripped in at the same rate. The appearance of pain within 10 minutes after shifting to the acid solution constitutes a positive response; the saline acid cycle should be repeated one or more times for verification.

The theory that gastric acid is the cause of the pain in patients with peptic ulcer serves as the basis for the *"acid test for peptic ulcer"* (Palmer test), which has proved helpful in patients who complain of typical ulcer symptoms but whose X-ray examination is equivocal or negative for peptic ulceration. The stomach, after overnight fasting, is evacuated with the aid of a Levin tube inserted through the nose. (It is advisable to determine the acid values of the evacuate, though this procedure has nothing to do with the test proper.) If the gastric aspiration is followed by pain, further steps are not taken until the pain has fully subsided. The patient, free from pain, then receives 400 ml. of an isotonic saline (or glucose) solution. After 45 minutes the stomach is emptied again (volume and pH of the collected material being recorded), and, under the same conditions as were used with the saline, 400 ml. of a 0.1 N HCl solution are permitted to enter the stomach by gravity from a second bottle held ready, this solution being

(Continued on page 99)

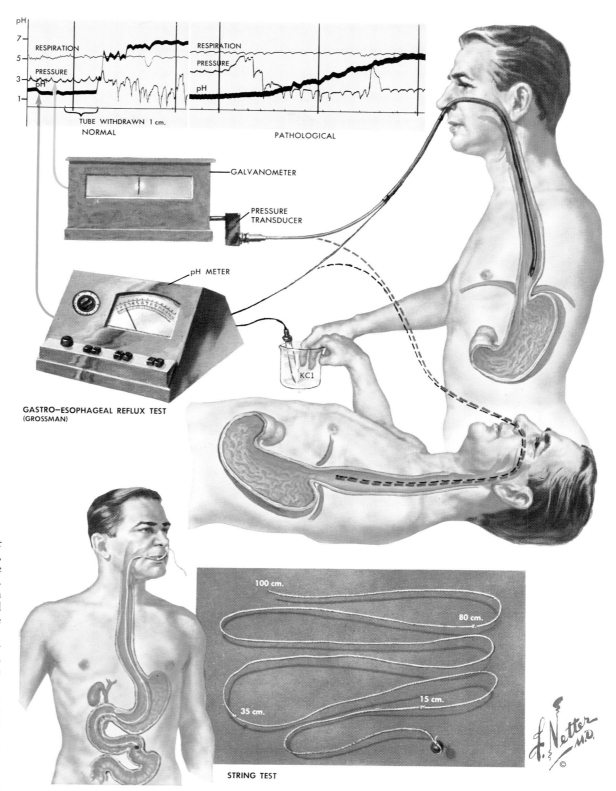

GASTRO—ESOPHAGEAL REFLUX TEST
(GROSSMAN)

STRING TEST

DIAGNOSTIC AIDS IN ESOPHAGEAL AND GASTRIC DISORDERS

(*Continued from page 98*)

allowed to remain in the stomach for another 45 minutes. If no pain develops, the procedure should be repeated twice before the result is considered negative. If the saline (or glucose) instillation produces as much pain as does the acid solution, the result is considered a "false positive".

In many cases of gastro-intestinal hemorrhage, the site of the bleeding remains a puzzle (see also page 175). A simple device has been suggested (Einhorn), which, in the hands of some authors, has proved most valuable, while others reported disappointing results. If the origin of the hemorrhage cannot be identified radiologically or endoscopically, an ordinary *string* about 100 cm. long, knotted at distances of 15 (approximate position of the pylorus), 35 (approximate position of the cardia) and 80 cm., is introduced with the aid of a lead shot or small bag filled with mercury attached to the end of the string and anchored by the teeth at the 80-cm. mark. The string is left overnight and withdrawn the next morning. The presence of a green-yellow discoloration near the end of the string, produced by the bile in the second portion of the duodenum, indicates that the string was in the correct position while in the canal. From a bloody staining of any segment of the string, conclusion may be drawn as to the site of the bleeding.

To detect a reflux of gastric content into the esophagus as a cause of esophagitis in patients with a positive Bernstein test, a procedure has been developed

(*gastro-esophageal reflux test;* Tuttle and Grossman) in which intraluminal pressure and pH are simultaneously recorded. To assure the presence of gastric pH 1 to 2 for the duration of the study (approximately 30 minutes), 300 ml. of 0.1 N HCl are introduced into the stomach of the fasting patient. An exploratory glass electrode on a long, flexible lead and a small-caliber, water-filled polyvinyl tube, held together with a fine thread or plastic band to maintain them at an even level, are passed through the nose into the esophagus. The tube is connected with a pressure transducer and this, in turn, with a galvanometer on which pressure changes can be both observed directly and recorded photographically, using a multichannel oscillograph. The glass electrode is attached to a pH meter with the circuit established by the patient's finger in a saturated KCl solution containing a calomel electrode. The location

of the diaphragmatic hiatus is determinable by observing the inversion point of the intraluminal pressure (thoracic inspiratory pressure, negative; intra-abdominal pressure, positive). Starting the examination with the glass electrode in the stomach and withdrawing it upward 1 cm. at a time, one obtains, in normal individuals, recordings such as are reproduced in the upper left corner of the illustration, showing the rapid change of pH toward neutrality when the pressure inversion point is passed. Acid regurgitation is diagnosed when pH of 3 or less is encountered over an area at least 4 cm. above the pressure inversion point as, *e.g.,* in the curves on the right. The test is performed in the supine position, in which regurgitation is more likely to occur. Presently available evidence indicates that gastro-esophageal reflux can be detected with this procedure in almost all patients with clinical, radiologic or endoscopic signs of esophageal inflammation.

GASTRIC ANALYSIS

For clinical purposes, a gastric secretory test reduces itself to the determination of the acid component. Gastric analysis may, in this context, be classified as qualitative or quantitative.

A *qualitative gastric analysis* is undertaken to ascertain whether the gastric glands can secrete acid. It is indicated in the differential diagnosis of pernicious anemia and gastric ulcer. Presence of HCl in the residual, basal or histamine-stimulated secretion almost certainly rules out pernicious anemia; persistent absence of acid in a case of gastric ulcer almost certainly rules out a benign lesion. Repeated failure to secrete HCl after histamine is termed absolute achlorhydria.

A *quantitative gastric analysis* seeks to determine the amount of HCl secreted by the stomach and is carried out by determining the basal secretion or the secretory response to insulin hypoglycemia. It is indicated (1) in cases of clinically suspected but radiologically undemonstrable duodenal ulcer, (2) in duodenal ulcer refractory to medical management, where a decision must be made regarding surgery and (3) as a test for completeness of vagotomy.

The technique of gastric analysis is as follows: After an overnight fast the patient is intubated (nasally, if possible) with a radiopaque tube, the position of which is then checked by fluoroscopy. The tip of the tube should be in the gastric antrum, and the tube should not be redundant or coiled in the stomach. (Any attempt to perform a *quantitative gastric analysis* without fluoroscopic control of the tube's position is a waste of time.) The residual gastric content is aspirated. A residuum in excess of 100 ml. is indicative of gastric retention, as is also the presence of food. The persistence of a pink color, on addition of Töpfer's reagent to the gastric fluid, indicates the presence of HCl and completes the qualitative test.

If the indicator, when added to the residual secretion, turns yellow (indicating a pH higher than 4), continuous gastric aspiration is started, using any device which will maintain a negative pressure of 40 to 50 mm. Hg; the patency of the tube should be checked every 5 minutes by injection of a few milliliters of air. The subject should be instructed to expectorate all saliva. If the objective is to ascertain whether the parietal cells secrete HCl, the continuously aspirated juice is tested with Töpfer's reagent at intervals of 15 minutes. If no acid has appeared in an hour, the analysis is pursued further by applying the histamine test (v.i.). If a quantitative gastric analysis is desired, it is necessary to titrate the specimens of gastric juice with a standard solution of NaOH. It is conventional to titrate first to the endpoint of Töpfer's reagent (change from pink to yellow) and to speak of the value so obtained as "free acid", then to con-

FLUOROSCOPIC CONFIRMATION OF POSITION OF LEVIN TUBE FOR GASTRIC ANALYSIS

40 mm. Hg

VACUUM PUMP

DETERMINE FOR EACH SPECIMEN

1. VOLUME

2. TITRABLE ACIDITY (TÖPFER'S REAGENT INDICATOR AFTER FILTRATION)

3. pH

100 ml.

50—

15 min.   15 min.   15 min.   15 min.   15 min.   15 min.

RESIDUUM

BASAL SECRETION

tinue the titration to the turning point of phenolphthalein for the "total acid". The difference between "free acid" and "total acid" is "combined acid"; these terms have no practical significance and should be abandoned. Titration of acid gastric juice with a standard solution of NaOH to the turning point of Töpfer's reagent neutralizes all but an inconsequential amount of the HCl, and the value so obtained represents, for ordinary purposes, the quantity of HCl secreted. The concentration of acid is expressed in milliequivalents per liter (mEq./l.) and the total quantity of acid (volume × concentration) as mEq. per unit of time (mEq./hr.). The determination of hydrogen ions in a concentration of 0.1 mEq./l. or less, which is beyond the range of Töpfer's reagent, requires the use of a pH meter and is applicable only in the special circumstance mentioned below.

The *histamine test* is indicated whenever no acid

is found in the residual and basal secretions. After the subcutaneous injection of histamine (0.01 mg. of histamine base per kg. of body weight) or Histalog® (0.5 mg./kg.), which is preferred by some authorities because its side effects are less severe, testing for acid continues at 15-minute intervals and is terminated with the first 15-minute specimen in which acid appears. If it has not appeared by the end of 90 minutes, a further attempt to verify the inability to secrete acid is made by the "augmented" histamine test, in which the injection of a much larger dose of histamine is made possible by the prior administration of an antihistamine drug. (This procedure is based on the fact that the antihistamines block all but the acid-secretory effects of histamine.) Thirty minutes after the administration of the antihistaminic, 0.04 mg. of histamine diphosphate per kilo is given subcutane-

(*Continued on page 101*)

GASTRIC ANALYSIS

(Continued from page 100)

ously; the continuously aspirated gastric content is tested at 15-minute intervals with Töpfer's reagent. When this reagent, added to the specimens, turns yellow, indicating a hydrogen-ion concentration with a pH above 4, it becomes necessary to determine the pH electrometrically with a pH meter before "absolute achlorhydria" can be pronounced.

More convenient but less reliable than the histamine test for qualitative gastric analysis is the so-called *"tubeless" gastric analysis,* in which an azure A resin compound is used. This chemical complex is a carbacryl-cation-exchange resin in which some of the hydrogen ions have been replaced by cations of the dye azure A. The application of this substance to the test of HCl secretion by the stomach is based on the fact that the azure A cations are displaced by hydrogen ions of the gastric acid releasing the dye, which is absorbed in the intestine and excreted in the urine, imparting to the latter a blue or blue-green color.

The fasting patient is given a gastric secretory stimulant orally or parenterally (caffeine salts, histamine) and at the time of their maximal secretory response, the resin is administered in aqueous suspension. The appearance of a blue color in the urine, collected for a standard period after the ingestion of the dye complex, indicates that the patient's stomach secretes HCl. This test yields about 3 per cent false positive and a similar number of false negative results. Where the result is negative, the implied achlorhydria must be verified by conventional gastric analysis. The occurrence of false positives impairs the value of the tubeless method as a screening test for achlorhydria.

The most important method of quantitative gastric analysis is the *measurement of the basal acid secretion.* The gastric secretion is continuously aspirated overnight or for at least 1½ hours in the morning. Although most ulcer patients secrete less than 5 mEq. HCl/hr. in the basal state, only exceptionally will a non-ulcer individual secrete in excess of that amount. If surgery is planned, the finding of an intense basal hypersecretion alerts the surgeon to the necessity for maximum measures aimed at reducing the acid-secreting potential.

Section of the vagus nerves sharply reduces the basal secretion; if it does not, particularly in the case of an unsatisfactory postoperative result, an *insulin hypoglycemia test* is undertaken as the definitive procedure for verifying vagal continuity. After a control gastric aspiration period of 1 hour, a blood sample is taken; 20 units of regular insulin are injected intravenously (15 units in patients weighing less than 60 kg.) and gastric aspiration is continued for 3 hours. A second blood sample is taken about 45 minutes after injection. Failure of the gas-

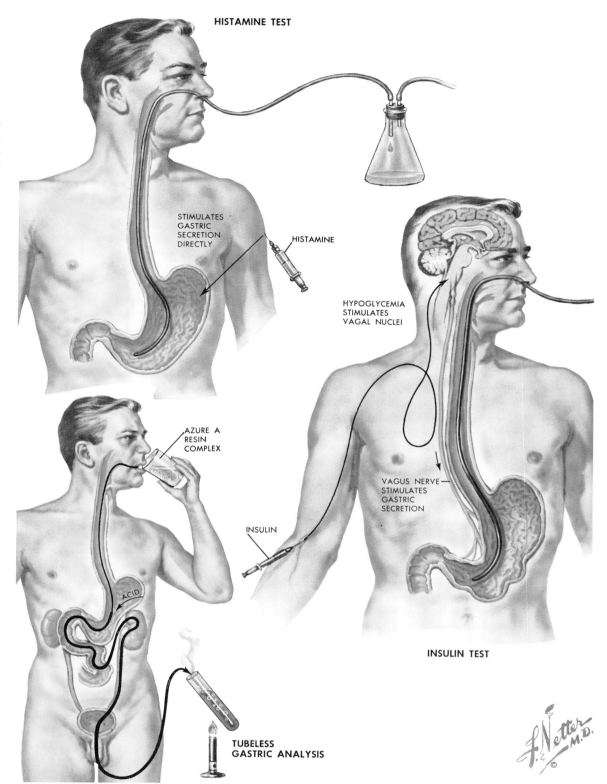

HISTAMINE TEST

STIMULATES GASTRIC SECRETION DIRECTLY

HISTAMINE

HYPOGLYCEMIA STIMULATES VAGAL NUCLEI

AZURE A RESIN COMPLEX

VAGUS NERVE STIMULATES GASTRIC SECRETION

INSULIN

ACID

INSULIN TEST

TUBELESS GASTRIC ANALYSIS

tric secretion to increase above the pre-insulin level during a hypoglycemia of at least 50 per cent of the control blood sugar value indicates complete vagotomy.

An additional quantitative method of gastric analysis, which is perhaps deserving of more widespread use, is the caffeine test (not illustrated). After the basal aspiration, 500 mg. of caffeine sodium benzoate in 200 ml. of water are introduced into the stomach through a Levin tube, which is then clamped for 30 minutes, after which the stomach is emptied completely and aspirated continuously until six 15-minute fractions have been obtained. A concentration of HCl in the last specimen exceeding 50 mEq./l. or an output of acid over the 90-minute period exceeding 6 mEq. is strongly suggestive of a duodenal ulcer.

Attempts have been made to employ the determination of uropepsinogen as a clinical test of gastric secretion, on the theory that the output of pepsinogen

in the urine is directly proportional to the secretion of pepsin into the stomach and, therefore, an index of the activity of the gastric glands. The majority of those who have concerned themselves with this problem have concluded that the amount of uropepsinogen excreted is not a reliable index of gastric secretion. While it is generally agreed that the average uropepsinogen values are significantly higher in duodenal ulcer patients than in normal individuals, the overlap of the two groups is too wide to make the test of diagnostic value. The uropepsinogen determination might be of interest in the diagnosis of pernicious anemia, and in a case with gastro-intestinal bleeding of undetermined origin. Absence of uropepsinogen would indicate atrophy of the glandular elements of the stomach and would support the suspicion of pernicious anemia. A very high value of uropepsinogen favors the probability of a duodenal ulcer.

CYTOLOGIC DIAGNOSIS

The diagnosis of upper gastro-intestinal malignancies in radiologically and endoscopically equivocal cases has been improved materially by the development of nonsurgical techniques for obtaining tissue from the suspicious areas for microscopic examination. The most extensively used of these methods is that of exfoliative cytology, or the examination of cellular material obtained from the lining of the esophagus, stomach or duodenum by lavage or abrasion. In the *lavage method* a Levin tube, with perforations appropriately placed, is passed under fluoroscopic visualization to the level of the suspected lesion. The area is irrigated by alternate introduction and withdrawal, with a syringe or some mechanical device, of normal saline or a digestant such as papain or chymotrypsin. The choice of solution is apparently not nearly as important as the rapid handling of the returns from the washings. These are collected in refrigerated containers, neutralized and centrifuged immediately, and the sediment is smeared on slides and fixed in alcohol-ether. After appropriate staining, the slides are studied by someone experienced in interpreting cytologic smears. The *preparation on the left* was obtained by saline lavage of the stomach and was reported as "reticulum cell sarcoma". The fixed tissue sections from the subsequently resected lesion were interpreted as "reticulum cell sarcoma with unusual features". The postoperative course was more suggestive of a highly anaplastic, small cell carcinoma, which, at autopsy, proved to be the correct diagnosis.

Abrasive devices for obtaining tissue for cytologic diagnosis include an intragastric brush, a net surrounding an inflatable balloon, and various types of sponges. The *intragastric brush* is introduced distal to the lesion and is rotated as it is withdrawn. Likewise, the sponge, or the net-covered balloon inflated within the stomach, is passed back and forth for the purpose of trapping abraded tissue in the interstices of the sponge or net. The material so obtained is processed by appropriate modifications of the usual methods of preparing histologic sections. The efficiency of these various exfoliative cytologic techniques is generally reported to be about the same by the protagonists of the respective methods, ranging from 50 to 75 per cent. With any of the recommended techniques, an occasional false positive diagnosis is reported.

Lavage of the duodenum has been rewarding, in the hands of several investigators, in the diagnosis of malignancies of the pancreas and biliary tract.

Aspiration biopsy by the *suction tube* provides a superior specimen of tissue for

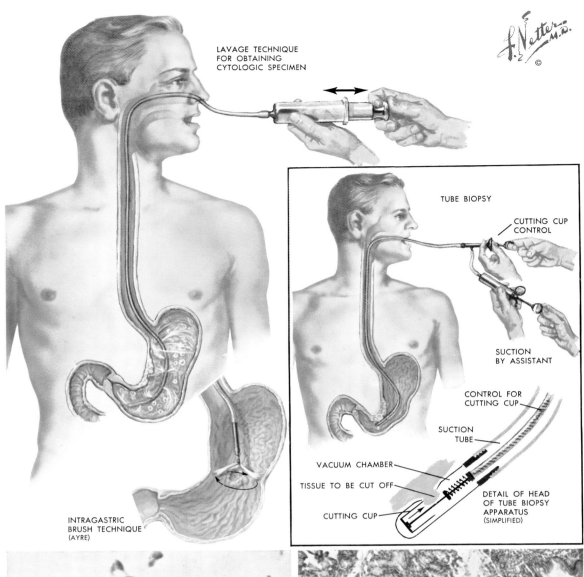

LAVAGE TECHNIQUE FOR OBTAINING CYTOLOGIC SPECIMEN

TUBE BIOPSY

CUTTING CUP CONTROL

SUCTION BY ASSISTANT

CONTROL FOR CUTTING CUP

SUCTION TUBE

VACUUM CHAMBER

TISSUE TO BE CUT OFF

CUTTING CUP

DETAIL OF HEAD OF TUBE BIOPSY APPARATUS (SIMPLIFIED)

INTRAGASTRIC BRUSH TECHNIQUE (AYRE)

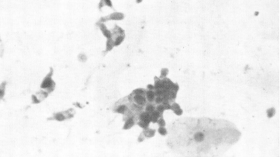

GASTRIC FLUID: LARGE CLUMP OF MALIGNANT GASTRIC EPITHELIAL CELLS WITH DENSE NUCLEI THAT VARY SOMEWHAT IN SIZE AND SHAPE; LARGE SQUAMOUS EPITHELIAL CELL AND ISOLATED BRONCHIAL EPITHELIAL CELLS WITH CLEARLY VISIBLE SURFACE CILIA
DIAGNOSIS: CLASS V—MALIGNANT GASTRIC EPITHELIAL CELLS

ASPIRATION (TUBE) BIOPSY OF GASTRIC MUCOSA: VILLOUS—TYPE METAPLASIA OF SURFACE GLANDS AND CLUSTERS OF BASALLY SITUATED METAPLASTIC ANTRAL—TYPE GLANDS
DIAGNOSIS: CHRONIC GASTRITIS

microscopic examination at the cost of less accuracy in obtaining the tissue from the site of the lesion. The cutting head of the suction tube is introduced through the mouth to the area of the lesion under fluoroscopic control, a maneuver which is, nevertheless, relatively "blind", since it is performed without any contrast material as a guide to the presumed site of the abnormality, which must be gauged by other landmarks such as the diaphragm or the spine. The yield is, accordingly, better in the diagnosis of gastritis than of neoplasms. When the tube is presumed to be in place, withdrawal of the piston of a large syringe communicating with the vacuum chamber will indicate, by the degree of resistance encountered, whether the aperture in the *cutting cup* is in contact with the wall of the lumen. If it is, a piece of tissue will be drawn into the cup, where it is amputated by a pull on the rod connected to the cylindrical knife-edge. The proce-

dure is repeated one or two times in adjacent areas before the tube is removed.

Control of the biopsy site is partially improved by taking the biopsy through a gastroscope equipped either with a biopsy forceps or with a suction tube.

The *suction-tube biopsy* in the accompanying illustration was obtained from the pyloric portion of the stomach in a case in which the X-ray appearance presented the problem of differentiating an infiltrating lesion from an antral gastritis. The relatively greater accuracy of placing the tube in the pyloric portion accounts for the particular value of the suction-tube biopsy in contributing to the clarification of antral lesions.

Photomicrographs kindly provided by Leo Kaplan, M.D., Director of Laboratories, Mount Sinai Hospital, Los Angeles.

Section V

DISEASES OF THE MOUTH AND PHARYNX

by

FRANK H. NETTER, M.D.

in collaboration with

MAX L. SOM, M.D., F.A.C.S.
Plates 27-33

LEO STERN, JR., D.D.S.
Plates 1-26

Congenital Anomalies of Oral Cavity

Congenital clefts of the face and mouth result from incomplete fusion of the embryonic facial segments. Their incidence varies, according to different authors, between 1 in 700 to 2000 births. The cause of these congenital malformations has not been clearly established. In 20 to 30 per cent of the cases, the same abnormality appeared in the same family in more than one generation. Besides this hereditary trend, dietary deficiencies, alcoholism, maternal infections, certain intra-uterine conditions and a variety of other situations have been said to play an etiologic rôle.

The cleft lip, cheiloschisis, better known as *harelip*, originates most often on the junction of the maxilla and median nasal process (later the philtrum) and may be *unilateral* or *bilateral*, ranging from a notching of the lip margin or merely a scarlike groove to a *complete cleft* extending into the nasal fossa. When confined to the lip, it remains a prealveolar cleft, but it may also involve the alveolar ridge and palate (classified as "alveolar" and "postalveolar cleft"). The median side of the cleft lip is thin, poorly developed and, at times, firmly attached to the bone. The lateral tissue is thick and well supplied with muscle. The nose is deviated, with a distinct flattening of the ala of the affected side, the margin lying at a lower level than the normal side. The columella is tilted. If not directly involved in the defect, the alveolar bone may be deformed in its midportion, owing to the deflection of the nasal septum. A flattening of both alae without other deviation or asymmetry is seen in bilateral clefts.

A cleft of the palate (palatoschisis or uranoschisis) may extend from the uvula forward and may involve part or all of the soft and hard palates. It is frequently associated with a cleft of the alveolar process (gnathoschisis), which, if complete, separates the premaxilla and the maxilla on one side, with the nasal septum attached to the palatal process of the opposite side. A bilateral alveolar cleft isolates the premaxilla, which is pulled upward and forward and continues as a median cleft of the palate. The nasal

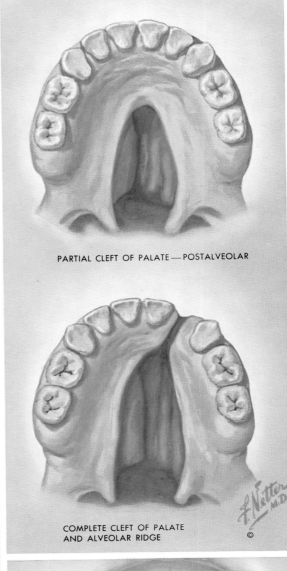

UNILATERAL HARELIP — PARTIAL

UNILATERAL HARELIP — COMPLETE, INVOLVING ALVEOLAR RIDGE

BILATERAL HARELIP

PARTIAL CLEFT OF PALATE — POSTALVEOLAR

COMPLETE CLEFT OF PALATE AND ALVEOLAR RIDGE

TORUS PALATINUS

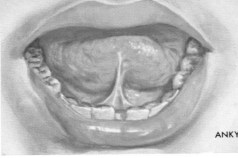

ANKYLOGLOSSIA

septum is free in the midline. The alveolar cleft either usurps the position of the lateral incisor or separates this tooth from the central incisor or cuspid. The dental arch tends to be fairly normal when the alveolar ridge is intact, but extensive clefts show irregular occlusion, with missing, rotating and misplaced teeth. The alveolar and postalveolar defect interferes with sucking, while swallowing of air with food and its regurgitation through the nose are deterrents to adequate nutrition. Intercurrent infection of the nasopharynx involving the Eustachian tube, otitis media, labyrinthitis or deafness are serious consequences. Undernourishment may account for chronic infections and poor growth of the child with a cleft palate. Later, because of air escape through the nose and failure of palatopharyngeal closure, speech defects result, which may sometimes be corrected by surgical repair alone but usually require

also careful training and correction of speech habits. The time of surgical intervention, around the second year, is considerably later than for cleft lip, which most surgeons elect to repair at 4 to 6 weeks of age.

Ankyloglossia, another congenital abnormality, is seen rarely as a fusion of the tongue and floor of the mouth but usually as an excessive lingual frenum attachment ("tongue-tie"). The tongue cannot protrude beyond the teeth but arches in the midportion. The deformity retards proper speech development. *Torus palatinus* (and similarly torus mandibularis) is a genetically and anthropologically (60 per cent occurrence in Eskimos) linked growth, or exostosis, which consists of very dense bone, with little or no spongiosa, in elliptical or nodular shape in the midline of the palate. It begins to develop in adolescence but may go unnoticed until it interferes with the construction of a denture.

ABNORMALITIES OF TEMPOROMANDIBULAR JOINT

The glenoid fossa of the temporal bone and the mandibular condyle constitute a compound, diarthrodial joint, separated by an articular cartilage and enclosed by a synovial membrane and capsular ligament (see page 5). The upper compartment (meniscotemporal articulation) permits gliding motions, while the lower compartment (meniscocondylar articulation) functions as a hinge. Muscle action (see pages 8 and 9) and the occlusal relations of the teeth are the major determining factors in movements of the joint, with the anatomy of the bony surfaces and the articular ligaments less important than in other joints.

Facial height and form depend largely on the proper growth of the mandible. While the maxilla grows by apposition against the anterior base of the cranium, the mandible develops vertically by an epiphyseal type of growth from the head of the condyle. Interference with the chondrogenic zone of the condyle has a disastrous effect on the facial profile. Growth arrest, partial or complete, may be the result of otitis media, radiation, arthritis, condylar fracture, or trauma by obstetric forceps. Complete arrest of mandibular growth or ankylosis occurring during childhood gives rise to *micrognathia,* a deformity in which the condyloid process is shortened with an obtuse mandibular angle, a stunted mental protuberance, and a concave lower border of the bone owing to the powerful action of the depressor muscles. A recessive, birdlike profile results.

Dislocation of the condyle may ensue from a blow on the ramus or chin when the mouth is open, from yawning, or from excessive manipulation of the jaw under general anesthesia. The dislocation is nearly always forward, the condyle resting anterior to the articular eminence. Backward displacement occurs rarely from a forceful blow, at the expense of the posterior attachment of the meniscus. The condyle then rests on the bony surface of the fossa, with a slight tilting of the mandible and an open position of the

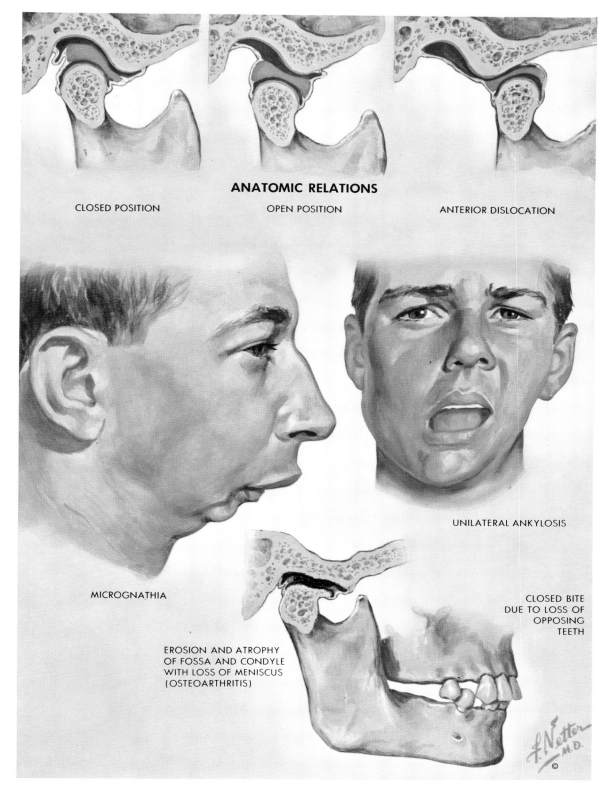

ANATOMIC RELATIONS

CLOSED POSITION   OPEN POSITION   ANTERIOR DISLOCATION

UNILATERAL ANKYLOSIS

MICROGNATHIA

CLOSED BITE DUE TO LOSS OF OPPOSING TEETH

EROSION AND ATROPHY OF FOSSA AND CONDYLE WITH LOSS OF MENISCUS (OSTEOARTHRITIS)

anterior teeth. Other dislocations are seen only with fractures of the condyle or base of the skull. Chronic injury to the joint ligaments as, *e.g.,* by malocclusion of the teeth, may lead to subluxation. A hypermobility of the condyle is accompanied by a "clicking" or "snapping" sound at the termination of opening. This sound is thought to be due to the condyle's slipping anteriorly past the meniscus and then striking the articular eminence. The same action occurs when the attachment of the external pterygoid muscle to the capsule has been lost through injury.

Fracture of the condyle is seen frequently as a result of a frontal blow on the chin. Displacement of the condylar head is sometimes caused by the trauma itself; more commonly, it is caused by the pull of the external pterygoid muscle (see pages 8 and 9) inward and forward. Following bilateral fracture of the condylar necks, the molar teeth close prematurely, while the incisors are still separated.

Ankylosis may result from injury or inflammation of the joint. Occasionally, extra-articular causes, such as fibrosis and cicatrization of the muscles attached to the mandible, cause a false ankylosis. This may happen in healing of extensive wounds of the face and in postradiation cases of mandibular carcinoma. In ankylosis proper, the cause can be a comminuted fracture of the condyle, a suppurative arthritis or osteomyelitis, intracapsular hemorrhage or rheumatoid arthritis. The ankylosis may be fibrous, with perceptible but slight movement, or bony. *Unilateral ankylosis* is characterized by a marked limitation of movement and a deviation toward the affected side on opening of the mandible. The uninjured condyle describes an arc about the injured condyle, which acts as a fulcrum. Muscles on the normal side hypertrophy; on the injured side they atrophy.

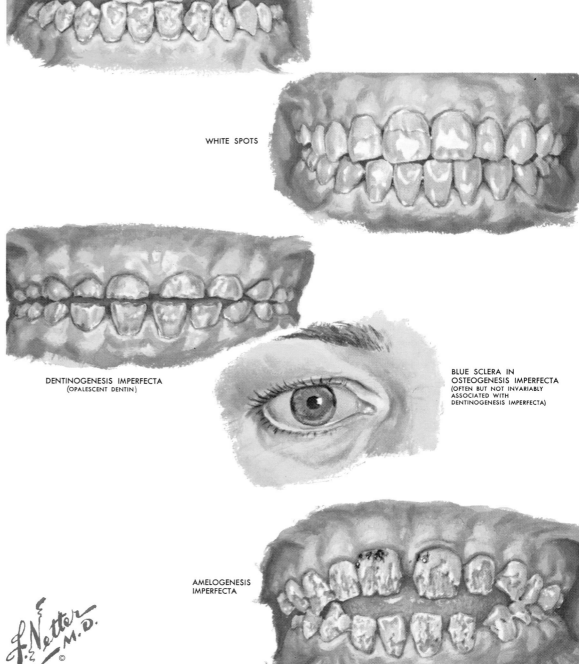

HYPOPLASIA OF ENAMEL

WHITE SPOTS

DENTINOGENESIS IMPERFECTA
(OPALESCENT DENTIN)

BLUE SCLERA IN OSTEOGENESIS IMPERFECTA
(OFTEN BUT NOT INVARIABLY ASSOCIATED WITH DENTINOGENESIS IMPERFECTA)

AMELOGENESIS IMPERFECTA

DENTAL ABNORMALITIES

The teeth exhibit many structural abnormalities which may be of significance for the general condition of the patient. Some furnish evidence of developmental interference by generalized diseases such as syphilis and rickets. Other less profound defects are simply chronologic signs of transient metabolic interference or produce minor cosmetic blemishes. Finally, some specific anomalies, such as amelogenesis imperfecta, result in disastrous wasting of tooth substance which impairs masticatory function unless restored by heroic dental treatment.

Hypoplasia of the enamel is produced by defective amelogenesis in the deciduous and permanent teeth and persists unchanged after the enamel is formed. It, therefore, differs fundamentally from caries, erosion and other acquired lesions. Enamel formation begins in the fifth intra-uterine month for deciduous teeth and in the fourth postnatal month for some of the permanent teeth, being completed at the age of from 4 to 7 years. The hypoplastic defects can usually be dated chronologically by the particular teeth in which they appear, since each has a different time of calcification. Rickets or other severe nutritional deficiencies or primary hypoparathyroidism during the first and second years of life may sometimes play an etiologic rôle. However, most of these hypoplasias are idiopathic and cannot be precisely explained.

The aspect of teeth with hypoplastic enamel ranges from shallow grooves on the smooth enamel to a number of deep grooves or areas of complete exposure of the underlying dentinal junction. Use of a dental explorer as a diagnostic instrument reveals a hard surface, in contrast to that of caries. The irregular outline and texture of the lesion distinguish it from a smooth abrasion or erosion of unknown origin. The mechanism of hypoplasia is believed to be either a temporary delay in calcification, with a resulting distortion and collapse of uncalcified matrix, or an actual degeneration of ameloblastic cells. Hypoplastic teeth are no more subject to caries than are normal teeth, but possibly a carious lesion will progress with greater rapidity.

White spots are opaque white patches on the enamel surface without loss of substance. The cementing substance between the enamel rods is lacking, probably also as a result of metabolic interference dur-

ing formation. The refractive property of the enamel layer is altered, but no further change is noted throughout life. This condition is not to be confused with fluorosis, or "mottled" enamel.

Amelogenesis imperfecta is a very rare hereditary hypoplasia of enamel. In one of the two types described, enamel is completely missing (agenesis), and, in the other, enamel matrix is laid down but fails to calcify. Both deciduous and permanent teeth are affected. Such enamel is soft and may be easily broken away from the dentin by normal wear or by an instrument. Consequently, the young individual may show intact crowns on recently erupted teeth, with progressing deterioration of the enamel on teeth which erupted earlier. In the older individual very little enamel is left, chiefly present at the cervical line. The soft dentin is whitish gray and rapidly discolors further, and is worn down to stumps in the course of

years of mastication. An open bite is frequently associated with the defect in amelogenesis.

In *dentinogenesis imperfecta* (*opalescent dentin*), another rare hereditary disorder, both deciduous and permanent dentition are affected. The crowns of the teeth are of normal dimension, but the roots are stunted, as viewed by X-rays. The pulp canals are markedly reduced in size or completely obliterated. The color of the teeth as they erupt ranges from slightly pink to darker bluish gray or brownish gray. This appearance is changed, however, by the tendency of the enamel to fracture and peel away owing to defective dentin, leaving an atypical, amber-brown dentin which is translucent or opalescent. The teeth show rapid wear. Sensitivity is lacking, because of continual deposit of secondary dentin in the pulp. A dystrophic arrangement of dentinal tubules and

(*Continued on page 107*)

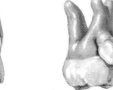

GEMINATION   ENAMEL PEARL   SUPERNUMERARY CROWN AND PORTION OF ROOT   FUSION OF TEETH   SUPERNUMERARY TOOTH BETWEEN ROOTS OF NORMAL MOLAR

DENTAL ABNORMALITIES

(Continued from page 106)

abnormal blood supply via canals which penetrate the dentinal substance and impart the brownish color are characteristic. This condition may be part of a generalized osteogenesis imperfecta, which is characterized by brittle bones and *blue sclerae*.

Gemination is the production of twin teeth from one enamel organ. The epithelium of the enamel organ invaginates as though to produce two separate teeth. If this abortive fission is symmetrical, the result is a bifid tooth, with fully developed crowns and confluent roots. Asymmetrical division gives rise to a smaller accessory tooth or component. When the gemination process is multiple, the designation "odontoma" should apply. A *fused tooth* is more common in the deciduous dentition, differing from twin teeth in that some physical pressure has caused a joining of young tooth germs (both enamel organ and dental papilla). If the fusion is late, only the roots may be joined, since the crowns have already developed. *Supernumerary teeth*, which are wholly formed, are usually due to hyperplasia of the dental lamina forming extra tooth germs. Such a tooth may be normal in shape, peg-shaped or of rudimentary size, lying *between the roots of a normal molar*. A *supernumerary cusp or root*, including the *enamel pearl*, on the other hand, is formed by local hyperplasia of the tooth germ, or in some cases of invagination of the dental epithelium as in geminated teeth.

Destruction of tooth surface by mechanical agency, whether from coarse abrasive foods, habits of chewing or grinding the teeth, tooth brushing or special occupational practices, such as holding nails between the teeth, is called abrasion. The term *attrition* is used for the more natural wear of incisal and occlusal surfaces, whereas abrasion from tooth brushing commonly affects the cervical parts of teeth on one side (the left side for right-handed individuals) and is most marked in the cuspid and bicuspid regions. *Erosion* is a chemical process which may, at times, be indistinguishable from abrasive lesions. Occasionally, habitual sucking of lemons or intake of acid substances, particularly hydrochloric acid as a medication, or lactic acid, as produced locally by lozenges and hard candies, results in surface erosion. More often, however, an alteration of the saliva, probably enzymatic in character, which appears in an affected individual in the

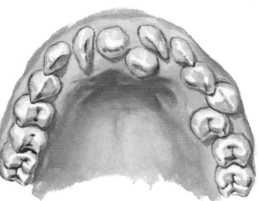

SUPERNUMERARY TEETH DISPLACING INCISORS

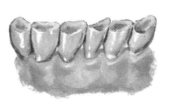

ATTRITION (INCISAL EDGES)

EROSION (CERVICAL AREA)

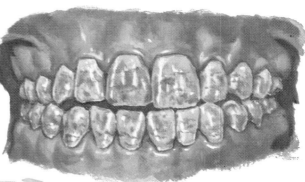

BROWN MOTTLING (FLUOROSIS)

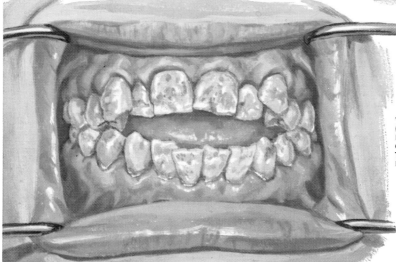

VITAMIN D DEFICIENCY (RICKETS): DEFORMITY OF JAWS, OPEN BITE, CROWDING OF TEETH, HYPOPLASIA AND PITTING OF ENAMEL

thirties or later, may cause wedge-shaped or spoon-shaped destruction on labial and buccal surfaces, particularly at the gingival margins. The lesions are usually smooth, similar to abrasions, but may be pitted and roughened in some cases.

Fluorosis, or *mottled enamel*, is an endemic lesion in geographic areas where the content of fluoride ion in the drinking water exceeds 2 p.p.m. It occurs only in individuals who are exposed to a higher than 2 p.p.m. fluorine content of the water during the years of enamel formation. After the age of 14 years, only the third molars might reveal mottling, if at all. For widespread fluorosis of all the teeth, exposure must be before the age of 6 to 7 years. The great interest in fluoride therapy via water supply in public health projects is based on the increased immunity to dental caries which has been ascertained in both endemic areas and those artificially treated with 1½ p.p.m.

of fluoride. With this concentration, no mottling of enamel appears, yet a caries reduction of up to 60 to 70 per cent has been observed. The clinical findings in endemic fluorosis vary as to degree. Slightly affected teeth will show small chalky spots, ranging to wider paper-white areas or striations. The surface is hard and glazed in mild defects. If the mottling is more severe, pitting and irregular marring or excoriation, with mottled color changes of chalky white and shades of brown from yellow to almost black appear.

In the course of rickets, severe changes in the developing dentition may occur. The rachitic syndrome includes enamel hypoplasia, poorly calcified dystrophic dentin, short roots and a delayed eruption and crowding of all teeth, sometimes associated with an open bite and underdevelopment of dental arches. Deformity of the mandible may also result from the pull of the masticatory muscles.

PERIODONTAL DISEASE

Disease of the periodontal tissues constitutes the chief reason, more prevalent even than dental caries, for the loss of teeth. It has been described as almost universally present among adults. Designated formerly by such terms as scurvy of the gums, Riggs's disease and pyorrhea alveolaris, it has not been until the last two or three decades that its diagnosis, classification and treatment have been systematically explored.

The manifestations include both inflammatory and dystrophic changes which may occasionally be distinct but usually reinforce one another. A *marginal periodontitis* is the sequel to a usually long-standing marginal gingivitis (see page 111) and generally includes all the signs of marginal gingivitis with an additional resorption of the alveolar *crestal bone* and of the adjacent *peridental membrane*. The formation of a periodontal pocket, being a pathologic alteration of the gingival attachment, is a pathognomonic sign of this condition. The epithelial lining of the gingival crevice is ulcerated, with a destruction of peridental membrane fibers and an inflammatory cell infiltrate in the corium, sometimes visible clinically as a purulent discharge. The epithelial attachment is displaced and takes successively deeper positions as the pocket increases. Beginning with a notching of the alveolar crest, bone resorption continues with a destruction of the cribriform plate (lamina dura). Under the influence of occlusal trauma, the pocket penetrates toward the apex of the root; such pocket formation is often described on roentgenographic evidence as "vertical" in type and indicates a more advanced stage of periodontal damage than does the simpler "horizontal" resorption. The local irritative factors governing pocket formation include deposits of calculi from the saliva and serum, food impaction, overhanging or poorly shaped fillings and other restorations, improper oral hygiene, mouth breathing, abnormal muscle and *high frenum attachments,* as well as other disturbances of gingival form or function.

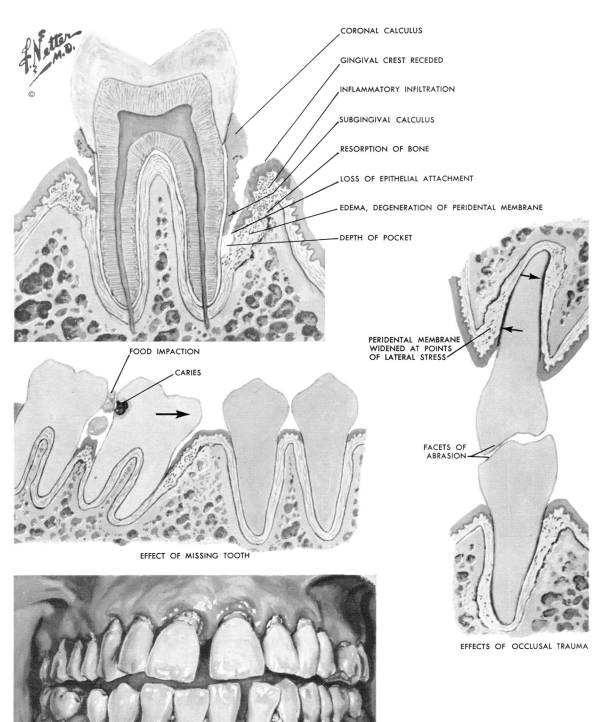

CORONAL CALCULUS

GINGIVAL CREST RECEDED

INFLAMMATORY INFILTRATION

SUBGINGIVAL CALCULUS

RESORPTION OF BONE

LOSS OF EPITHELIAL ATTACHMENT

EDEMA, DEGENERATION OF PERIDENTAL MEMBRANE

DEPTH OF POCKET

FOOD IMPACTION

CARIES

EFFECT OF MISSING TOOTH

PERIDENTAL MEMBRANE WIDENED AT POINTS OF LATERAL STRESS

FACETS OF ABRASION

EFFECTS OF OCCLUSAL TRAUMA

ADVANCED PERIODONTITIS: MIGRATION OF TEETH, GINGIVAL COLOR CHANGES AND HYPERPLASIA, CALCULUS, HIGH FRENUM ATTACHMENT

Furthermore, complex dystrophic changes may occur. Periodontosis, for example, is an unusual noninflammatory disease, beginning in young individuals, marked by progressive loosening and migration of teeth with deep infrabony pockets. Much more common are the various derangements caused by *occlusal trauma,* which are being increasingly identified as the result of grinding (bruxism), clenching or similar habits producing repetitive and excessive contacts of tooth on tooth. To such nonfunctional stresses may be added the effects of improper tooth form or position, overloaded abutment teeth under prosthetic replacements, or *abrasion of teeth.* Here, lateral stresses are augmented, with injury and eventual widening of the peridental membrane and mobility of the tooth.

A *missing tooth* is a familiar example of the combination of irritative and dystrophic factors. Initiated by an irritant such as calculus, tilting and forward drifting of a tooth next to the gap permit an open contact, with food impaction causing an interproximal pocket, usually with caries of the distal tooth surface. The stress of occlusion on such a tooth may, in addition, cause acceleration of pocket formation on the mesial aspect.

Migration of teeth, a late symptom in periodontitis, is a consequence of open contacts, wedging of food particles, extrusion of teeth through the pressure of granulation tissues and other traumatic relationships in the deranged occlusion. Mobility of the teeth becomes marked as bone resorption increases the ratio of dental parts supported by bone to those not supported. The gingiva in this phase of periodontitis is typically soft and spongy, duskier in color than normal, with retraction of the margin and abundant accretions of calculus.

ODONTOGENIC INFECTIONS

Their Spread and Abscess Formation

The most frequent causes of inflammatory swellings of the jaws, the middle and lower thirds of the face and the upper part of the neck are infections of the teeth, with the pulp canal or the periodontal membrane as the primary focus. The *dento-alveolar abscess* takes first place with regard to frequency. It is usually the end result of dental caries; more rarely, it originates in a tooth devitalized by trauma. The abscess may develop very acutely and burrow through bone to lodge under the periosteum, which it then perforates to induce an intra-oral or a facial abscess. In other instances, a more chronic inflammatory process leads to an organized granuloma at the root apex, which may remain dormant for years, evolve slowly into a sterile cyst or, at a period of lowered resistance, fulminate into an acute alveolar abscess. While the abscess is confined to the bone, pain and extreme tenderness of the involved tooth are the characteristic symptoms. By the pressure of edema, the tooth is extruded from its socket, so that each contact with the teeth of the opposing jaw aggravates the pain.

The periodontal abscess is the second common odontogenic infection arising from an ulcerated periodontal crevice (pocket), which is created by the loss of attachment (*poor contact*) between tooth on one side and investing gingiva, periodontal membrane and bone on the other. This periodontitis, as the process should be designated (instead of "pyorrhea"), occurs almost universally and with increasing severity in older age groups and is the most prominent etiologic factor in the loss of teeth. *Calculous deposits,* traumatic occlusion, *irritating filling margins* and other factors may play a contributing rôle. A third odontogenic infection, the *pericoronal abscess,* originates in a traumatized or otherwise inflamed flap of gingiva overlying a partly erupted tooth, usually a lower third molar.

Odontogenic infections involve the soft tissues chiefly by *direct continuity* (by routes indicated by arrows and figures). Lymphatic spread plays a secondary rôle, while the hematogenous dissemination is rare as a route for facial abscesses. Bacteremia, however, is common and has been demonstrated as a transient phenomenon arising from chewing or manipulation of apically or periodontally infected teeth. Local extension follows the line of minimal resistance and depends on the particular tooth and the anatomic relationship of bone, fascia and muscle attachment. Where the mus-

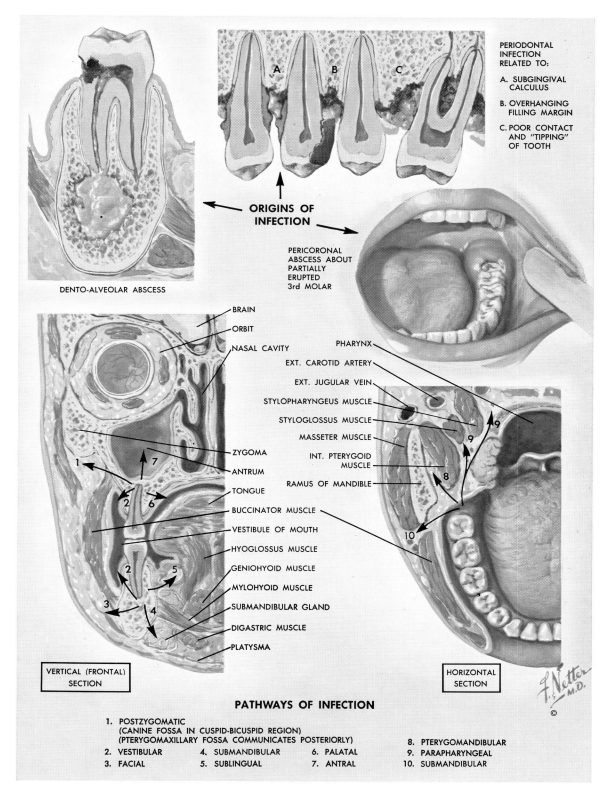

ORIGINS OF INFECTION

DENTO-ALVEOLAR ABSCESS

PERIODONTAL INFECTION RELATED TO:
A. SUBGINGIVAL CALCULUS
B. OVERHANGING FILLING MARGIN
C. POOR CONTACT AND "TIPPING" OF TOOTH

PERICORONAL ABSCESS ABOUT PARTIALLY ERUPTED 3rd MOLAR

BRAIN
ORBIT
NASAL CAVITY
ZYGOMA
ANTRUM
TONGUE
BUCCINATOR MUSCLE
VESTIBULE OF MOUTH
HYOGLOSSUS MUSCLE
GENIOHYOID MUSCLE
MYLOHYOID MUSCLE
SUBMANDIBULAR GLAND
DIGASTRIC MUSCLE
PLATYSMA

PHARYNX
EXT. CAROTID ARTERY
EXT. JUGULAR VEIN
STYLOPHARYNGEUS MUSCLE
STYLOGLOSSUS MUSCLE
MASSETER MUSCLE
INT. PTERYGOID MUSCLE
RAMUS OF MANDIBLE

VERTICAL (FRONTAL) SECTION

HORIZONTAL SECTION

PATHWAYS OF INFECTION

1. POSTZYGOMATIC (CANINE FOSSA IN CUSPID-BICUSPID REGION) (PTERYGOMAXILLARY FOSSA COMMUNICATES POSTERIORLY)
2. VESTIBULAR
3. FACIAL
4. SUBMANDIBULAR
5. SUBLINGUAL
6. PALATAL
7. ANTRAL
8. PTERYGOMANDIBULAR
9. PARAPHARYNGEAL
10. SUBMANDIBULAR

cle layers act as a barrier, extensive cellulitis may spread along the fascial planes of the head and neck. Infections from the maxillary teeth may perforate the cortical bone of the palate, the vestibule or the regions separated from the mouth by attachments of the muscles of facial expression or the buccinator muscle. Those from the incisor teeth tend to involve the upper lip; from the cuspids and premolars, the canine fossa; and from the molar teeth, the infratemporal space or mucobuccal fold. The *vestibular abscess* is generally localized and not accompanied by excessive edema, owing to the softness of the tissues and lack of tension. In the advanced stage a shiny fluctuant swelling is visible at the region of the root apex or somewhat below it. *Abscess (postzygomatic) of the canine fossa* usually bulges into the buccal sulcus but is chiefly marked by swelling of the infraorbital region of the face and the lower eyelid. The

upper lid, the side of the nose and nasolabial fold and the upper lip may be involved by edema.

Infections of the mandibular teeth may give rise to swellings of the *vestibule* or the sublingual, submental or submandibular space. *Abscess of the submandibular region* is encountered with infections of the premolar and molar teeth. The classic sign is a large visible swelling below the mandible, extending to the face and distorting the lower mandibular border, extremely tender and accompanied by trismus. Submandibular space abscess may easily pass into the sublingual space (5) along the portion of the gland which perforates the mylohyoid muscle. This results in elevation of the floor of the mouth and displacement of the tongue to one side. The submental area may be invaded by passage of pus past the digastric muscle, resulting in a general swelling of the entire subman-

(Continued on page 110)

ODONTOGENIC INFECTIONS

Their Spread and Abscess Formation

(Continued from page 109)

dibular region. Dento-alveolar abscess from a lower molar tooth is capable of producing the most serious and fulminating infections of the submandibular (4), pterygomandibular (8) and parapharyngeal (9) pathways. A pterygomandibular abscess results in deep-seated pain and extreme trismus, with some deviation of the jaw owing to pterygoid muscle infiltration. Infection in this space may, in exceptional cases, enter the pterygoid and pharyngeal plexuses of veins and result in a cavernous sinus thrombosis. A parapharyngeal abscess causes bulging of the pharynx, with equally marked trismus.

The onset of a facial cellulitis is heralded by edema of the soft parts, often quite extensive and without discernible fluctuation. Pain increases with pressure and induration. As abscess formation progresses, the central area reveals pitting edema and eventually becomes shiny, red and superficially fluctuant. Pain and tenderness are related to pressure and induration. Temperature of 38.5 to 40° C., leukocytosis and severe toxemia are characteristic. Trismus occurs when the elevator muscles are affected by inflammation or reflex spasm due to pain. In some cases, rather than the typical abscess production, a chronic cellulitis follows the acute phase, with persistent, deeply attached swelling. A phlegmon may be apparent from the onset, with a brawny, indurated distention of muscular and subcutaneous layers, devoid of exudate and showing no tendency to localize.

Ludwig's angina, a purulent inflammation, begins as a phlegmon in the submandibular space, usually after a molar tooth infection or extraction, and spreads with great rapidity to occupy the submandibular region, bounded inferiorly by the hyoid bone. The floor of the mouth and tongue are raised through infiltration of extrinsic and intrinsic muscles. The hard, dusky swelling descends to the larynx, where edema of the glottis, combined with the pressure of the tongue against the pharynx, interferes with respiration. In addition to the usual flora of odontogenic infections (alpha, beta and gamma streptococci and occasional gram-negative bacilli), the bacterial picture in true phlegmon tends toward anaerobic organisms, or facultative anaerobes, and gangrene-producing mixed groups such as the fusospirochetal combination.

Osteomyelitis may produce cellulitis or abscess similar to the odontogenic variety. Its chief incidence is as a complication following a traumatic extraction,

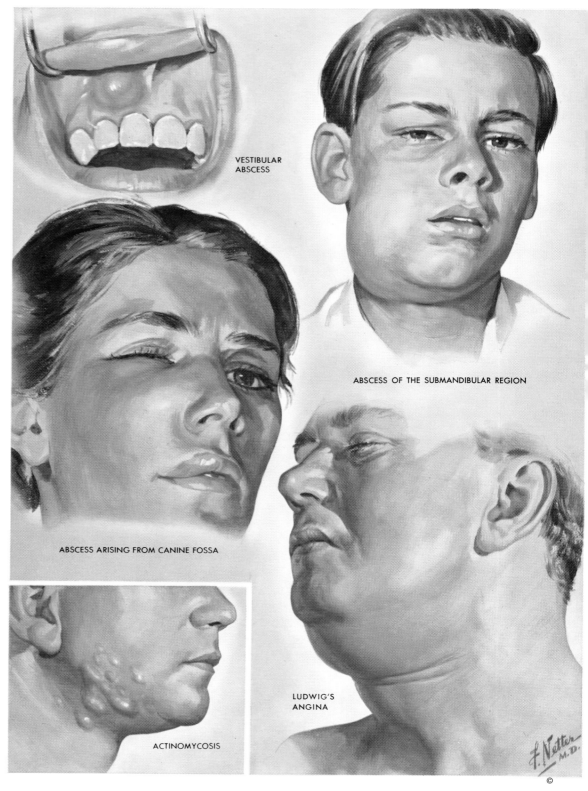

VESTIBULAR ABSCESS

ABSCESS OF THE SUBMANDIBULAR REGION

ABSCESS ARISING FROM CANINE FOSSA

LUDWIG'S ANGINA

ACTINOMYCOSIS

F. Netter M.D.

particularly if performed in the presence of acute infection, or a comminuted fracture involving the roots of teeth. Occasionally, it is the result of an abscess contiguous to a large area of bone, or a specific tuberculous or syphilitic infection. It begins most typically in the lower third molar region. Sclerotic or dense bone is more easily deprived of nutrition through trauma and is consequently infected by ever-present organisms of the mouth. Symptoms include those of cellulitis, with intermittent, deep, boring pain, and sequestrum and involucrum formation, seen radiographically in late stages. Wide radiolucent areas of bone, apparently involved by infection, surprisingly return to normal, following adequate drainage and minimal interference with sequestration.

A fracture of the mandible or maxilla is always compound where teeth are present, causing the line of fracture to be contaminated by oral organisms. This alone seldom produces infection, but projection of a tooth root in the line of fracture is usually responsible for suppuration. An externally compounded fracture is more prone to develop sepsis than is the usual variety.

Actinomycosis is a specific infection which occurs centrally in the jaws or peripherally in the soft tissues, where it forms an indurated swelling with multiple fistulae of the skin, resembling a chronic odontogenic abscess. The mode of inoculation is unknown, whether from exogenous Actinomyces bovis or from oral saprophytes, which are potential pathogens. Diagnosis is chiefly made by a smear of the exudate, which contains peculiar granular yellow bodies ("sulfur granules"), and the specific organism, the ray fungus (Actinomyces bovis), which causes the disease. Culture of the organism is unreliable, and biopsy may be required to establish the diagnosis.

GINGIVITIS

Marginal gingivitis is chiefly caused by local irritating factors, such as calcareous deposits on the teeth, food impaction, rough or overhanging filling margins and other dental restorations, malalignment of teeth, open contacts or other morphologic faults causing improper function, and hygienic neglect. These factors are, of course, complicated by such conditions as allergies, mouth breathing and pregnancy. Marginal gingivitis is the first stage in a complex periodontal syndrome which is further characterized by pocket formation and inflammation of the investing tissues (periodontitis) and, finally, by the periodontal abscess (see page 109). Clinically, the gingiva is conspicuous for a shiny pink or red or even cyanotic surface, for edema and a strong bleeding tendency of the margins and papillae of the gum. The graceful festoon of the gingiva is altered into irregular lines, while visible accretions are often seen distending the free margin from the teeth.

Hypertrophic gingivitis describes a frequent variation of the marginal type of inflammation, depending upon the individual response and the chronicity. An increase in size of the papillae is more noticeable than that of the free margin of gum and is especially related to accretions of calculus on the teeth. Hormonal alterations, as in pregnancy, will increase the degree of hypertrophy (see page 118). A different sort of enlargement is seen in diffuse, idiopathic fibromatosis of the gingiva, which is free of inflammation, normal in color and presents a uniform proliferation of gingiva in a firm, bulging mass throughout the jaws, similar to Dilantin gingival hyperplasia (see also page 116).

Necrotizing, ulcerative gingivitis, or fusospirochetal gingivitis, has been known by many other names, such as Vincent's or Plaut-Vincent's infection and trench mouth. It is a most common oral infection in young adults. Formerly considered to be highly communicable, necrotizing gingivitis is presently believed to be rather the result of a lowered local tissue resistance to certain organisms which are indigenous to most mouths. Predisposing causes are both general and local. Of the former it is known that avitaminosis B and C, gastro-intestinal disease and blood dyscrasias are of major importance. Yet in the average case emotional stress, fatigue and consumption of alcohol and tobacco frequently set the stage. Local causes include all conditions promoting growth of anaerobic organisms: gum flaps over third molar teeth, crowded and malposed teeth, inadequate contact areas, food-impaction areas and poor oral hygiene.

The flora of necrotizing, ulcerating stomatitis includes typically one or more types of spirochetes and the fusiform bacillus. A vibrio and coccus may be included, and some authors believe that this complete "fusospirochetal complex"

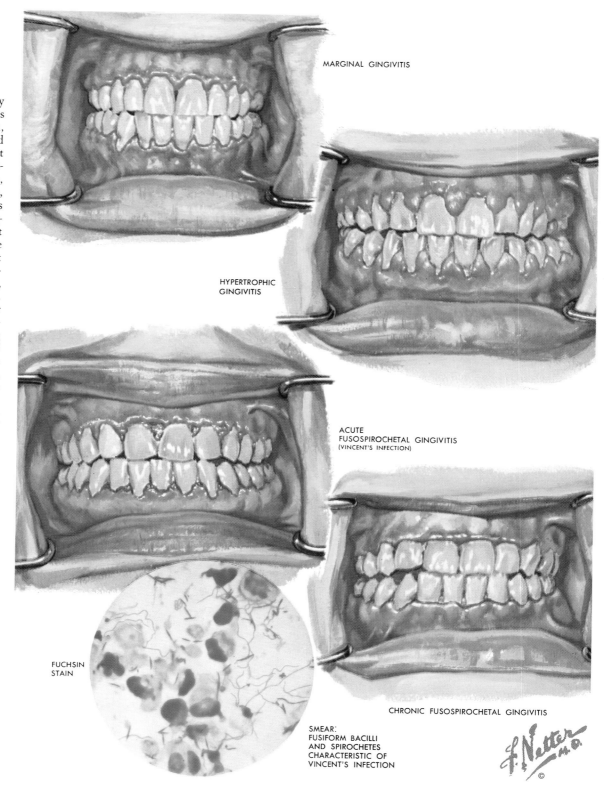

MARGINAL GINGIVITIS

HYPERTROPHIC GINGIVITIS

ACUTE FUSOSPIROCHETAL GINGIVITIS (VINCENT'S INFECTION)

FUCHSIN STAIN

CHRONIC FUSOSPIROCHETAL GINGIVITIS

SMEAR: FUSIFORM BACILLI AND SPIROCHETES CHARACTERISTIC OF VINCENT'S INFECTION

is required to produce the clinical symptoms, which vary as to severity. Ulceration and pseudomembrane formation are the specific lesions; the acute form is of rapid onset and may present an elevated, rarely high temperature, except in young or debilitated patients. Malaise, rapid pulse and other general toxic symptoms may dominate the picture. Submandibular lymphadenopathy is variable. Severe pain, a strong characteristic fetid odor and gingival bleeding are marked; objectively, these are related to flat, punched-out, grayish ulcers, which erode the tips of the papillary gingivae and spread to the margins, which are covered by a thin diphtheriticlike membrane. On slight pressure, bleeding may occur from all affected areas. In severe cases the lesions spread to the tongue, palate, pharynx and tonsils, with profuse salivation, thickly coated tongue and bleeding.

Chronic necrotizing gingivitis is a milder form of

this disease and is either present from the outset or is a slowed-down phase of the acute form. Subjective symptoms are much reduced. The first awareness is of bleeding when brushing the teeth. Careful retraction of the papillae may be necessary to reveal the typical necrosis. Pain is usually absent. Typical odor develops later, as destruction proceeds slowly. The response to therapy is far slower in the long-established cases, and recurrence is a constant hazard. As the architecture of the gingiva is altered, anaerobic areas are created and food retention is abetted, so that therapy against the infection alone is of only momentary value and must be directed to a restoration of proper gingival form.

The photomicrograph is reproduced by the courtesy of the Bacteriology Laboratory, Overlook Hospital, Summit, New Jersey.

MANIFESTATIONS OF TONGUE

As a consequence of the easy accessibility to clinical inspection, the tongue, in the course of medical history, has played a rather special rôle as a diagnostic indicator (see also page 95). Fascinated also by the great variety of aspects the tongue may assume in local and systemic diseases, physicians have in the past attributed to it an unduly exaggerated significance. Nevertheless, a careful observation of this organ has rightly remained one of the most important resources in physical diagnosis. The degree of moisture or dryness of the lingual mucosa may indicate disturbances of fluid balance. Changes in color, the appearance of edema, swelling, ulcers and inflammation or atrophy of the lingual papillae may represent signs of endocrine, nutritional, hemopoietic or metabolic disorders or infectious diseases (see pages 118, 119 and 120) or metallic poisoning (see page 116). On the other hand, it should be recognized that the tongue participates with the gingivae and the buccal mucosa in localized pathologic processes of the oral cavity, and that a number of conditions exist in which the surface or the parenchyma of the tongue itself is exclusively involved.

Fissured tongue must be included in the group of congenital lingual defects to which belong also ankyloglossia (see page 104), thyroglossal cyst, a lingual thyroid, a cleft or bifid tongue, as well as a congenitally small or large or hypermobile tongue. The fissured tongue, sometimes also called grooved or scrotal tongue, is characterized by deep depressions or furrows, which run mostly in a longitudinal direction starting near the tip and disappearing gradually at the posterior third of the dorsum. Both the length and depth of the furrows vary and can best be demonstrated by stretching the tongue laterally with tongue blades. It has often been observed that the fissures form a leaflike pattern, with a median crack larger than the other furrows. In general, the larger grooves run parallel, with smaller branches directed toward the margin of the tongue. The mucosal lining of the crevices is smooth and devoid of papillae. Only seldom does this congenital condition give cause for subjective symptoms and, if it does, the complaint may concern mild pains on eating acid or spicy foods. Sometimes, it happens that a fissured tongue is asso-

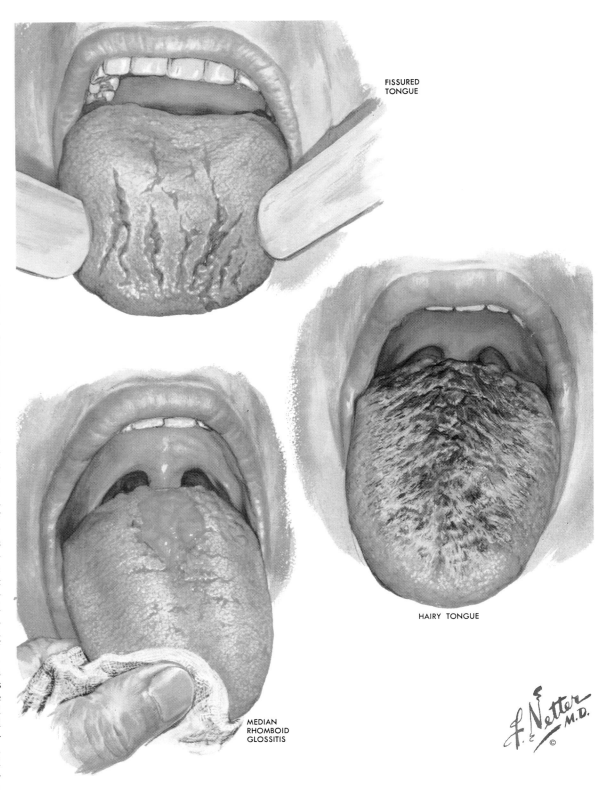

FISSURED TONGUE

MEDIAN RHOMBOID GLOSSITIS

HAIRY TONGUE

ciated incidentally with macroglossia and with a geographic tongue, although these conditions have no intrinsic relation to each other. In the past, the two terms, geographic tongue and fissured tongue, have often been confused.

Hairy tongue, or black tongue, is an acquired discoloration. Thick, yellowish, brownish or black furry patches, made up of densely matted, hypertrophied filiform papillae, cover sometimes more than half of the dorsum linguae. The cause of this discoloration has not been established, though a variety of explanations have been offered in a speculative fashion. One school of thought assumes that the color derives from a pigment produced by bacteria or yeastlike organisms, or from an alteration of the normal pigmentation of the epithelial cells. Others consider that the phenomenon results from a hyperkeratosis of the papillae or a chemical staining of keratin, which con-

tains large quantities of sulfur-bearing amino acids and undergoes chemical changes when in contact with tannin, iron salts and other agents. The true black tongue has no relation to the niacin-deficiency blacktongue seen in dogs. Since many examples of idiopathic hairy tongue are seen, it is tempting to label as "pseudohairy tongue" the coloration seen secondary to various drugs and in bleeding states. Prolonged intake of many medicaments produces the identical histochemical and histopathologic picture. The most common incitants are strong oxidizing mouthwashes (perchlorate or peroxide), which may possibly oxidize the iron in hemoglobin. Various antibiotic troches can, however, produce a similar picture. The condition is usually painless and symptomless, but an accompanying stomatitis from antibiotics is often painful.

(Continued on page 113)

MANIFESTATIONS OF TONGUE

(Continued from page 112)

Median rhomboid glossitis is a misnomer, because it is not an inflammatory process but a developmental lesion resulting from failure of the lateral segments of the tongue to fuse completely before interposition of the fetal tuberculum impar. It is an oval or rhomboidal, red, slightly elevated area, about 1 cm. in width and 2 or 3 cm. long, contrasting in color with the surrounding parts of the dorsum. This area is devoid of papillae. Sometimes it may be nodular, mammillated or fissured. Except for an occasional secondary inflammation, it causes no subjective symptoms. Frequently, however, this condition gives rise to cancerophobia, and it is important that the character of the lesion be promptly recognized to relieve the fear.

Geographic tongue, otherwise labeled erythema migrans, Butlin's wandering rash, and many other names, is a chronic superficial desquamation of obscure etiology seen most often in children. It may, however, recur at intervals throughout life or persist unchanged in degree. The rash is confined to the dorsum of the tongue and appears, rarely, on its inferior surface. The dorsal surface is marked with irregular, denuded grayish patches, from which, at times, the papillae are shed to reveal a dark-red circle of smooth epithelium bordered by a whitish or yellow periphery of altered papillae, which have changed from normal color and are about to be shed in turn. The circles enlarge, intersect and produce a map-like configuration. The lesions appear depressed, compared with the papillated surface, and clearly delimited. Continued observation, which reveals the migratory character of the spots, is necessary to be sure of the diagnosis. The geographic tongue may sometimes be fissured or lobulated at the margin, where it contacts the teeth.

Megaloglossia is, on rare occasions, an isolated congenital anomaly. An acute form is caused by septic infections and by giant urticaria. In chronic form it is a result of lymphangioma or hemangioma, or a secondary effect of Mongolism, acromegaly or myxedema. (It can also be produced by tumors, syphilis and tuberculosis.) In myxedema the tongue enlarges, resulting in thick speech and difficulty of mastication and swallowing. The margins are typically lobulated from the pressure or confinement against the teeth.

Luetic glossitis (see also page 114)

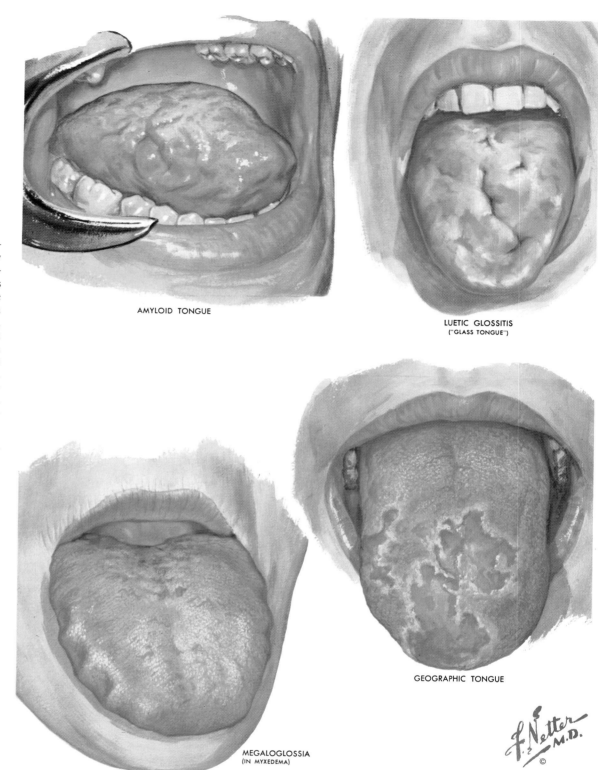

AMYLOID TONGUE

LUETIC GLOSSITIS
("GLASS TONGUE")

MEGALOGLOSSIA
(IN MYXEDEMA)

GEOGRAPHIC TONGUE

has been variously called bald or glazed luetic tongue, sclerous or interstitial glossitis, or lobulated syphilitic tongue. The clinical appearance depends on the extent of gummatous destruction, which may be superficial or deep, causing an endarteritis with a smooth, atrophic surface. Hyperkeratosis may also be evident. On palpation various degrees of fibrous induration are detected in the relaxed tongue. The surface is thrown into ridges, grooves and lobulations, with a pattern of scars which may assume a leukoplakic appearance. The induration and scarring are direct results of the gummas. The smooth, depapillated, "varnished" surface is, strictly speaking, an atrophic symptom seen in advanced forms of anemias, vitamin B deficiency, sprue, Plummer-Vinson's syndrome and prolonged cachectic states.

An *amyloid tongue* is usually a part of a generalized amyloidosis (see other CIBA COLLECTION volumes). Only occasionally are isolated amyloid deposits found in the base of the tongue without a generalized disease. The tongue, as illustrated here, has been heavily infiltrated, together with the liver, spleen and other mesodermal organs, in a generalized secondary amyloidosis resulting from a multiple myoma. Amyloid deposit causes a hyaline swelling of connective tissue fibers, with accumulation of waxlike material and obliteration of vessels through thickening of their walls. Clinically, the tongue is enlarged and presents a mottling of dark-purple areas with translucent matter. Furrows and lobules cover the denuded dorsum. The diagnosis is easily ascertained by biopsy specimen, which will show the typical brown color when exposed to Lugol's solution, a color which turns blue when sulfuric acid is added. Lugol's solution also displays the diagnostic reaction if introduced into a small lingual incision in situ.

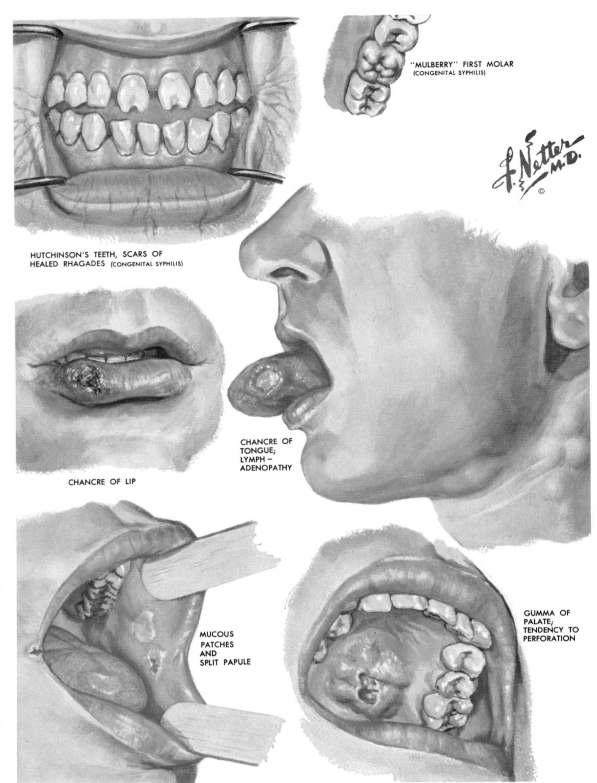

"MULBERRY" FIRST MOLAR
(CONGENITAL SYPHILIS)

HUTCHINSON'S TEETH, SCARS OF
HEALED RHAGADES (CONGENITAL SYPHILIS)

CHANCRE OF LIP

CHANCRE OF TONGUE; LYMPH–ADENOPATHY

MUCOUS PATCHES AND SPLIT PAPULE

GUMMA OF PALATE; TENDENCY TO PERFORATION

SYPHILIS OF ORAL CAVITY

The primary lesion of syphilis is the chancre (see CIBA COLLECTION, Vol. 2, page 38); 5 to 10 per cent are extragenital and mostly around the oral cavity. *Chancre of the lip* is usually a single lesion, only occasionally multiple. The erosive type may resemble a minute herpetic vesicle, with slight crusting and a tendency to ooze. The hypertrophic type is larger and more indurated. The ulcerative type presents further alteration by secondary infection. The lesion is painless or only slightly painful. The crusting differs from a herpetic lesion by being darker in color. Lymphadenopathy is always present and is usually unilateral, irregular in shape, hard, movable and slightly painful. The chancre abounds with spirochetes, but distinction by darkfield examination from the common oral spirochetes is sometimes difficult. *Chancre of the tongue,* usually located near the tip, makes its appearance as a circular erosion surrounded by a firmly indurated, elevated and reddened wall of tissue. As a consequence of secondary infection, the necrotic ulceration increases. The accompanying *lymphadenopathy,* however, results from the spirochetal invasion. The gingiva, the buccal mucosa, the palate and the tonsillar region may also be the site of chancre.

From 4 to 6 weeks after the appearance of the chancre, the syphilitic infection becomes generalized (cf. CIBA COLLECTION, Vol. 2, pages 70, 132 and 149). *Mucous patches,* the oral signs of generalized syphilis, are found on the tongue, buccal mucosa, pharynx and lips. When occurring at the commissure of the lips, the lesion appears as a split papule. The macular syphilids are brightred areas of erythema with a concomitant beefy redness of the fauces, dryness and hoarseness constituting an acute pharyngitis. Annular red and gray macules may present a ringlike network on the roof of the mouth and pharynx. The mucous patches or erosive syphilids are covered by an exudative, grayish, thin membrane. At times, the mucous patches become

hypertrophic and manifest themselves as slightly raised areas, which can coalesce to cover large parts of the mucosal surface. The mucous patches contain numerous treponemata.

Participation of the buccal cavity in late syphilis is very common. The tongue often presents multiple gummas in the form of pea-size nodules on the dorsum. Ulceration and necrosis heal by forming stellate and grooved scars typical of luetic interstitial glossitis (see page 113). Gummatous infiltration may be so extensive as to cause macroglossia. The *palate* is involved with variously sized *gummas,* which invariably ulcerate. On the hard palate this process results in perforation between the nasal and oral cavities. The velum also may perforate or can be partially destroyed by more scattered lesions.

Prenatal syphilis presents postrhagadic scarring about the oral and anal orifices. The original acute

lesions occur in the first few weeks of life as deep, oozing, crusted fissures or *rhagades, typically radiating from the commissures of the lips,* most prominently on the lower lip. The Hutchinsonian triad, which becomes evident months or even years after birth, includes specific hypoplasia of the permanent incisor teeth, eighth nerve deafness and interstitial keratitis. It is rare, however, to find all these symptoms together. The dental aberrations (*Hutchinson's teeth*) are seen in perhaps one of five cases of congenital syphilis. The Hutchinsonian upper incisor (less frequently the lower) is "peg-shaped" or "screw driver-shaped" in appearance, owing to a dwarfing of the middle denticle, with a notched incisor surface and bulging of the lateral denticles. The tip of the upper cuspid may be missing. The so-called *"mulberry"* molar is characterized by a constricted pattern of cusps, with shrunken and poorly covered fissures.

INFLAMMATIONS OF SALIVARY GLANDS

POUTING OF ORIFICE OF STENSEN'S DUCT

PAROTITIS (Obstruction or Ascending Infection)

SUBMANDIBULAR SIALADENITIS

CALCULUS IN WHARTON'S DUCT. PROBE INSERTED AND DROP OF PUS EXUDING

The major salivary glands and the accessory mucous glands are subject to functional abnormalities as well as inflammations. Ptyalism, or excessive salivation, is associated with the use of several drugs, especially mercurial salts (see page 116). On the other hand, xerostomia, or dryness of the mouth, is seen in febrile states, obstructive breathing from enlarged adenoids or tonsils, Sjögren's syndrome, vitamin deficiencies (see page 119) and other conditions. Inflammation of the major glands is usually attended by swelling and may be a feature of a generalized syndrome. Epidemic parotitis or Hodgkin's or leukemic infiltration should be considered diagnostically whenever more than one gland is involved or when a local cause is not obvious.

The *submandibular gland* may be the site of an acute or subacute infection, causing pain on palpation. The swelling differs from that of an alveolar abscess by being deeply seated, not complicated by trismus and rather fixed beneath the mandible but not obliterating its border, with the overlying skin relatively movable. The orifice of Wharton's duct is reddened, and its course is tender and edematous. Pus may sometimes be expressed by milking the duct. Swelling of the submandibular gland is most often due to obstruction in the form of a salivary calculus, which may be too small or nonopaque to be seen in the roentgenogram. Precipitation of calcium salts is probably initiated by irritation of the duct and stasis of saliva, aided by the presence of a matrix of filamentous colonies of saprophytic actinomyces or other organisms.

The *parotid gland* is subject to similar acute and chronic swellings superimposed on recurrent obstruction of its duct. It may also become infected by an ascending pyogenic infection of Stensen's duct in debilitated or postoperative patients. In this "terminal parotitis" the onset is sudden, with severe pain, fever and swelling of the parotid gland. It has been suggested that the drying of the secretions by atropine during general anesthesia is, in some cases, contributory. The mortality before sulfonamides and antibiotics was approximately 40 per cent. Obstructive parotitis, in contrast to submandibular adenitis, is usually not associated with calculus formation. An inflammatory disturbance in the duct or catarrhal constriction causes characteristic recurrent swelling. Complete obstruction predisposes to abscess formation, with reddening of the skin and a tense, fluctuant swelling of the parotid space. Repeated parotitis may lead to stenosis of the interlobar ducts or main excretory duct.

The most frequent and, because of its complications, most important disease specifically involving the parotid gland is the highly contagious viral infection known as mumps or epidemic parotitis. The glandular swelling in this disease is usually (70 per cent of the cases) bilateral, has a doughy or elastic consistency, reaches its maximum in 24 to 48 hours and lasts about 7 to 10 days. Microscopically, the glands are heavily infiltrated by lymphocytes and show a destruction of acinar cells in varying degree. The danger of this disease lies in the complications, which include epididymo-orchitis (cf. CIBA COLLECTION, Vol. 2, page 82), oöphoritis, meningo-encephalitis, deafness, ocular lesions and neuritis of the facial and trigeminal nerves.

EFFECTS OF CHEMICAL AGENTS ON ORAL MUCOSA

Aspirin burn is a frequently encountered local lesion which manifests pain. The irritation of topically applied acetylsalicylic acid can produce a surface necrosis with blebs, which will slough away, leaving a superficial erosion. The onset is rapid, as is healing.

The pale bluish-to-heavy-black *"lead line"* (Burton's line or halo saturninus), coursing along parts or all of the gingival margin, is a symptom of lead absorption but not necessarily of lead intoxication. Its nature and biochemical genesis have not been definitely established, but available evidence favors the view that the material forming the line consists of lead sulfide which has precipitated in the capillaries or surrounding tissue, when the lead compounds circulating in the blood react with hydrogen sulfide. The latter is liberated by bacterial action from organic matter deposited around the teeth as a consequence of poor oral hygiene. The "lead line" has been seldom, if ever, observed in a clean or edentulous mouth. It is more distinct in those regions with heavy deposit around the teeth or with inflammatory processes, even involving the adjacent cheek or lips. Secondary invasion of fusiform and spirochetal organisms often occurs, producing a marked gingivitis. A metallic taste, a heavily coated tongue and increased salivation, together with systemic signs (headache, nausea, pallor, colic, etc.), are indications of more advanced or definite plumbism.

Mercurialism, as the chronic poisoning by mercury or mercury salts is called, is nowadays as rare as is plumbism. It is seen only as the result of occupational hazards and accidental exposure to mercury vapors. The oral manifestations, consisting essentially of ptyalism and a necrotizing stomatitis, are caused mainly by the toxic action of mercury salts excreted in the saliva. The salivary flow is greatly increased and of a thick mucinous consistency. A strong metallic taste accompanies the gingival stomatitis, which is more extensive than in other metal poisonings. Interdental papillae are bloated, bluish red and ulcerated. The tongue is swollen, lobulated, often ulcer-

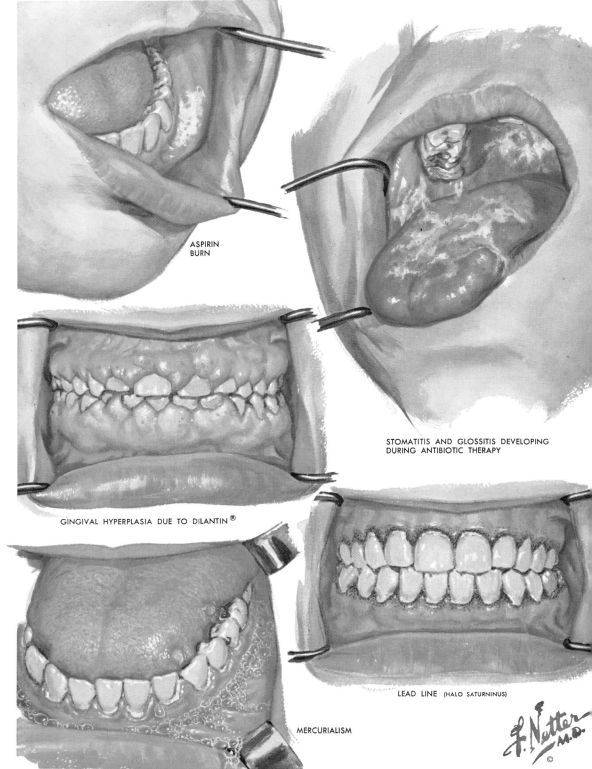

ASPIRIN BURN

STOMATITIS AND GLOSSITIS DEVELOPING DURING ANTIBIOTIC THERAPY

GINGIVAL HYPERPLASIA DUE TO DILANTIN®

MERCURIALISM

LEAD LINE (HALO SATURNINUS)

ated and furry. Foul odor and lymphadenitis are marked. Lips are dry and swollen. The ulcerations become widespread in the alveolar bone, with periostitis or exfoliation of the teeth. The palate and pharynx may also be involved.

Gingival hyperplasia develops in a great percentage of individuals receiving the anticonvulsive drug *Dilantin.* Edentulous mouths do not reveal the disturbance, emphasizing the rôle of local irritants and oral hygiene. All gradations of hyperplasia are observed, beginning with tumescence of the interdental papillae. The consistency is fibrous, without edema, inflammation or color change. The swellings may further proliferate to cover the crowns of the teeth with sessile, lobulated growths which are light pink in color and sharply defined from the surrounding gum.

Stomatitis as a result of antibiotic therapy is becom-

ing more widely recognized and prevalent. A black hairy tongue is not uncommonly the result of topical treatment with penicillin or other antibiotics. Troches and lozenges are most prone to sensitize the tissues directly, producing a generalized, beefy-red glossitis and stomatitis which, if severe, are accompanied by erosion, desquamation, bullous formation and, more rarely, ulceration. When the same agent is taken systemically, the stomatitis usually recurs immediately. Systemic administration of antibiotics may also produce stomatitis without previous sensitization, which is observed chiefly with the wide-spectrum antibiotics administered orally. Generalized gastro-intestinal symptoms are mirrored in the mouth by a denudation of the tongue and fiery-red coloration of all tissues. *Thrushlike lesions* may be observed, and, occasionally, monilia are identified in smear. White encrustations occur in the cheeks, palate and tongue.

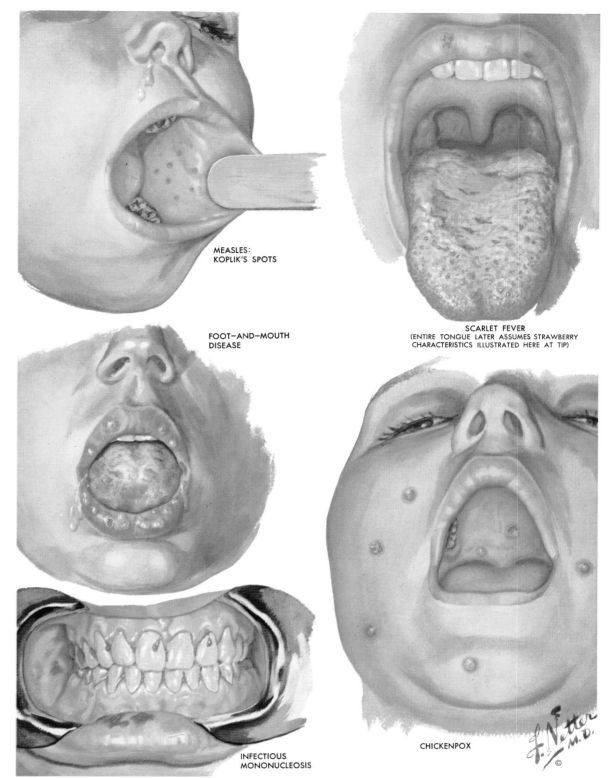

MEASLES:
KOPLIK'S SPOTS

FOOT—AND—MOUTH
DISEASE

SCARLET FEVER
(ENTIRE TONGUE LATER ASSUMES STRAWBERRY
CHARACTERISTICS ILLUSTRATED HERE AT TIP)

INFECTIOUS
MONONUCLEOSIS

CHICKENPOX

ORAL MANIFESTATIONS IN SYSTEMIC INFECTIONS

Oral manifestations can be observed in almost every generalized systemic infectious disease. Only the most characteristic ones are illustrated on this page.

Measles (rubeola) produces a pathognomonic eruption of the mouth in the prodromal stage before any cutaneous lesions have become evident. About the second day after the first signs of the disease (coryza, conjunctivitis and fever), the palate and fauces become intensely red, and the typical Koplik's spots appear on the buccal or labial mucous membranes as isolated rose-red spots with a pale bluish-white center. They are best seen in ultraviolet light. At the onset the buccal mucosa is normal in color. Soon the eruptions become diffuse, with rose red predominating and the bluish spots more numerous, until the coalescence of all spots produces an even redness, with myriad white specks. The cutaneous rash, which is dull red and macular, follows the first Koplik's spots by 2 to 3 days. The oral mucosa assumes normal color before the skin rash has disappeared.

If one examines the mouth at the time the typical vesicular eruption of *chickenpox* starts to appear, one will nearly always find in the mouth, mostly at the soft palate, isolated small vesicles, which may be of diagnostic help. These eruptions in the oral cavity may appear even somewhat prior to those on the skin. The thin vesicles, with a reddened halo, rupture quickly to form a shallow erosion with gray tags of epithelial debris. Usually, the size is that of a pinhead, but it may be larger. It resembles a solitary aphtha but is generally not so painful.

The oral symptoms of *scarlet fever* originate in the throat, which is red and swollen, as are the tonsils and palate and, occasionally, the gingivae. The tongue is next involved with a heavy, grayish, furry coating through which enlarged, red papillae are scattered. The edges of the tongue and its tip are vivid red.

Within 3 or 4 days the dorsum has desquamated, with enlarged variously placed papillae, presenting the so-called strawberry tongue.

Foot-and-mouth disease, or epizootic stomatitis, is an acute, highly contagious viral infection, confined chiefly to cloven-footed animals. The disease occasionally is transmitted to humans either by the consumption of unsterilized milk from cows suffering from the disease or by direct contact with the saliva of infected animals. After an incubation time of 2 to 5 days, the disease begins with slight fever and malaise. The oral symptoms follow in a day or two, with dry, swollen, reddened membranes. The tongue is coated and enlarged. Some days later, yellow vesicles appear and rupture. Salivation and fetid odor are prominent. The vesicles enlarge and then appear also on the hands and, occasionally, the toes. Fever and lymphadenopathy increase for 10 to 12 days,

after which they subside spontaneously and rapidly.

Infectious mononucleosis, or glandular fever, a communicable disease of probably viral but not yet definitely established etiology, presents a picture of fever and lymphadenitis, with increase of mononuclear, nongranular cells in the blood. Malaise, prostration, stiffness of the neck and gastro-intestinal symptoms may appear, with abrupt onset, followed by considerable lymph node swelling and tenderness. In the early stage, usually with the onset of the fever, a reddened pharynx is seen (see page 130), with scattered petechiae of the buccal and labial mucosa and of the soft palate. The oral signs alone are not a reliable indicator, but in association with the lymphadenopathy, they should direct suspicion to the disease, and then a heterophil antibody agglutination test (Paul-Bunnell reaction) may be performed which will establish the diagnosis.

ORAL MANIFESTATIONS RELATED TO THE ENDOCRINE SYSTEM

The oral mucosa, particularly of the gingivae and tongue, frequently exhibits changes in pregnancy, menstruation, dysmenorrhea, puberty and menopause. In *puberty* a marginal type of gingivitis is not unusual. Bleeding on slight trauma is the incipient sign. Hyperemia may produce a generally deeper raspberry color of the entire gum margin, with varying degrees of hyperplasia in the interdental papillae. Poor oral hygiene, leading to collections of materia alba, is often a contributing cause.

In *pregnancy* a chronic marginal gingivitis (see page 111) is fairly common, beginning in the second month and often continuing after term. Symptoms range from slight hyperplasia and bleeding to mulberrylike swellings or fungoid proliferations (so-called pregnancy "tumor", see page 124). All fibrous epulides occurring prior to pregnancy are markedly stimulated in growth. Clinically, the gum shows proliferation of a granulation type of tissue, which appears edematous and turgid. Histologically, one may observe hydropic degeneration of the epithelium, loss of keratin and proliferation of rete pegs, with infiltration and fibrinous exudate in the corium.

The oral symptoms during *menstruation* are similar but more transient. Hemorrhages from the oral mucosa, sometimes termed a vicarious menstruation, have been reported, and so have edema, gingival soreness and desquamation. Oral herpes is frequently associated with menstruation. *Menopause* is often accompanied by alterations in taste, burning, dryness and soreness of the oral mucosa, especially of the tongue. Objective signs include papillary flattening, fusion and glazing, similar to vitamin B deficiency states, occasionally resembling the acute redness and pebbly appearance of the mild pellagrous tongue (see page 119). Atrophy and paleness, typical of the Plummer-Vinson syndrome, have been described. A special form of *desquamative gingivitis* is sometimes associated with menopause, causing recurrent denudation of gingivae or even the buccal mucosa, which occasions great soreness.

Increased pigmentation of the skin and mucosal membranes is one of the most

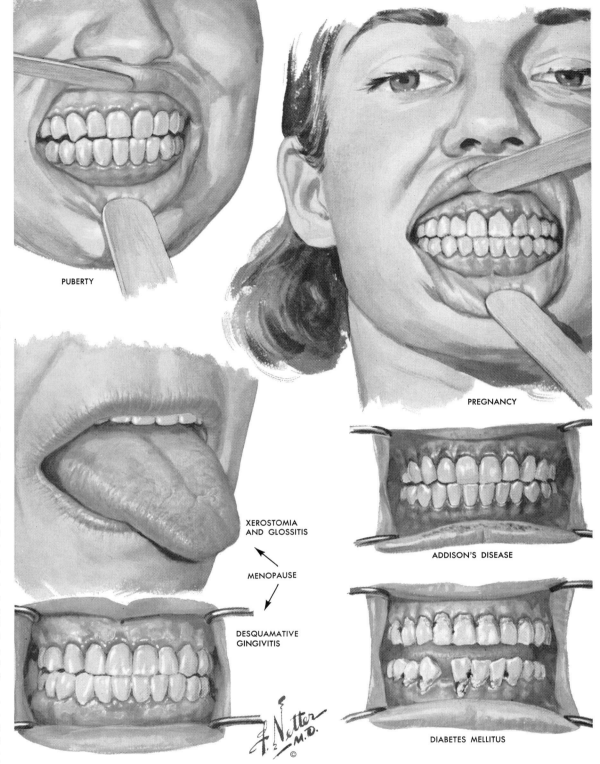

PUBERTY

PREGNANCY

XEROSTOMIA AND GLOSSITIS

MENOPAUSE

ADDISON'S DISEASE

DESQUAMATIVE GINGIVITIS

DIABETES MELLITUS

striking and earliest signs of *Addison's disease*. This pigmentation is caused by a deposition of melanin and appears only in chronic primary deficiency of the adrenal cortex. It does not develop in those cases in which the adrenal cortex has lost its function secondary to an insufficiency of the anterior lobe of the pituitary. In the oral cavity melanin may be deposited in the mucosa of the lips, of the buccal parts, of the tongue and of the gingivae, in which it sometimes may appear as a color festoon along the gingival cuff. The color of the pigmentation varies from a pale brown to a dark blue, depending upon the race or complexion of the patient as well as upon the duration and severity of the disease. In view of the individually varying normal pigmentation of the oral mucosa, the important diagnostic feature is not the coloration of the mucosa as such, but its change within a certain time. The increase in pigmentation in the

oral mucosa is usually observed by the patient himself. Finally, it should be remembered that Addison's disease is not the only pathologic condition responsible for a change in the coloration of the oral mucosa. Though produced by other mechanisms, increased deposits of dark pigments occur also in hemochromatosis, malaria, liver cirrhosis, alkaptonuria, argyrosis and other conditions.

Diabetes mellitus, in a controlled state, seldom produces characteristic lesions of the mouth. When the disease is uncontrolled and severe, the oral symptoms may be striking. In such cases the mucosa is deeply reddened and dry, and an abundance of calcareous deposits and soft detritus around the teeth may be seen. Infection in this state progresses rapidly, and abscesses develop. Pronounced gingival recession, periodontal bone loss, ulceration and loosening of teeth are other associated phenomena.

ORAL MANIFESTATIONS IN NUTRITIONAL DEFICIENCIES

The oral mucous membranes respond with perhaps the greatest sensitivity of all bodily tissues to nutritional deprivation, whether involving total water, proteins, minerals or vitamins; but it is only in a few deficiency states that the pathologic manifestations are so characteristic as to be diagnostic. It should be emphasized in passing that clinical malnutrition is often observed from a combination of factors other than dietary: decreased absorption due to gastro-intestinal disease or the effect of medications, failure of storage, increased elimination or metabolic demand, toxic destruction of body protein, and so forth. In general, the changes of the oral mucosa seen in states of undernourishment are the result of multiple deficiencies, since the essential enzyme components (vitamins) occur in close association in nature. The B complex group, for example, is water soluble and appears, as is well known, in yeast, lean meat, grain and other foods. Deficiency in one or another member of this group results only from unusual conditions of diet, or in experimental studies in animals wherein specific changes are induced by elimination of one factor, *e.g.*, black-tongue in dogs fed on a nicotinic acid-free diet.

Ariboflavinosis undoubtedly results from a multiple vitamin deficiency, yet, as a clinical syndrome, presents certain features which can be attributed specifically to lack of riboflavin (formerly vitamin B₂ or G). This is evident from controlled observations in man and from easily reproducible experiments in animals kept on a riboflavin-free diet. The oral lesions in ariboflavinosis begin with a pallor of the labial mucosa and the skin at the corner of the mouth, followed by a maceration of the epithelium and the formation of fissures and crusts. These angular fissures and superficial ulcerations are termed cheilosis (formerly perlèche). The association of conjunctivitis, corneal opacities and increased vascularization, photophobia and signs of dermatitis in the nasolabial regions, together with cheilosis, may be considered pathognomonic for ariboflavinosis, particularly so if, simultaneously, signs of a glossitis can be observed. The most striking features on the tongue are a "purplish-magenta" discoloration, which, however, is not seen in all cases, and a pebbly appearance which results from early edematous enlargement of the fungiform papillae. The filiform papillae tend to atrophy, and the gingivae may

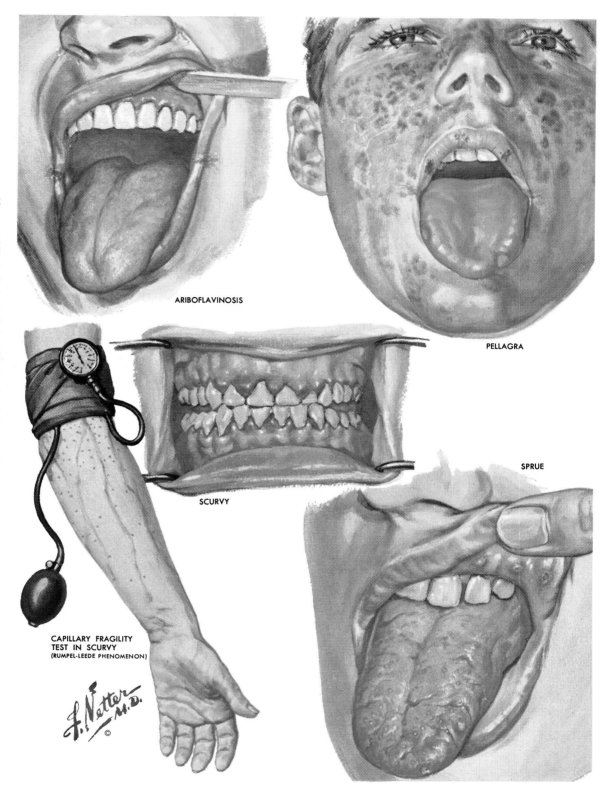

ARIBOFLAVINOSIS

PELLAGRA

CAPILLARY FRAGILITY
TEST IN SCURVY
(RUMPEL-LEEDE PHENOMENON)

SCURVY

SPRUE

be colored more deeply red than is normally seen.

Pellagra is presently thought to be a disease caused by a lack of several vitamins of the B group but essentially of nicotinic acid and, probably also, by a lack of the essential amino acid tryptophan. Soreness of the tongue and mouth may be one of the initial signs, but the fully developed changes of pellagrous tongue appear at a later stage. The papillae of the lateral margins and tip are first affected, the changes progressing to involve the entire tongue and all mucous membranes. The color at this time is scarlet red. Increased soreness and salivation are accompanied by edema, with indentations from the teeth and often ulcerations, in which fusospirochetal organisms abound. Later, the tongue becomes bald and more beefy red in color (bald tongue of Sandwith). The papillary changes involve, first, hypertrophy, flattening and coalescence (producing furrows), then atrophy.

An old-rose color of the gingivae, with readiness of bleeding, is one of the earliest signs of *scurvy*, or vitamin C (ascorbic acid) deficiency, provided that the patient is not edentulous. In later stages the gingival papillae become enlarged, bluish red and spongy, the teeth become loose, salivation increases and an oral fetor appears, owing to the development of a mixed fusospirochetal infection. The bleeding tendency of the gingivae is part of a generally increased capillary fragility, which may be ascertained by producing the Rumpel-Leede phenomenon.

Sprue produces oral symptoms which are prominent in the diagnosis. A burning of the oral mucosa and tongue appears after episodes of diarrhea, with fatty, light-colored stools. Numerous vesicles may form; a scarlet color and aphthous lesions and fissures make "sprue tongue" closely resemble a pellagra tongue.

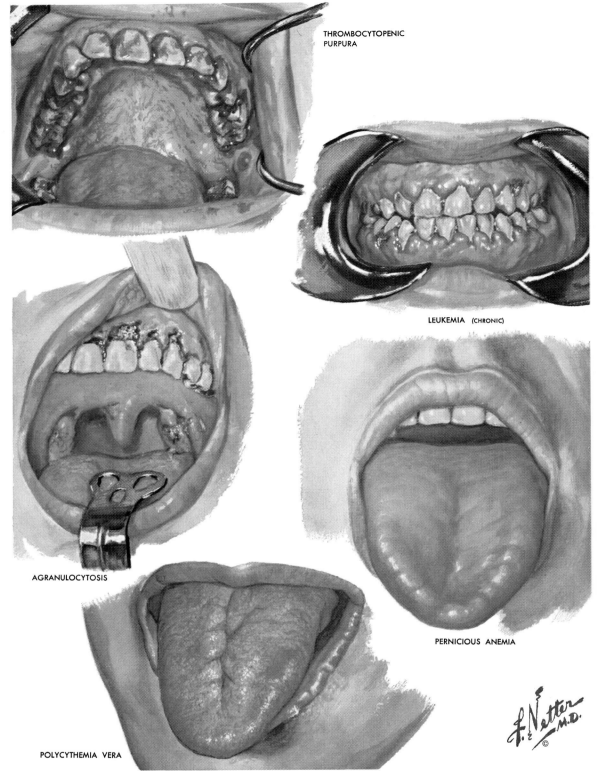

THROMBOCYTOPENIC PURPURA

LEUKEMIA (CHRONIC)

AGRANULOCYTOSIS

POLYCYTHEMIA VERA

PERNICIOUS ANEMIA

Oral Manifestations in Blood Dyscrasias

Though oral manifestations in blood dyscrasias make their appearance usually after the disease has progressed considerably, still a good percentage of first diagnoses can be made by correct interpretation of a complaint of bleeding or of color or textural changes of the oral mucosa.

The prominent oral signs of *thrombocytopenic purpura* include widespread capillary oozing from the gingival margin of all the teeth. From adherent clots a fetid odor may emanate. Spontaneous hemorrhages of greater severity may arise, especially in areas of inflammation. Petechial spots also appear as purplish-red patches on the lips and other mucosa. Erosion and ulcerations are seen only in debilitated, advanced cases.

In the acute phases of *agranulocytosis,* ulcerative lesions of the mouth and pharynx, with dysphagia, are a frequent finding and sometimes the first source of complaint. The disease may be acute or chronic (cyclic and recurrent); it may be primary or else the sequel of known infection, hormonal dysfunction or drug idiosyncrasy. Since the myeloid cells are arrested in maturation, the mucous membranes are subject to rapid invasion of bacteria. With sudden onset the oral mucosa is involved by necrotic ulcers, which show little or no surrounding erythema. All types of gingivitis and stomatitis with gangrenous areas have been observed, which are apt to appear particularly about the pharynx, tonsils and hard palate. The severity varies greatly, with ptyalism and oral fetor prominent in full-blown cases.

The frequency of oral lesions in *chronic leukemia* is appreciable and varies considerably in severity. Beginning insidiously, pallor of the mucous membrane may be followed by soft hypertrophy and ulceration of the gingivae, with spontaneous bleeding, and fusospirochetal infection in necrotic papillae, producing a foul odor. A blackish, pseudo-membranous exudate may cover the tongue, gingivae and fauces. Enlargement of the gingiva begins usually in the lower interior region. Teeth may loosen, and pulpal liquefaction or abscessed pulps with odontalgia may appear. In the lymphatic form the lymphoid structures of the floor of the mouth and tongue, together with the submandibular lymph nodes, may become enlarged. In general, the acute leukemias produce symptoms more severe than do the chronic.

In *polycythemia vera* (erythremia, or Vaquez's disease) the skin and oral tissues show a vivid purplish-red discoloration. Superficial vessels are distended and the gingivae are swollen and bleed frequently. Petechiae are often noted.

In *pernicious anemia* the oral mucosa accepts a pale or greenish-yellow color, except for the tongue which is bright red. The latter is in a state of chronic inflammation, characterized by irregular, fiery-red patches resembling a burn, near the tip and the lateral margins (Hunter's or Moeller's glossitis). A sensation of burning, itching or stinging is always present, and the patients complain of paroxysmal pain or tenderness to food intake or to cool, as well as hot, fluids. These symptoms appear in the early stages of pernicious anemia, sometimes before the hemogram reveals the disease. They also may continue when all other pathognomonic signs indicate a remission. With present-day knowledge and specific treatment of this disease, the later stages of the oral manifestations (gradual loss of the papillae, progressive atrophy of the tongue) in pernicious anemia are not often seen, being encountered only in neglected cases. All the changes of the tongue must be carefully distinguished from other forms of glossodynia and glossopyrosis, from allergic lesions, from the lingual manifestations in syphilis and from geographic tongue (see page 113).

ORAL MANIFESTATIONS IN VARIOUS SKIN CONDITIONS

A great number of pathologic conditions of the skin present oral manifestations which may precede or accompany or even arise independently of the cutaneous eruption. In general, such lesions do not bear strict comparison with the homologous skin lesions, because of the considerable difference in moisture, temperature, exposure to trauma, lack of a keratin layer and the presence of secondary infection. In differential diagnosis the prevalence of purely local lesions of a vesicular or bullous type, *e.g.*, recurrent aphthous ulcers, should be kept in mind.

One of the familiar dermatoses in which the oral mucosa may participate is *lichen planus*. The diagnosis of this disease of unknown etiology is easily made when the typical skin eruptions — the purplish, polygonal or angular papules — are present. In a majority of cases, however, the oral lesions precede those of the skin surfaces, and, not infrequently, the disease may remain confined to the mouth. Most often, the cheek mucosa displays the characteristic fine, lacelike pattern of bluish-white lines and small, pinhead-size, elevated papules, although the tongue, palate and gingiva may be similarly affected. The latter locations, as compared with the cheek, usually show coarser plaques and aggregated papules. The lips are least commonly involved. Occasionally, an erosive form may be observed, which is painful and characterized by a caked, whitish material which covers a red, easily bleeding base. The radiating and interlaced grayish-white lines are the most significant signs in the diagnosis. Differentiation from syphilis, moniliasis and glossitis migrans is easily made; but from other local leukokeratoses this is sometimes very difficult, and biopsy becomes then a helpful adjunct. The histopathologic picture in lichen planus shows moderate keratosis or parakeratosis, "saw-tooth" arrangement of the rete pegs and a very typical band of lymphocytes chiefly concentrated beneath a vague basal cell zone. This lymphocytic infiltrate is sharply demarcated from the rest of the stroma.

Pemphigus begins in over 50 per cent of all cases with manifestations of the oral mucosa, where large, painless vesicles or bullae develop. The thin-walled blebs rupture in a short time, leaving a superficial ulcer rimmed with tattered, grayish shreds of thin membrane. Signs of inflammatory reactions are absent in the early stages but may present themselves later in the form of a slightly red halo. The onset is insidious, chronicity and recurrence being typical even when unaccompanied by skin signs. As the disease progresses, confluent areas become raw and oozing, and salivation, pain and bleeding increase; mastication and swallowing are impaired.

Erythema multiforme exudativum may affect, along with the skin, the mucous membranes of the mouth, eyes and anogenital regions. The earliest vesicular lesions in the mouth are sometimes indistinguishable from pemphigus. A diffuse bullous stomatitis ensues, with heavy yellowish pseudomembrane, marked variation in size of the lesions, and often a bluish-red areola around them. The lips, usually, are swollen, ulcerated and covered with hemorrhagic crusts. A great variety of local and general diseases must be considered in making the diagnosis, which, of course, is easier to establish when skin and other mucous membrane manifestations are present simultaneously. The severity of the disease varies. Recurrence is common and tends to be seasonal. The etiology is unknown, though, at least in a few cases, a sensitivity to drugs or specific foods may play a rôle.

Disseminated lupus erythematosus, though for long considered to be a dermatologic condition, is classified today under the group of collagen diseases. Oral lesions are present in about 15 per cent of the cases and consist of red patches of irregular outline, which may become eroded, atrophic and, later, scarred. White pinhead spots are discernible about the periphery. The sites of predilection are the cheeks, palate and lips.

The photomicrograph is reproduced by the courtesy of the Division of Oral Pathology, The Mount Sinai Hospital, New York.

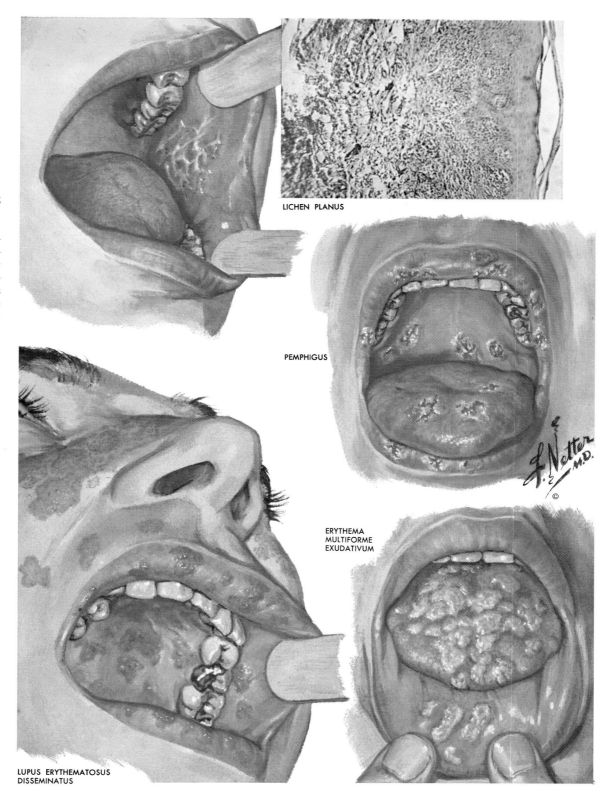

LICHEN PLANUS

PEMPHIGUS

ERYTHEMA MULTIFORME EXUDATIVUM

LUPUS ERYTHEMATOSUS DISSEMINATUS

CYSTS OF JAW AND ORAL CAVITY

Nonepithelialized cysts of the mandible or maxilla may result from trauma with intermedullary hemorrhage, or they may be manifestations of monostotic and polyostotic fibrous dysplasia (disseminated or localized osteitis fibrosa) and generalized osteitis fibrosa, also called cystic osteodystrophy (von Recklinghausen's disease). Since the latter conditions are systemic disorders of the bones or of the endocrine system (primary or secondary hyperparathyroidism), they will not be discussed in this volume. The lesions are more often solid than fluid in content and are recognized as cysts chiefly by their roentgenographic appearance.

The epitheliated cysts of the jaws are etiologically divided into radicular, follicular and facial cleft cysts. The *radicular cyst* has an inflammatory basis and evolves from a granuloma at the root apex of a tooth devitalized by caries or trauma. Bacteria and toxins of the infected pulp canal stimulate proliferation of epithelial remnants left in the periodontal membrane from Hertwig's sheath, after it has been ruptured and fragmented by the developing tooth. Eventually, this epithelium lines the necrotic center of the granuloma and thickens, tending to isolate the inflammatory process. A fibrous capsule develops outside the epithelial sac, while the lumen increases by transudation of fluid. Round cell infiltration of the cyst membrane, including the adjacent connective tissue and cellular debris, pus, macrophages and cholesterol crystals are usually found histologically. Even if the tooth with the granuloma is removed, the cyst remains and may even expand more rapidly as a sterile lesion.

The *follicular cyst* arises from the enamel organ epithelium of the dental follicle. The cause of stimulation is unknown. Infection is present only when contiguous teeth are coincidentally abscessed. The pathogenesis of follicular cysts begins with retrograde changes and edema in the enamel organ, which, by expansion, assumes various shapes above the developing crown. A *simple follicular cyst* forms before enamel is excreted, arresting tooth maturation or growing entirely separate from the tooth. A *dentigerous cyst* arises at a later phase, after amelogenesis, and gradually envelops

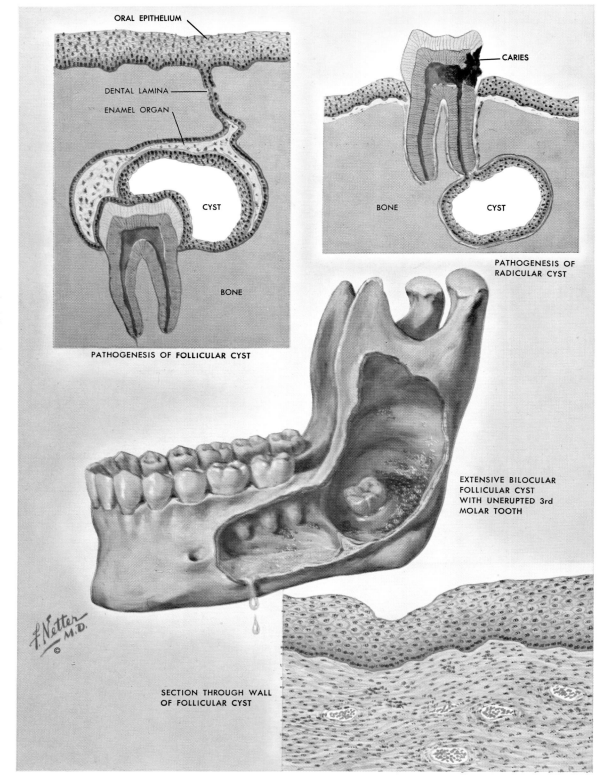

PATHOGENESIS OF FOLLICULAR CYST

PATHOGENESIS OF RADICULAR CYST

EXTENSIVE BILOCULAR FOLLICULAR CYST WITH UNERUPTED 3rd MOLAR TOOTH

SECTION THROUGH WALL OF FOLLICULAR CYST

the crown, thus interfering with eruption. The tooth may be forced by the cyst fluid to a site remote from its normal position in the jaw. A follicular cyst is usually unilocular, but multilocular forms occur. The most frequent location is the mandibular third molar region. Until the cyst attains a large size and expands the cortical plate of bone, the cyst may remain unrecognized. The buccal, palatal or alveolar bone may then bulge outward, or the maxillary sinus or nasal cavity may be invaded. The wall of the cyst becomes parchment-thin and yields a crackling sound on palpation. Owing to the pressure of the cyst and the crowding of roots, the adjoining teeth are tilted when viewed roentgenographically, while unerupted teeth are displaced in toto. Teeth are not devitalized, nor is resorption of roots encountered. A smooth, encapsulating layer of cortical bone, a unilocular shape and the absence of root erosion distinguish a cyst from an

invasive neoplasm, ameloblastoma, benign giant cell tumor and osteitis fibrosa localisata or generalisata. However, a cyst secondarily infected from an adjacent tooth shows an obliterated capsule and appears infiltrative. Also, a few cysts may be multilocular and cannot be completely distinguished from an ameloblastoma without biopsy examination. A layer of compact bone borders the cyst sac, which is composed of fibrous connective tissue lined with epithelium. The latter is stratified squamous, ranging to considerable thickness, or in some cysts may be simple columnar. The fluid content is clear and straw-colored, with an iridescent sheen imparted by cholesterol crystals, or thick and cheesy from epithelial and hemorrhagic debris.

Facial cleft cysts, also called fissural cysts, form at the junction of the embryonic segments which fuse to make up the jaws. They may be found at the

(Continued on page 123)

CYSTS OF JAW AND ORAL CAVITY

(Continued from page 122)

median fissure of the palate, maxillary bones or mandible (midline or median cyst), or at the naso-alveolar junction. The *nasopalatine cyst,* because it is formed in the incisive canal or the incisive foramen from remnants of the fetal nasopalatine communication, may be grouped with the facial cleft cyst. Possibly irritation or mucous secretions play an etiologic rôle in the more superficial type. Ordinarily, a nasopalatine cyst presents no clinical swelling, unless it is very large, and is detected only on roentgenographic examination. A radiolucent area appears in the midline between the apices of the central incisor teeth and is often misinterpreted as a radicular cyst (see above). The size varies from slight enlargement of the incisive fossa to one of a few centimeters, involving a higher part of the incisive canal. If a retention of serous or mucoid secretion produces a swelling in the region of the interincisive papilla, drops from the two tiny orifices on the side of the papilla may be expressed. Secondary infection may occasionally ensue, producing a fluctuant swelling of the palatal mucosa, resembling a dento-alveolar abscess. Mucopurulent discharge then appears at the incisive outlets on pressure. In edentulous mouths, resorption of the alveolar ridge may expose a nasopalatine cyst which escaped previous detection.

Cysts of the oral mucous membranes are retention cysts of the mucous glands or their ducts or, occasionally, the sublingual salivary gland. The *mucocele* may appear on the inner surface of the lips or cheeks, especially at a level parallel to the occlusal plane, where chewing injuries cause obstruction of the mucous ducts. A round, translucent, sometimes bluish swelling may range from a very minute size to a centimeter. In the tongue, the glands of Blandin and Nuhn (see page 11) may form more deeply seated mucoceles which reach a considerable size, presenting a swelling on the anterior ventral surface.

The *ranula,* so called because of its resemblance to a frog's belly, is a rather loose term applied to cystic swellings of the floor of the mouth. A common error is to attribute a ranula to obstruction of the submandibular (Wharton's) duct, which in the presence of a typical ranula

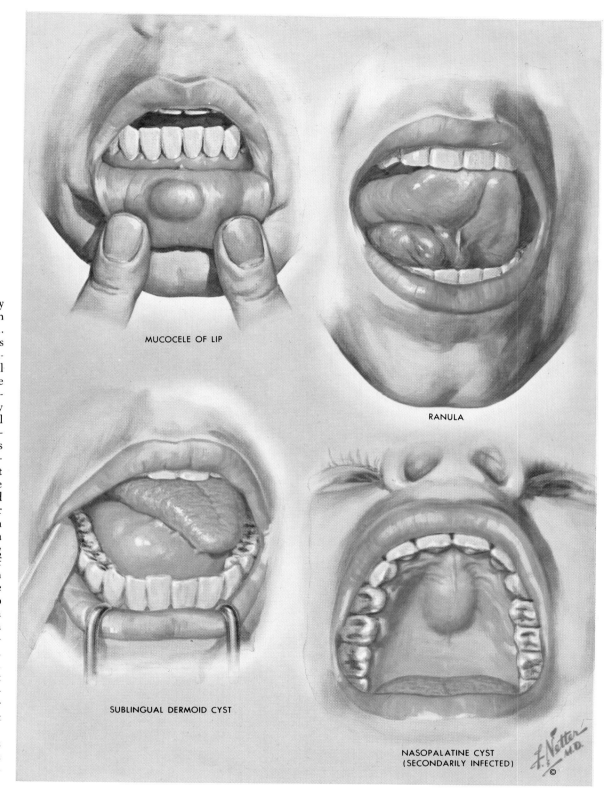

MUCOCELE OF LIP

RANULA

SUBLINGUAL DERMOID CYST

NASOPALATINE CYST
(SECONDARILY INFECTED)

is found patent. The most frequent cause is the occlusion of an excretory duct of the sublingual gland. In a few cases a ranula may arise from the incisive glands in the midline or from the ciliated epithelium-carrying cysts (Bochdalek's "glands") deriving from the primitive thyroglossal duct. A typical ranula begins in the lateral anterior floor of the mouth immediately beneath the mucous membrane. It is usually slow-growing, but rapidly developing cystic swellings (acute ranulas) are also known. The color is bluish gray, with numerous small vessels well outlined. Palpation gives a decided impression of fluid confined by an elastic membrane; the wall may rupture spontaneously but soon refills. As it reaches large proportions it crosses the midline and shows a division marked by the frenum, also displacing the tongue and impeding speech. A ranula will sometimes bulge downward toward the chin, since a portion of the sublingual

gland perforates the mylohyoid muscle (see page 11).

Dermoid cysts, owing their origin to inclusion of ectodermal structures by the mesoderm during the embryonic development of the head, usually become visible only in the second or third decade of life. They are located in the midline beneath the chin or between the geniohyoid muscles deep in the floor of the mouth, or in a lateral position beneath the angle of the jaw. The structure of the cyst consists of a fibrous capsule lined with a stratified, squamous epithelial membrane, with a cheesy or semisolid mass containing sebaceous material and hair filling the lumen. Theoretically, teeth and other appendages may be present. The dermoid may reach large proportions and protrude in the neck or beneath the tongue as a soft or semifirm, doughy lump which pits on pressure and is not fluctuant. The color tends to be waxy or yellowish when the mucosa is thin enough to reveal it.

BENIGN TUMORS OF ORAL CAVITY

Tumors of the oral cavity are very diversified. Only the more frequent neoplasms can be discussed here. A *fibroma* may be found on the gingiva, lips, palate and buccal mucosa. It is hard or soft, pale or reddish, depending on the density of collagen and the abundance of vascular elements. The gingival fibroma (fibrous epulis) is usually derived from the periosteum. It is sessile or pedunculated, well defined and slow growing.

The *papilloma* is soft and pedunculated or, when arising from an area of leukoplakia, hard with a warty, keratinized epithelium. The epithelial projections may grow beyond the basal layer and may occasionally curl inward into the stroma and become fixed at their base, in which cases they are potentially malignant. They are found in the same areas as the fibromas and also on the tongue.

The *hemangioma*, either cavernous or capillary in structure, is seen especially on the tongue but arises in any part of the mouth from the endothelium of blood vessels. It may be congenital or familial, or it may develop at a later period in life. Multiple hemangiomas can occur anywhere in the mucous membrane of the intestinal tract, but the lip, tongue, gum and rectum are sites of predilection. The color is light red to dark purple, with a tendency to blanch on pressure. Some large hemangiomas appear more globular than flat, even definitely lobulated on their free mucosal surface, and also tend to displace bone by osteolysis. Extension occurs through endothelial proliferation along the nourishing blood vessels, usually more widespread than is apparent on clinical inspection. This is a surgical danger, and fatal hemorrhage has been reported from incidental minor procedures such as tooth extractions.

The *benign giant cell tumor*, or *epulis*, is a not uncommon gingival or, more rarely, an intra-osseous growth, which originates from the periodontal membrane or periosteum and has a tendency to recur unless this tissue is widely excised. The superficial form is apparently an

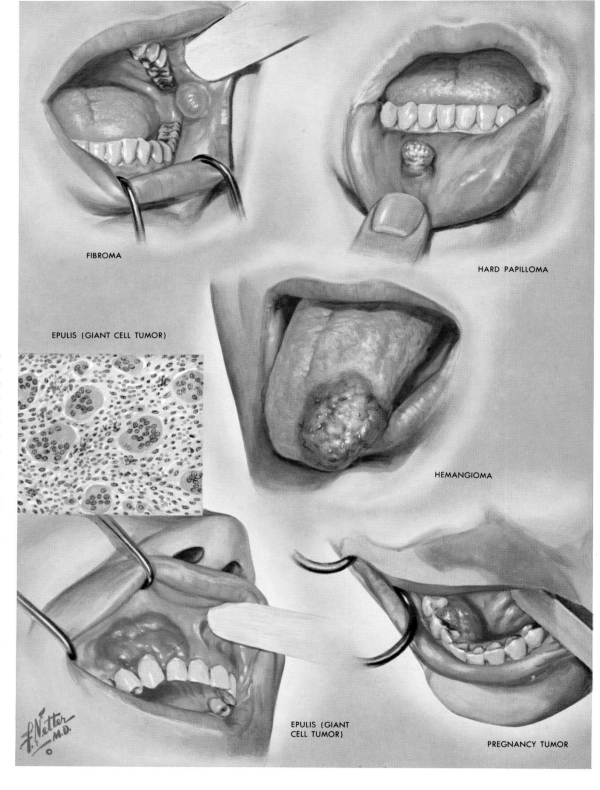

FIBROMA

HARD PAPILLOMA

EPULIS (GIANT CELL TUMOR)

HEMANGIOMA

EPULIS (GIANT CELL TUMOR)

PREGNANCY TUMOR

exaggerated granulation process, with numerous giant cells eroding the bone trabeculae; older lesions contain more adult fibroblasts and less hemorrhages. Extravasation of erythrocytes releasing hemoglobin, which is transformed to hemosiderin, explains the occasional brown color. The central giant cell tumor may show features of resorptive inflammation but behaves like a neoplasm and may be identical with the giant cell tumor of the long bones, though it has, contrary to older concepts, little relation to giant cell sarcoma. The tumor can, however, infiltrate bone and displace teeth. It is nonencapsulated but does not metastasize. Essentially, it is composed of spindle cells with a varying amount of collagen fibers, hemorrhagic debris and multinucleated cells. Occasionally, a giant cell tumor on the gum or in the bone is a manifestation of hyperparathyroidism.

The so-called *pregnancy "tumor"* is a hyperplasia,

developing in the course of a chronic gingivitis (see also pages 111 and 118), which is not infrequently observed in pregnant women but sometimes also with other hormonal alterations, *e.g.*, puberty. Bleeding, particularly of the interproximal papillae, with light-raspberry to dusky-red coloration, is an early sign, followed by a hypertrophic swelling of the papillary gingiva, ranging from a slight bloating to a tumor of 1 to 2 cm. It may envelop more than one tooth. The growth regresses with proper oral hygiene and adjusted toothbrush technique, though surgery may be required because of constant hemorrhages. Generally, the tumor disappears after term, if not too large.

The *ameloblastoma*, sometimes termed adamantinoma or adamantoblastoma, is an epithelial neoplasm occurring chiefly in the mandible (region of the third molar, ramus, premolar, in that order of frequency)

(Continued on page 125)

BENIGN TUMORS OF ORAL CAVITY

(Continued from page 124)

and belongs to the group of odontogenic tumors (as do the myxoma and cementoma) (not illustrated). According to generally accepted belief, the ameloblastoma originates from remnants of the enamel organ or dental lamina, but from less differentiated cells (pre-ameloblasts) than those producing a follicular cyst (see page 122). The tumor is mostly polycystic, sometimes monocystic and occasionally solid. It is this solid form which on rare occasion has been found to metastasize. The growth of this otherwise benign tumor is very slow. Microcystic infiltration, roentgenologically revealed by tiny locules or notching, enlarges the jaw which is often only represented by a tiny bony capsule distending the surrounding tissue. Eventually, expansion into the orbit, antrum and even cranium may take place. The most common variety, microscopically recognizable, is the ameloblastic type, characterized by follicles resembling the enamel organ, with its outer layer of cylindrical cells and stellate reticuloma in the center. Occasionally, solid strands of undifferentiated cells or sheaths of stellate cells or an accumulation of squamous and prickle cells may be found. A microscopic descriptive grading of ameloblastoma is necessary for proper management of each case and for the choice between local or radical removal. The recurrence rate of ameloblastoma is extremely high, but true malignancy is extremely low.

Made up of mixed ectodermal and mesodermal tissue, the *odontoma,* also odontogenic in origin, may be a hard or soft tumor, depending upon the presence or absence of calcified accretions. The hard odontoma is composed of abnormally arranged enamel, dentin and cementum, in a soft fibrous matrix which is gradually replaced by the calcified elements, leaving a capsule. *Complex odontomas* contain a bizarre conglomeration of hard structures without finite shape; *compound odontomas* include both rudimentary and apparently normal supernumerary teeth, at times numbering

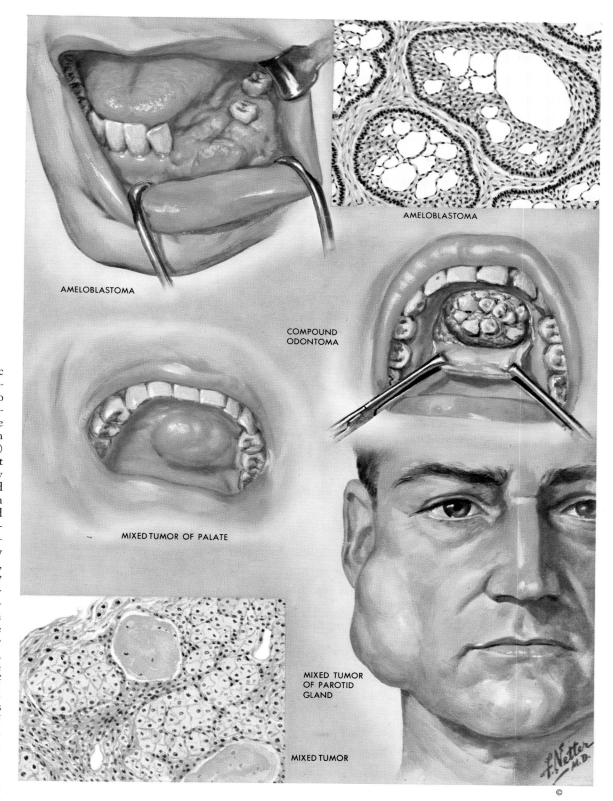

AMELOBLASTOMA

AMELOBLASTOMA

COMPOUND ODONTOMA

MIXED TUMOR OF PALATE

MIXED TUMOR OF PAROTID GLAND

MIXED TUMOR

several dozen. These structures may erupt and imitate the normal dentition.

Myxoma of the jaw (not illustrated), deriving from embryonal tissue of the dental papilla, is also a benign odontogenic tumor, as is the cementoma, a special form of fibroma, which appears usually at the apices of the lower anterior teeth. Multiple cementomas appear only in women, suggesting an estrogenic influence.

Osteoma (not illustrated) is a compact osteogenic tumor, and fibro-osteoma is diffuse. Both are slow-growing benign neoplasms, prompting conservative (cosmetic) surgical approach when leading to deformities.

Involving most frequently the major salivary glands but also the mucous glands of the palate, lip or cheek mucosa, the *mixed tumors of the salivary gland* are composed of glandular or squamous epithelium, fibrillar connective tissue, mucoid deposit and cartilage in varying proportions. Whether the tumor genesis is epithelial or mesenchymal is still controversial. For some time considered an adenocarcinoma, the mixed tumor is now recognized as a slow-growing, in most cases benign neoplasm (occurring principally in young adults), with a fibrous capsule. However, it may be scattered with tumor cells which penetrate beyond the capsule limits. The likelihood of malignancy is highest in the *mixed tumor of the parotid glands,* which is also the most frequent (70 per cent) location. It begins, as a rule, in the lower portion of the gland and gradually enlarges to present an ovoid or rounded mass, which, if developing into the depth of the parenchyma, tends to be hard and lobulated and may cause thinning of the skin or may, by pressure or infiltration, involve the facial nerve. Recurrences after removal are frequent.

LEUKOPLAKIA

Leukoplakia of the oral mucosa is a chronic inflammatory process, which may persist for many years and which may, in some forms, ultimately degenerate and become a squamous cell carcinoma. Predisposing factors include age, sex and race, since it is found usually in mid-life or after, almost exclusively in males and seldom in Negroes. Generally, it is assumed that continued irritation, both mechanical and chemical, is the most frequent direct cause. Mechanical irritation may be brought about by malpositioned or broken teeth, poorly fitting crowns or fillings, or faulty dentures. Galvanism has been implicated, and syphilis, avitaminosis and alcoholism have been thought to be contributory conditions. The majority of investigators, however, assign the most important rôle to the distillation products of tobacco and to the mechanical and thermal effects, particularly deriving from pipe smoking. The chewing of betel nut (a mixture of the areca nut, shell lime and leaves of the pepper species) has been observed to produce leukoplakia.

The alteration of the mucosa starts with an inflammatory reaction in the corium, followed by an epithelial thickening and cornification, producing whitish, opaque plaques. The lesions are not painful but may, in advanced cases, produce a sensation of dryness or burning. The whitish patches may be located in practically all regions of the oral cavity, but over half are on the buccal mucosa. The early sign of the chronic inflammation, a mild erythema, is rarely, if ever, noticeable. In later stages one observes, according to older clinical descriptions, three types of leukoplakia, which may be helpful for the diagnosis but have little direct relation to the histologic changes in the corneum. In the first type the lesions are pearly white or of grayish opacity, smooth and checkered or tessellated. The second or *raised-plaque type* is characterized by thicker, more irregular lesions of a harsh, leathery texture. With increasing cornification the surface of the plaques becomes warty and nodular, and this has been called the papillomatous or verrucous type.

Leukoplakia of the cheek is usually found parallel to the line of occlusion, sometimes extending from the corners of the mouth as a pattern of fanlike radiating lines. On the *tongue* the white markings are tessellated ("parquet tongue") and appear most frequently on the anterior two thirds of the dorsum or on the

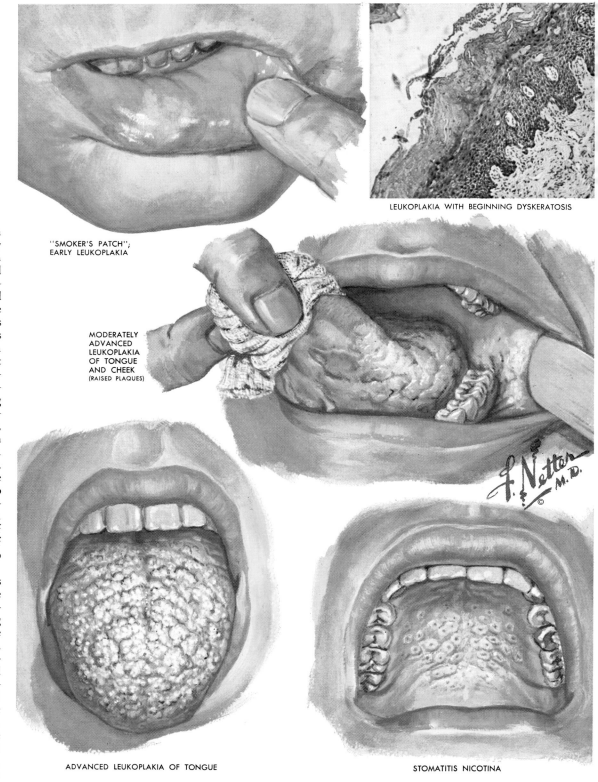

"SMOKER'S PATCH"; EARLY LEUKOPLAKIA

LEUKOPLAKIA WITH BEGINNING DYSKERATOSIS

MODERATELY ADVANCED LEUKOPLAKIA OF TONGUE AND CHEEK (RAISED PLAQUES)

ADVANCED LEUKOPLAKIA OF TONGUE

STOMATITIS NICOTINA

lingual margins. In the verrucous stage the lingual papillae are matted together, forming a cohesive mass. A boardlike consistency, with leathery strips of keratinized nodules, is characteristic of the corresponding stage of leukoplakia in the cheek. Desquamations with erosions or ulcerations or an indurated fissure may develop, and these alterations should be considered almost indicative of a malignant degeneration.

A favorite site of leukoplakia is the lower lip, where a barely discernible whitish plaque ("smoker's patch") appears, which at first may be removed by rubbing but becomes more permanent and thickened with time. The *leukoplakia of the palate* is somewhat peculiar in so far as it may manifest itself as an overall grayish-white discoloration or as more discrete plaques or rings around the orifices of the palatal mucous glands, which, in time, may become enlarged and nodular, owing to chronic obstruction. The cen-

tral duct orifices appear then as red centers in a white field. This condition is known as *stomatitis nicotina*.

Diagnosis of leukoplakia requires differentiation from syphilis, thrush, carcinoma, lichen planus and traumatic scars. Lichen planus presents a very similar picture, although the delicacy of the lacy markings, the skin lesions and its presence in females help identify it. A biopsy is most indicative although not always definitive. The histologic features are hyperkeratosis, accentuation of the stratum granulosum and moderate dyskeratosis of the prickle cells with hyperchromatic nuclei, particularly in the cells of the basal layer, a characteristic which helps in differentiation from lichen planus.

The photomicrograph is reproduced by the courtesy of the Division of Oral Pathology, The Mount Sinai Hospital, New York.

MALIGNANT TUMORS I

The variety of malignant tumors of the mouth and jaws is limited. *Squamous cell carcinoma* comprises 90 per cent of all malignancies, with adenocarcinoma and malignant salivary tissue tumors seen on occasion. Sarcoma, malignant lymphoma and melanoma are rare. Oral cancer, which occurs in males five times as frequently as in females, represents 4 per cent of all malignant tumors in man.

Among factors recognized to predispose the oral tissue structures to *epidermoid* cancer are:

1. Syphilis (particularly of the tongue)

2. Leukoplakia of the infiltrative variety

3. Nutritional deficiencies (avitaminosis B, Plummer-Vinson syndrome, etc.)

4. Actinic exposure (farmer's and sailor's skin)

5. Chronic irritation of mechanical or, more especially, chemical origin (tobacco, betel nut, etc.).

Luetic glossitis (see page 114) is clearly correlated with carcinoma, since one third of patients with a lingual cancer have positive serologic tests for syphilis. (Under no conditions does a positive test for syphilis obviate the need for a tissue examination.) In leukoplakic lesions (see page 126) the tendency toward malignant growth is high if the cells of the prickle cell layer show disorientation with dyskeratosis. Fissuring and papillomatous formation are clinical danger signs.

Epidermoid carcinoma develops in the following order of frequency: lower lip, tongue, gingiva, floor of mouth, cheek and palate. It is almost never found centrally in the jaws, except by extension from the soft tissues or antrum. The initial lesion in the soft tissues is usually a deceptively benign ulcer, without marginal induration or pain. The *incipient carcinoma of the lip*, as illustrated, is a granular ulcer with tiny, reddish lobulations like the surface of a strawberry, which is quite characteristic for this site. This early lesion arises frequently in an area of hyperkeratosis and also in areas of atrophy. It may also begin as a nodule or as a papillary projection in dense, chronic leukoplakia. Epidermoid carcinoma of the lip is favorably situated for early detection and has also the advantage of relatively late lymph node involvement — two factors which contribute toward a more favorable cure rate.

The lesion of the *retromolar gingiva* illustrates another early *tumor*, which tends, however, to remain undetected if the individual does not submit to careful oral examination. It is situated in an area where secondary infection is commonplace and may, therefore, be confused with simple pericoronitis (see page 108).

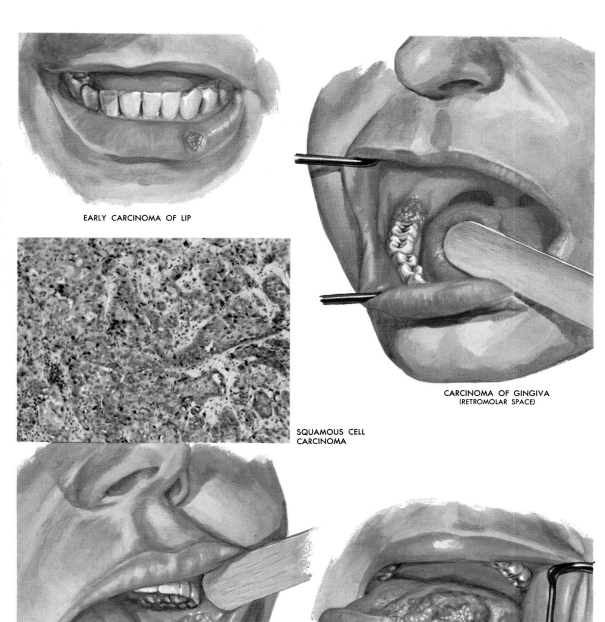

EARLY CARCINOMA OF LIP

SQUAMOUS CELL CARCINOMA

CARCINOMA OF GINGIVA
(RETROMOLAR SPACE)

CARCINOMA OF CHEEK

CARCINOMA OF TONGUE
(ON LEUKOPLAKIA)

In view of the lymph drainage to the submandibular and cervical lymph nodes, a lesion in this place presents an early danger. As an oral cancer progresses, its fixation in the adjacent tissues becomes deeper and is attended by central necrosis, causing a varying amount of surface sloughing and secondary infection. The fairly advanced *carcinoma of the cheek* is warty and lobulated, with ulceration not a prominent feature. Pain is, therefore, minor or absent.

The *large carcinoma of the tongue*, which penetrates deeply into the parenchyma, arises from a preexisting leukoplakia and is usually secondarily infected and painful. Increasing infiltration of contiguous structures restricts movement of the tongue and jaws.

The prognosis of oral carcinoma is dependent on its location and duration, and particularly is influenced by whether cervical lymph node involvement has occurred early or late. The cure rate is most favorable for lesions of the lip, with prognosis poorest for lesions of the posterior tongue and floor of mouth.

The *histopathologic picture* in epidermoid carcinoma varies considerably, tending to well differentiated forms on the lip and, frequently, the gingiva. Others are more highly anaplastic, especially those of the posterior tongue. In the former type, columns of cells can be traced clearly into the stroma. These vary in size and shape and display large, deeply staining nuclei. The prominent features are many keratinized cells and epithelial pearls. Nucleoli are prominent, and mitosis is variable. The stroma is highly inflamed, and eosinophils are frequently found in considerable number.

The photomicrograph is reproduced by the courtesy of the Division of Oral Pathology, The Mount Sinai Hospital, New York.

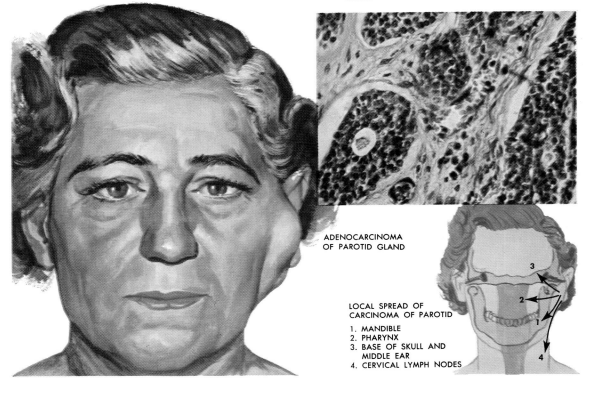

ADENOCARCINOMA
OF PALATE

LYMPHOSARCOMA OF
PALATE AND GINGIVA

LYMPHOSARCOMA

ADENOCARCINOMA
OF PAROTID GLAND

LOCAL SPREAD OF
CARCINOMA OF PAROTID

1. MANDIBLE
2. PHARYNX
3. BASE OF SKULL AND
   MIDDLE EAR
4. CERVICAL LYMPH NODES

MALIGNANT TUMORS II

Adenocarcinoma is rare in the oral cavity. When it develops from embryonic epithelium associated with small mucous glands, it arises chiefly in the palate and, in a few cases, on the lip, tongue and cheek. It is also encountered as a primary tumor of the major salivary glands, particularly the parotid. The adenocarcinoma begins as a deep-seated nodule beneath the mucosa, which may break through the surface and ulcerate at a late stage. Pain is usually not a feature of the early onset, and inflammation is far less evident than in the squamous cell variety. The palatal bone is invaded diffusely, as shown by a moth-eaten, ragged outline on the roentgenogram. Alveolar bone and antrum may be involved by extension, with loosening of teeth, which is sometimes the first symptom noticed by the patient. Metastasis is common.

Primary malignant tumors of the salivary glands may be discussed as a supplement to the description of mixed salivary tumors (see page 125). With regard to the parotid gland, it has been estimated that of all tumors of this gland about 20 per cent are malignant. Of these the greater part are primary malignancies; the remainders are malignant transformations of mixed tumors, adenomas and cysts. Primary malignant tumors may represent any embryonal cell type present in the gland. They include adenocarcinomas as well as undifferentiated, squamous cell and atypical spindle cell carcinomas, but a few sarcomas have also been reported. *Adenocarcinoma of the parotid gland* is pictured here as a primary tumor which presents a hard, non-encapsulated swelling, beginning in the uppermost part of the gland or in the retromandibular lobe and growing rapidly to distend the face. The intensity of pain, in such cases, may vary and may become excruciating from the extreme pressure on sensory nerves. The adjacent tissues are infiltrated, and the mass appears, on palpation, to be implanted on the ramus of the mandible, with fixation of the overlying skin. Infiltration of the masseter and other muscles results in trismus and, in one third of the cases, early facial nerve involvement. The pharynx or the base of the skull or the middle ear may be involved by direct

extension. Roentgenograms reveal a destructive lesion of bone, with a diffuse periphery. Regional lymph node metastasis is an early feature of this tumor, and metastasis via the blood stream is not uncommon in undifferentiated forms. The histopathologic picture of adenocarcinoma of the parotid gland may reproduce clearly the ducts or acini, or may be composed of strands and groups of mucus-producing cells enclosing lumenlike structures (cylindroma). The stroma often shows mucoid or hyaline degeneration.

Lymphosarcoma, as well as other varieties of lymphoblastomas, may be observed occasionally in the oral cavity. It takes origin from lymphoid tissue in the submucosa, favorite sites being the palate and pharynx. Typical features of this type of tumor are the rapid growth and the early extension into neighboring tissues and the metastases to all regional lymph nodes. Extremely rapid and early metastases may

account for the frequently noted characteristic of apparently multiple sites of origin, such as in separate parts of the maxilla simultaneously or at close time intervals.

Hodgkin's disease and lymphatic leukemia may also produce hyperplastic growths on the palate, gingiva and other locations. While the histopathologic appearance of Hodgkin's disease usually distinguishes it from lymphosarcoma, the nodule of lymphatic leukemia presents the same picture in tissue section as that of lymphosarcoma — a monotonous infiltration of lymphocytes. The lack of epithelial reaction and the monotony of cell type sets the lesion apart from an inflammatory growth with which it may be confused.

The photomicrographs are reproduced by the courtesy of the Division of Oral Pathology, The Mount Sinai Hospital, New York.

MALIGNANT TUMORS III

Jaws

Malignant tumors involving the jaw bones are nearly always epidermoid carcinomas, which are formed from peripheral epithelium and invade the bones secondarily. Malignant transformation of a benign neoplasm, particularly of a mixed tumor of salivary tissue, is sometimes seen. Metastases of primary carcinoma of the thyroid, breast or prostate to the jaws via the blood stream are very rare, and so are malignant primary tumors of odontogenic, osteogenic or other origin.

Though *osteogenic sarcoma* is the most common and most malignant of bone tumors, only 2 to 3 per cent of all cases appear in the jaw bones. Trauma is believed to play a rôle in its etiology, as evidenced by clinical histories and experimental production in animals. It is a solitary growth, which differentiates it from various tumors of nonosteogenic origin (*e.g.*, endothelioma, multiple myeloma). The maxillary tumor illustrated has caused wide, mottled destruction of bone, as revealed by roentgenographic findings. The classic "sun-ray" pattern, as known in the long bones, is seldom seen in the jaws, although new bone formation may be noted. The swelling has involved the entire maxilla and a portion of the palate and is invading the antrum. Pain, paresthesia, swelling, tenderness and displacement of teeth, with disturbed mastication, are associated symptoms. Blood-stream metastasis can be an early phenomenon.

The histopathologic picture shows immature cells, which are pleomorphic and hyperchromatic, with some admixture of stroma, myxomatous tissue, cartilage and osteoid tissue. Pathologic descriptions sometimes refer to osteolytic, osteoblastic and telangiectatic (vascular) types. The osteoblastic variety tends to grow more slowly than the vascular type.

Fibrosarcoma may be formed peripherally and invade the jaws, or centrally from either tissues of the tooth germ or other mesenchymal enclavements or connective tissue elements of the nerves and blood vessels. In the case of rapidly advancing osteolytic lesions, clinical recognition is usually delayed until loosening of the teeth, encroachment on the antrum or nose, or perforation of the cortical plate has occurred. No evidence of periosteal activity is noted, as is sometimes the case with osteosarcoma. Frequently, proud flesh in the socket of an extracted tooth is the first symptom of

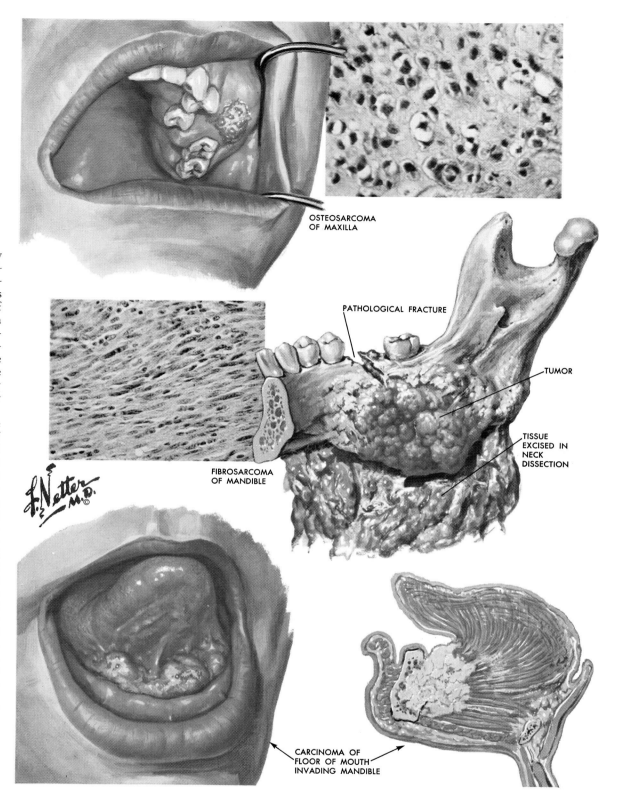

OSTEOSARCOMA OF MAXILLA

PATHOLOGICAL FRACTURE

TUMOR

TISSUE EXCISED IN NECK DISSECTION

FIBROSARCOMA OF MANDIBLE

CARCINOMA OF FLOOR OF MOUTH INVADING MANDIBLE

danger. In the *mandibular tumor,* chosen for illustration, pathologic fracture was caused by the widespread destruction of medullary bone. The tumor mass has perforated the lingual wall of the mandible, with invasion of soft tissues in the floor of the mouth and neck. Roentgenographic examination showed a blurred, diffuse osteolytic area, denoting an invasive rather than an expansile growth. The microscopic picture reveals spindle-shaped cells, with anaplasia and varying amounts of intercellular collagenous tissue; in the rapidly growing forms, a plump cellular shape, with frequent mitoses, and little intercellular material are present.

Carcinoma invading the mandible is illustrated in a lesion of the anterior *floor of the mouth.* The tumor here is a Grade III malignancy, causing an early infiltration of cortical bone, with progress along the Haversian canals and destruction of a large portion of cancellous bone. At the same time, extension occurs through the lymph channels to involve the submandibular and cervical nodes, as well as the soft tissues contiguous to the tumor. The base of the tongue has become fixed and immobile. A fungating tumor mass is observed in the floor of the mouth, which is secondarily infected and extremely painful, with a foul exudate and odor. Radiosensitivity of carcinoma in the floor of the mouth has been noted to be somewhat higher than that of the anterior tongue or cheek, yet the prognosis is poor in this location because of the proximity of bone and the difficulties of satisfactory irradiation, as well as the early appearance of lymph node metastases.

The photomicrographs are reproduced by the courtesy of the Division of Oral Pathology, The Mount Sinai Hospital, New York.

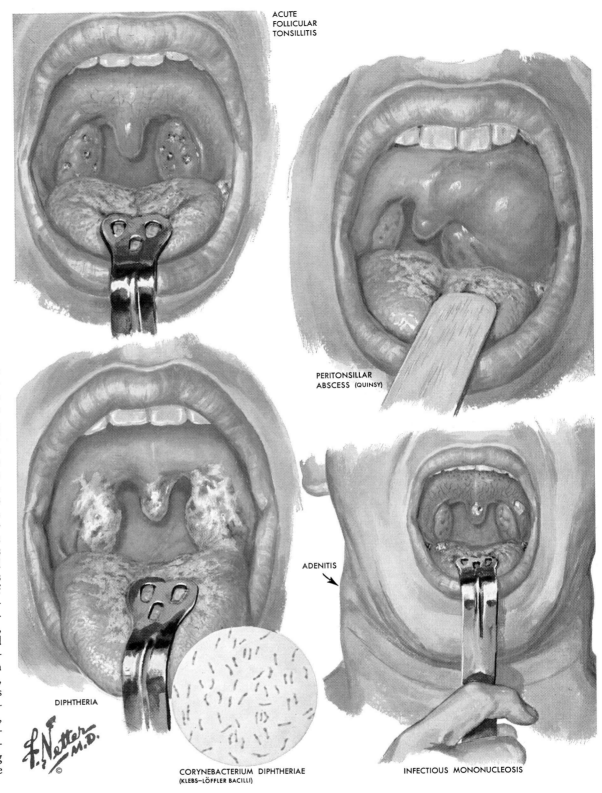

ACUTE FOLLICULAR TONSILLITIS

PERITONSILLAR ABSCESS (QUINSY)

DIPHTHERIA

CORYNEBACTERIUM DIPHTHERIAE (KLEBS–LÖFFLER BACILLI)

ADENITIS

INFECTIOUS MONONUCLEOSIS

INFECTIONS OF PHARYNX

Acute follicular tonsillitis, certainly one of if not the most frequent illness encountered in the practice of medicine, is essentially caused by streptococci of Group A, though in recent years an antibiotic-resistant strain of staphylococci has dramatically attained an increasing pathogenetic significance. It is a disease which predominantly occurs in early life and is more prone to affect patients with hypertrophic tonsils and a history of recurrent infections. After an incubation period varying from 1 to 10 days, the symptoms, such as headache, chills, pain in the throat and fever (101-104° F.), may set in quite abruptly. The tonsils are enlarged and inflamed with a cheesy, rarely coalescing exudate, which is visible in the tonsillar crypts. The infection is usually bilateral; the local lymph nodes (see pages 27 and 28) are tender and enlarged. Edema of the uvula produces a thick, muffled speech and pooling of saliva in the oral cavity. The neighboring adenoid tissue (lingual and pharyngeal tonsils, see pages 16 and 19, respectively) is very frequently involved in the inflammatory process of the infection. The disease may break out as an epidemic, especially in hospital wards, in which case the causative organism is almost invariably a hemolytic streptococcus. Sulfonamides and antibiotics, both used discriminately after determining the optimal sensitivity of the offending bacteria against them and excluding an allergic sensitivity of the patient, are most effective.

Scarlet fever (see also page 117) is, according to modern concepts, a special form of an acute follicular tonsillitis caused by a more infectious streptococcus, producing an erythrogenic toxin which is responsible for the exanthema and enanthema.

A local complication of acute follicular tonsillitis, but also of chronic tonsillar infection, is a suppurative process of the peritonsillar area. Such a *peritonsillar abscess,* also known as "quinsy", may begin to develop during the acute stage of the tonsillitis, but more often it becomes manifest when the patient is seemingly recovering from the acute throat infection. Soreness on swallowing, signs of trismus, marked edema of the uvula, which later becomes displaced to

the side opposite to the abscess, ipsilateral earache and increasing tenderness of the lymph nodes are the early characteristic signs, followed by a visible bulge of the anterior pillar of the fauces and soft palate. Occasionally, the swelling may occur in the posterior pillar and displace the tonsil forward. Palpation with the finger and the feeling of fluctuation in the swelling establishes the diagnosis. Spontaneous rupture or surgical drainage brings rapid relief, and antibacterial therapy will help cure this· disease.

Diphtheria, caused by Corynebacterium diphtheriae (Klebs-Löffler bacillus), is characterized by a membranous inflammation of the pharyngeal mucosa (though many other mucosal surfaces may be a primary site of the infection too). The membrane, a raised, yellowish-white patch, which may later become brownish and putrid, leaves a raw, bleeding surface if detached. The process is not limited to the

tonsillar crypts, as in follicular tonsillitis, but may involve the tonsillar pillars, soft palate, nose and larynx. The diagnosis can always be made by a smear from the exudate, in which the Corynebacterium diphtheriae can be identified morphologically or, more reliably, by culture in specific mediums. Antitoxin therapy is the treatment of choice, if necessary supported by penicillin after exclusion of an allergy against this antibiotic. Severe cases involving the larynx, necessitating tracheotomy, have become rare.

With the anginal type of glandular fever (*infectious mononucleosis,* see also page 117), small discrete patches surrounded by an area of erythema are dispersed throughout the throat. They disappear as the infection subsides but may last from 2 to 3 weeks and may recur. Although the adenopathy is generalized, the cervical glands are most often predominantly involved.

ALLERGIC PHARYNGITIS
(AS OFTEN SEEN AFTER
USE OF ANTIBIOTIC OR
OTHER THROAT LOZENGES)

ALLERGIC CONDITIONS OF PHARYNX

ANGIONEUROTIC EDEMA
OF SOFT PALATE AND UVULA
(QUINCKE'S EDEMA)

ANGIONEUROTIC EDEMA
OF ARYTENOID REGION

Manifestations of an allergic background may present themselves in the pharynx as independent disorders or may occur in association with allergic symptoms in the skin and elsewhere.

Angioneurotic edema, an acute, circumscribed, noninflammatory swelling of the mucosa of the pharynx, may occur without warning or apparent cause and can produce alarming and dangerous symptoms. It is not unusual to learn, in taking the family history, that relatives of the patient are afflicted with allergic diseases or that the patient himself suffers from asthma and certain skin disorders. Attacks may be precipitated by exposure to cold, extreme fright or ingestion of certain foods or drugs. The allergic edema involves not only the exposed mucous membranes but the deeper connective tissues. The involved surfaces are suddenly distended by an edematous fluid of a purely serous variety without inflammatory reaction. Such swellings can occur in the palate, uvula or aryepiglottic folds and in the arytenoids. Fatal cases involving the entire laryngeal mucosa have occurred. The edema is characteristically supraglottic, but isolated involvement of the epiglottis and aryepiglottic folds may also produce sudden threatening symptoms of asphyxia. The patient usually complains of an abrupt difficulty in deglutition or respiration associated with a sensation of a swelling or lump in the throat.

In *Quincke's edema* the uvula, soft palate and tonsillar pillars become distended with a pale edema, which protrudes into the pharynx and touches the tongue. Swallowing is impaired, and air hunger may supervene. If the supraglottic structures are involved, a sense of suffocation may be so oppressive that the patient has the feeling of impending death. The general treatment is similar to that of other allergic conditions, namely,

avoidance of the precipitating agent if possible and specific hyposensitization. Calcium preparations are administered in the belief that they decrease the permeability of the blood vessels and prevent abnormal passage of fluids through the capillaries, although the pharmacologic evidence for such an effort is anything but convincing. Local vasoconstrictors may be employed with the hope of shrinking the mucosa and relieving the air hunger. Antihistaminic drugs, on the other hand, should be given freely and may be very effective in relieving the edema. Corticosteroids have been helpful in lessening the edema. In severe and urgent cases, where no response to medication is prompt, an emergency tracheotomy may be resorted to as a lifesaving procedure. In most allergic conditions an associated eosinophilia will be helpful in confirming the diagnosis.

Allergic pharyngitis is now frequently seen as a

result of the use of antibiotic therapy and throat lozenges. Isolated superficial ulcerations, varying a few millimeters in diameter, surrounded by a small area of erythema, can be seen distributed throughout the soft palate, tonsillar pillars, buccal mucosa, undersurface of the tongue and lips. These, as a rule, have a whitish membranous covering. They may result from an antigen present in the local lozenge, such as an antibiotic or menthol frequently included in these lozenges. More often, these ulcerations result from administration of the broad-spectrum antibiotics, which produce them either as a manifestation of allergy to the drug or as a fungous infection incident to the antibiotic effect of these drugs on the normal flora in the oral cavity. The use of antihistaminics and steroids will usually give prompt relief, but, here again, avoidance of the offending drug should be impressed on the patient.

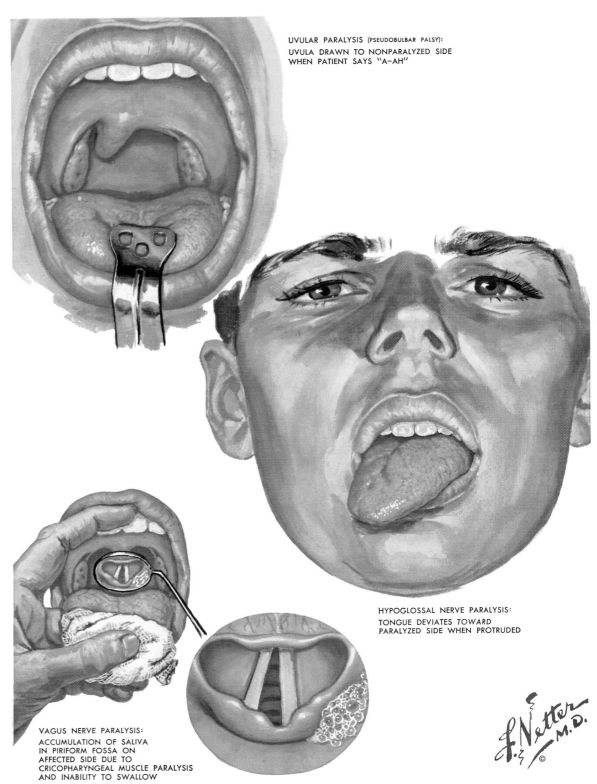

UVULAR PARALYSIS (PSEUDOBULBAR PALSY):
UVULA DRAWN TO NONPARALYZED SIDE
WHEN PATIENT SAYS "A–AH"

HYPOGLOSSAL NERVE PARALYSIS:
TONGUE DEVIATES *TOWARD*
PARALYZED SIDE WHEN PROTRUDED

VAGUS NERVE PARALYSIS:
ACCUMULATION OF SALIVA
IN PIRIFORM FOSSA ON
AFFECTED SIDE DUE TO
CRICOPHARYNGEAL MUSCLE PARALYSIS
AND INABILITY TO SWALLOW

Neurogenic Disorders of Mouth and Pharynx

The motor innervation to the pharynx and almost all sensory supply is through the pharyngeal plexus (see pages 29 and 30), which is formed by branches of the ninth and tenth cranial nerves. Because of overlapping in the innervation of these nerves and because, when a disturbance of their conduction occurs, the objective findings are similar, they are generally considered together.

Normally, the *uvula* hangs in mid-position, and in case of a *unilateral paralysis*, it deviates to the healthy side. This can be demonstrated when the patient utters: "A-AH". In bilateral, peripheral or nuclear (bulbar) palsy, the uvula does not move at all on attempted phonation or reflex stimulation. On the other hand, in supranuclear (pseudobulbar) palsy, the lower motor neuron reflex is preserved, and the uvula will move on tickling or stimulation with a tongue depressor, but it will not move on willful effort. The loss of pharyngeal reflex can be tested by irritation with a tongue depressor. Deglutition can be examined by having the patient swallow a few mouthfuls of water and by observing the upward excursion of the larynx. In paralysis of the soft palate, one notices nasal regurgitation or spasmodic coughing, because the fluid is propelled into the nasal cavity which is incompletely shut off during the act of swallowing. Nasal and palatal speech, aphonia and dyspnea, and difficulty in swallowing are the essential signs of a vagus paralysis. Since *vagal paralysis* leaves the superior pharyngeal constrictor muscle without innervation, retention of barium and distention of the involved piriform fossa can be demonstrated in such an instance by X-ray examination. Furthermore, it is possible to observe the pooling of the saliva in the postcricoid region and in the involved piriform fossa by mirror laryngoscopy. The vagal paralysis may be peripheral, as in a postdiphtheric condition, or it may be part of a jugular foramen syndrome, or it may have an intracranial origin, as occurs in amyotrophic sclerosis, thrombosis of the posterior inferior cerebellar artery, syringomyelia, or true bulbar paralysis so frequently seen in poliomyelitis. Paralysis may also result from supranuclear involvement (upper motor neuron), as seen usually in multiple vascular lesions producing the so-called "pseudobulbar paralysis". Normally, the tongue, which is innervated by the twelfth *hypoglossal nerve,* can protrude far out in the midline. In *unilateral paralysis* of this nerve, the tongue deviates to the paralyzed side. In complete bilateral paralysis the tongue cannot protrude at all and lies flat in the mouth. Unilateral or bilateral paralysis may be associated with atrophy and fibrillation, both indicative of peripheral involvement. Articulation, except for the pronunciation of labials, is impaired. In vagal paralysis the recurrent laryngeal nerve on the same side is always involved. This produces hoarseness owing to fixation of the vocal cord. In bilateral paralysis the cords either assume the cadaveric position or may become fixed in the midline, producing dyspnea and requiring emergency tracheotomy. Paralysis of the recurrent laryngeal nerve may result from a great variety of causes (trauma during surgery of the thyroid gland, pressure by metastatic carcinoma of the lymph nodes in cases of lung or breast cancer, from aneurysm of the aorta, lymphoma, extension of carcinoma of the thyroid gland and of the esophagus, etc.).

BENIGN TUMORS OF FAUCES AND ORAL PHARYNX

PAPILLOMAS OF SOFT PALATE AND ANTERIOR PILLAR

MIXED (SALIVARY GLAND) TUMOR OF PHARYNGEAL WALL

HEMANGIOMA OF PHARYNGEAL WALL

NEUROFIBROMA OF PHARYNGEAL WALL

The great majority of benign tumors of the oral pharynx are of connective tissue origin; small epithelial *papillomas of the tonsillar pillars and soft palate,* though not rare, are less often seen, because they are generally symptom-free and are detected only accidentally on routine examination. These small papillary masses can be removed at their base with a forceps, and after cauterization they almost never return.

Small adenomas of the soft palate and the posterior pharyngeal wall are also seldom seen and are best treated by excision.

The more frequent types of tumors are the sessile, connective tissue tumors of angiomatous origin. *Hemangioma* of the oral pharynx is usually congenital but may go unnoticed until later in life. The bluish-purple discoloration of the tumor through the overlying distended mucosa is characteristic and permits the diagnosis without further microscopic examination. The mass is soft and collapsible on pressure. Many of these tumors are symptom-free, and only rarely do they produce bleeding. Hemangiomas of the pharynx are occasionally associated with similar lesions on the lip, tongue, cheek, and elsewhere in the gastro-intestinal tract. No therapy is indicated unless the lesions attain such size as to produce disturbing symptoms. Various methods of treatment, such as radiotherapy, radium pack, application of carbon dioxide snow, instillation of sclerosing solutions and coagulation with diathermy, have been practiced, but generally without satisfying results. Surgical excision,

with an attempt to find and ligate the afferent and efferent vessels, seems to be the best approach.

Mixed tumors of the pharyngeal wall present as smooth, rather firm, submucosal bulges. They are occasionally seen in the retrotonsillar region behind the soft palate or on the posterior pharyngeal wall, or in the substance of the soft palate itself. Diagnosis may be made by needle biopsy. More frequently, excisional biopsy of the whole tumor with a safe margin of mucosa on the free edges not only establishes the diagnosis but may effect a permanent cure. Mixed tumors have a tendency to recur unless they are widely excised. If the tumor is broken or incompletely removed, recurrence is an all too frequent event.

Neurofibroma of the hypopharynx presents as a sessile, nodular, submucosal tumor frequently extending in a linear fashion along the posterior or lateral

pharyngeal wall. These tumors may be associated with diffuse neurofibromatosis. They are encapsulated tumors which protrude into the hypopharynx. Diagnosis may be suspected from aspiration biopsy, but excisional biopsy with a wide margin of mucosa is more reliable.

Other, less frequent types of tumor of connective tissue origin, occasionally seen in the oral pharynx, include the lipomas, myoblastomas (especially on the posterior aspect of the tongue), and fibromas of the pharyngeal mucosa. Rarely, a myoblastoma may develop as a result of a trauma and submucosal hemorrhage. These tumors, characterized by polygonal cells with highly granular cytoplasm, can be felt as a deep mass below the mucosa. They are not as firm as carcinoma and have no tendency to ulcerate. All these neoplasms are best treated by local excision, which establishes the diagnosis and effects a cure.

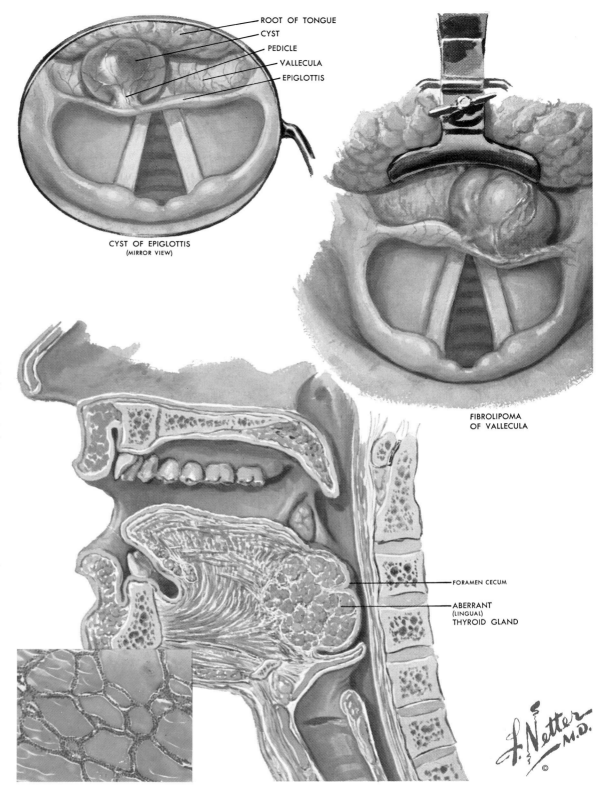

CYST OF EPIGLOTTIS
(MIRROR VIEW)

FIBROLIPOMA
OF VALLECULA

BENIGN TUMORS OF VALLECULA AND ROOT OF TONGUE

In the *vallecula and root of the tongue*, small connective tissue *tumors* of benign character may exist for a long time before they attain a size which interferes with the deglutition of solid food. Occasionally, the first complaint of the patient may be a difficulty in breathing when assuming a certain position of the head, mostly because these benign tumors are pedunculated and compromise the airways when the tumor mass is dislodged by a change in position of the head. These tumors are smooth, soft and covered by an intact mucosa. The most common of them is the retention *cyst of the epiglottis*, which may be detected during a casual mirror examination. The cyst may be freely movable in view of its pedunculated attachment to the mucosal surface of the epiglottis. Removal by forceps under indirect laryngoscopy is adequate.

A *fibrolipoma of the vallecula* may not be discovered until threatening symptoms of suffocation are present. The tumor mass is usually rounded, of a yellowish tinge and covered by a smooth mucosa. The mass has a sessile attachment to the lingual surface of the epiglottis, which it displaces posteriorly, thereby overhanging the aditus of the larynx. The benign nature of the tumor is usually self-evident. Removal can best be effected by suspension laryngoscopy. The tumor can be grasped and its attachment severed from the wide base to the epiglottis with scissors or diathermy snare.

Neuroma of the vallecula (not illustrated) is rare but may attain a large size before becoming apparent. The symptoms, again, are referable to the size of the tumor and may result in either dysphagia or difficulty in breathing.

An *aberrant lingual thyroid gland* may be present for a long time before it is diagnosed. It makes its appearance as a smooth bulge in the posterior surface of the tongue, starting in the region of the foramen cecum and extending posteriorly to the lingual surface of the epiglottis. The mass presents a smooth surface which is soft to the touch and covered by an intact mucosa. Sometimes the tumor may attain a size so large as to produce a major impediment in breath-

ing, by virtue of its extension inferiorly and/or by depressing the epiglottis into the laryngeal vestibule. The diagnosis should always be entertained when a smooth tumor of the base of the tongue is encountered. The diagnosis is often made by exclusion. The administration of radioactive iodine and demonstration with the Geiger counter of its being taken up in the region of the protruding mass will establish the diagnosis. Biopsy is usually not rewarding, because one must penetrate the deep mucosa of the base of the tongue in order to get to the substance of the thyroid tissue. If the mass produces no symptoms, therapy is probably not indicated.

Microscopically, the aberrant lingual thyroid presents usually the picture of a normally functioning thyroid gland, which should be left intact whenever possible, because in about half of the cases it is the only functioning thyroid tissue in the body, the

thyroid residues in the normal location being nonfunctional (also demonstrated by I[131] uptake). If the mass is so big that it endangers respiration, therapeutic doses of radioactive iodine suffice to cause a subsidence of the tumor and to create a hypothyroid state, which must be treated accordingly. Only in children does the use of I[131] seem inadvisable, because it still remains to be determined whether any deleterious effect results in later life from the use of this radioactive element. Adenomatous tissue, which can be found in the lingual thyroid gland and is also often found in the normally located thyroid, is best removed by lateral pharyngotomy and submucosal resection.

In the base of the tongue, other tumor masses may occur which require removal. Myoblastoma is a common finding and responds to surgical extirpation. Amyloid tumors of the tongue and chondromas have been described and are less amenable to therapy.

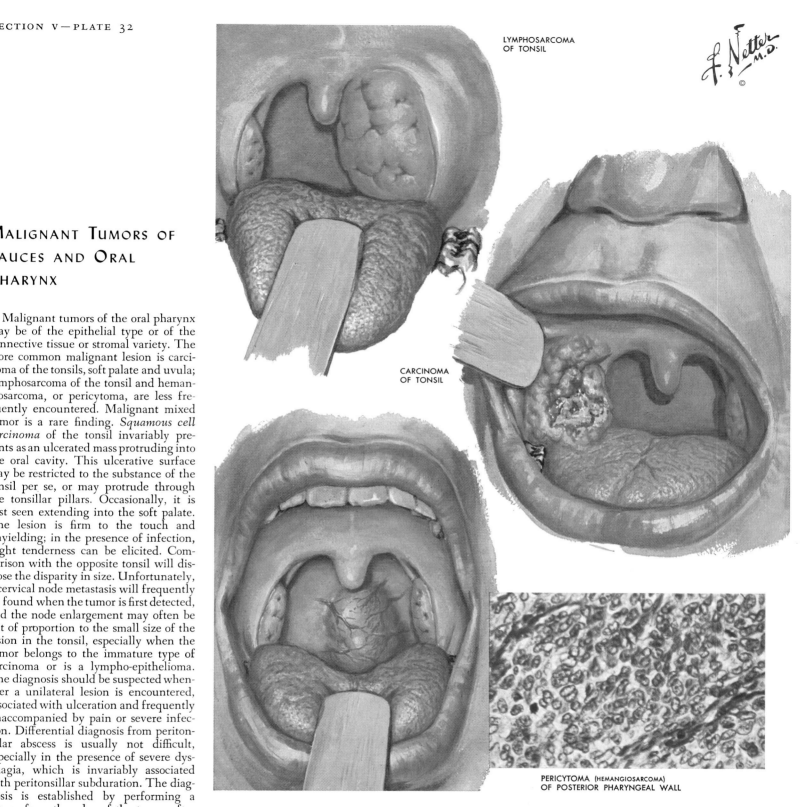

LYMPHOSARCOMA
OF TONSIL

CARCINOMA
OF TONSIL

PERICYTOMA (HEMANGIOSARCOMA)
OF POSTERIOR PHARYNGEAL WALL

MALIGNANT TUMORS OF FAUCES AND ORAL PHARYNX

Malignant tumors of the oral pharynx may be of the epithelial type or of the connective tissue or stromal variety. The more common malignant lesion is carcinoma of the tonsils, soft palate and uvula; lymphosarcoma of the tonsil and hemangiosarcoma, or pericytoma, are less frequently encountered. Malignant mixed tumor is a rare finding. *Squamous cell carcinoma* of the tonsil invariably presents as an ulcerated mass protruding into the oral cavity. This ulcerative surface may be restricted to the substance of the tonsil per se, or may protrude through the tonsillar pillars. Occasionally, it is first seen extending into the soft palate. The lesion is firm to the touch and unyielding; in the presence of infection, slight tenderness can be elicited. Comparison with the opposite tonsil will disclose the disparity in size. Unfortunately, a cervical node metastasis will frequently be found when the tumor is first detected, and the node enlargement may often be out of proportion to the small size of the lesion in the tonsil, especially when the tumor belongs to the immature type of carcinoma or is a lympho-epithelioma. The diagnosis should be suspected whenever a unilateral lesion is encountered, associated with ulceration and frequently unaccompanied by pain or severe infection. Differential diagnosis from peritonsillar abscess is usually not difficult, especially in the presence of severe dysphagia, which is invariably associated with peritonsillar subduration. The diagnosis is established by performing a biopsy from the edge of the tumor after preliminary cocainization. Careful examination for extension of the tumor into the nasopharynx and the hypopharynx must be made before deciding on the type of therapy. The method of treatment is essentially radiotherapy to the primary lesion and then elective neck dissection after the primary tumor has been controlled. Owing to the relatively high radiosensitivity of this tumor type, therapy with cobalt[60] has been successful in a number of cases. If this treatment fails to effect a cure, the so-called "commando operation" or radical neck dissection, with partial mandiblectomy (ascending portion of ramus) in continuity with the tumor and the tonsillar region should be performed.

Lymphosarcoma of the tonsil presents as a huge bulge into the oral pharynx, in which the mucosal surfaces are almost always intact. The tumor is located within the tonsillar substance itself, producing a widening of the tonsillar tissue between the crypts. About 50 per cent of the cases of lymphosarcoma of the tonsil occur as an isolated type of lymphosarcoma and may not become generalized lymphosarcomatosis for many years. Cervical node enlargement on the ipsilateral side is, however, quite common. Here again, a biopsy deep to the mucosa will establish the diagnosis. Bleeding may be brisk and is controlled by pressure. The treatment of choice is radiotherapy. A certain proportion of these cases of lymphosarcoma of the tonsil remain isolated, and a 5-year cure is obtainable, but the great majority of cases will be, sooner or later, complicated by generalized lymphosarcomatosis.

Hemangiosarcoma of the oral pharynx, especially *pericytoma,* is a rare condition. The tumor presents as a bulge submucosally on the posterior or lateral pharyngeal wall. The mucosal blood vessels appear distinct, and the mass is firm to the touch. The diagnosis can be made only by adequate biopsy deep to the mucosa. While lymph node metastasis occurs, it is not as frequent as metastasis to the lungs. Radiotherapy is generally ineffective in these lesions, and the greatest hope for cure rests with wide surgical excision, occasionally associated with skin graft replacement for the mucosal surface excised with the tumor.

A malignant mixed tumor of the hypopharynx is occasionally seen where there has been rapid growth of a pre-existing smooth, firm tumor. The diagnosis is usually made only after excision of the tumor (performed transorally) by histologic examination.

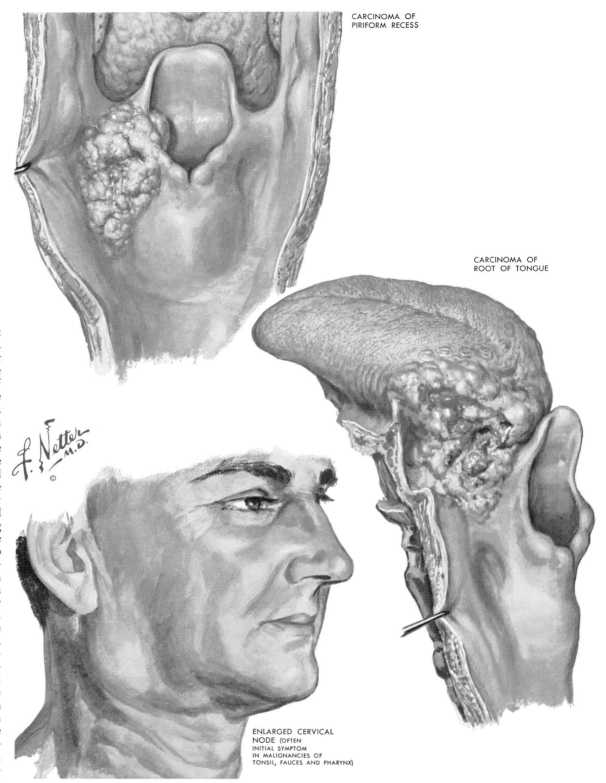

CARCINOMA OF
PIRIFORM RECESS

CARCINOMA OF
ROOT OF TONGUE

ENLARGED CERVICAL
NODE (OFTEN
INITIAL SYMPTOM
IN MALIGNANCIES OF
TONSIL, FAUCES AND PHARYNX)

MALIGNANT TUMORS OF HYPOPHARYNX

Malignant tumors of the hypopharynx are predominantly of epithelial origin. *Carcinoma of the root of the tongue* or of the immobile portion of the tongue has proved to be the most serious type of lesion which occurs in this region. The first symptoms are pain on swallowing, otalgia on the same side, discomfort in the throat and, finally, difficulty in breathing. The ulcerative, infiltrative form of such a carcinoma is the more treacherous and produces early cervical node metastasis, while the proliferative type presents itself as a bulge on the root of the tongue and is readily visible and easily palpable. It is often surprising how advanced the lesion appears to be before producing symptoms sufficient to bring the patient to the physician. Palpation of the base of the tongue will often permit recognition of a firm mass, even when it is not detectable on ordinary examination with the tongue depressor. Many of these carcinomas are of the immature or undifferentiated type, explaining their tendency to early metastasis. The tumor may extend into the vallecula and displace the epiglottis toward the laryngeal lumen, causing some hoarseness and, occasionally, difficulty in breathing in the reclining position. Pain on swallowing usually prompts the patient to seek medical advice. On mirror examination, an ulcerative growth may be visible, which is frequently covered with debris and whitish exudate. The tumor may extend into the tonsillar pillars and floor of the mouth. Although usually confined to one side, it may extend across the midline. Grasping and extending the tongue with a piece of gauze, the posterior third of the tongue may be visualized, and after thorough cocainization a representative biopsy should be taken for diagnostic purpose. Where the lesion extends more posteriorly into the vallecula, a biopsy can best be obtained by indirect or direct laryngoscopy. The therapy of carcinoma of the tongue is the least rewarding of that of carcinoma anywhere in the body. Surgical extirpation often necessitates total laryngectomy, hemiglossectomy, partial mandiblectomy and radical neck dissection. The therapy of choice, according

to recent experience, seems to be cobalt radiation, followed within a period of 4 to 6 weeks by an elective neck dissection on the side of the lesion. Residual growth should be treated with radium implantations, which are occasionally effective.

Carcinoma of the piriform fossa is an extrinsic laryngeal lesion. The tumor may arise on the medial wall of the piriform fossa and extend on to the aryepiglottic fold and epiglottis, or it may have its origin on the lateral wall of the piriform fossa and extend on to the lateral wall of the pharynx and down into the mouth of the esophagus. These lesions produce symptoms only in a late stage of the disease. The vocal cords are not compromised, and hoarseness is a relatively late symptom. Dysphagia may also occur only late, since the pathway left free at the opposite piriform fossa is usually adequate for deglutition. The first symptom of the presence of this lesion may be

the appearance of a cervical node on the same side of the neck. Diagnosis is best made by mirror examination followed by biopsy, which can be obtained by either indirect or direct laryngoscopy. Tomography of the larynx, especially in the anterior-posterior position, will often show an obliteration of the piriform fossa on the involved side. The lesions are invariably of the squamous type carcinoma, with a high percentage of undifferentiated or immature type. Therapy consists of wide excision, including total laryngectomy in continuity with radical neck dissection and hemithyroidectomy on the same side. Radiotherapy has been generally ineffective but should be tried, especially in the immature type of carcinoma. If ulceration persists, and if the tumor does not seem to subside soon after a radiation trial period, institution of surgery with laryngectomy and neck dissection is inevitable.

Section VI

DISEASES OF THE ESOPHAGUS

by

FRANK H. NETTER, M.D.

in collaboration with

MAX L. SOM, M.D., F.A.C.S.
Plates 1-6, 8-19

BERNARD S. WOLF, M.D.
Plate 7

CONGENITAL ANOMALIES

Congenital atresia of the esophagus and tracheo-esophageal fistula are the most common anomalies encountered in the newborn infant. The formation of these anomalies must be attributed to the fact that in early fetal life the so-called "laryngotracheal groove" runs length-wise on the floor of the primitive gut and that during that period esophagus and trachea are one tube, which, by the ingrowth of mesoderm, divides into two tubes between the fourth and twelfth weeks of embryonal development. The early esophageal lumen is first closed by proliferation of the epithelial lining cells but is later re-established by vacuolation. Some disturbance in this normal developmental growth may inhibit the mesoderm to dissociate the trachea and esophagus completely, resulting in a congenital tracheo-esophageal fistula, or the vacuoles may fail to coalesce, leaving a solid core of esophageal cells which is responsible for an atresia. In the great majority of anomalies, the upper portion of the esophagus ends as a blind pouch at the level of the second thoracic verte-bra, and the lower segment of the esopha-gus enters the trachea just above its bifurcation. The upper segment of the esophagus becomes dilated and hyper-trophied as a result of the ineffectual attempts of the fetus to swallow. The dis-tal segment of the esophagus may be of normal size but tapers proximally, so that its lumen may be reduced to 3 or 4 mm. at its communication with the trachea. The symptoms are noted soon after birth, and the patient seems to produce an excessive amount of saliva accompanied by spells of choking and cyanosis, which increase with attempts to feed the infant. Roentgen examination will establish the diagnosis. The exact location of the obstruction, in congenital atresia usually 10 to 12 cm. from the mouth, may be determined by introducing a rubber cath-eter under fluoroscopic control. The out-line of the abnormality can be clearly visualized by instillation of an appropri-ate contrast medium (½ to 1 ml. of Lipiodol® or Ethiodol®).

Congenital anomalies of the esophagus are frequently associated with anomalies of other organs of the body, and some of these are incompatible with life unless corrected surgically, if at all possible. The congenital atresia manifests itself in a number of different ways, the more common of which are illustrated. Very frequently, the proximal portion of the *esophagus ends as a blind pouch* (1a and 1b). A fibrous cord extends from the distal part of this pouch to the upper portion of the distal esophagus which, in turn, communicates with the trachea or, less frequently, with a bronchus (*broncho-esophageal fistula*). In another variety of congenital atresia (2) no com-munication, *i.e.*, fistula between esopha-gus and respiratory tract, has developed;

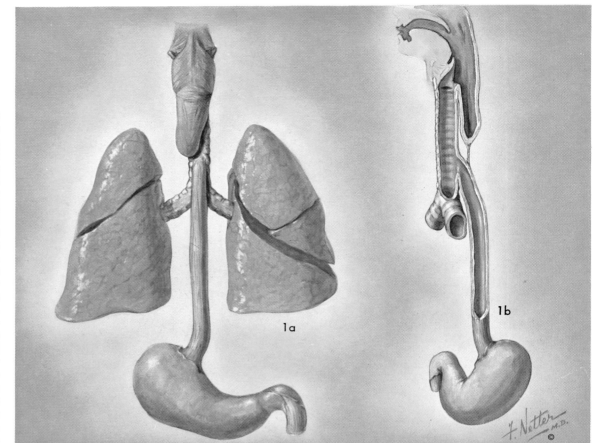

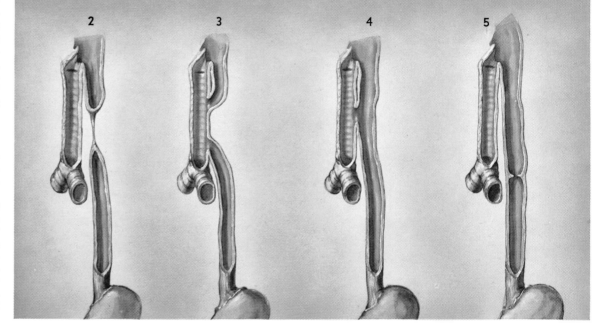

only a fibrous cord connects a *blindly ending pouch at the proximal part* of the esophagus with its lower part and, in rare cases, even the fibrous cord may be miss-ing, so that both blind pouches end freely without connection. In other instances (3) the proximal por-tion, as well as the distal part, of the *esophagus may open into the trachea*. A congenital tracheo-esopha-geal fistula may also exist any distance along the posterior wall of the trachea when the lumen of the esophagus is completely normal (4). Finally, with a perfectly normal trachea and no communication between it and the gullet, a congenital atresia may be produced by a *stenosing web* somewhere along the course of the esophagus (5).

Pediatricians and obstetricians must be alerted to these anomalies, because symptoms will be observed soon after birth. The patient should be kept in the incubator, which provides for an influx of oxygen, controlled temperature and humidity. A soft rubber catheter should be introduced into the pharynx for constant suction. Slight Trendelenburg position will facilitate aspiration of the mucus. Intravenous feed-ing of a 5 per cent solution of dextrose in distilled water is mandatory to maintain or restore the infant's nutri-tional status, so that an operation, the only rational treatment, may be performed at the earliest possible moment. A variety of operative procedures have been described, the principles of which are, essentially, closure of the fistula if present and anastomosis of the esophageal ends. A gastrostomy for temporary feeding may be necessary but can usually be avoided, and feeding can be maintained after the fourth day by the normal alimentary route. A considerable improvement in the survival rate of infants with atretic esophagus and tracheo-esophageal fistula has

(*Continued on page 139*)

CONGENITAL ANOMALIES

(Continued from page 138)

been achieved in the past decade. Strangely enough, infants in the first 48 hours of life stand major surgical procedures well.

Difficulty in swallowing caused by the presence of webs at or near the cricopharyngeal fold may be well treated by dilation with bougies.

A different type of congenital stenosis in the thoracic esophagus is caused by incomplete cannulization of the distal portion of the esophagus, which leads to manifestations typical of stricture formation in the esophageal lower third. The symptoms, beginning in early infancy, are usually dysphagia and regurgitation of solid food but, as a rule, are noticed only when ingestion of solid food begins. Esophagoscopy reveals a stricture or flap usually located near the cardiac end of the stomach. Gradual dilation with bougies usually proves successful.

A congenital *shortness of the esophagus* — having recently come into prominence as a result of extensive research (Brown, Kelly and Findlay) and because of its significance in later life — is caused by an inadequate elongation of the esophagus, which interferes with its following the descent of the diaphragm at the moment of birth and first respiration. If, owing to some unknown developmental defect, the esophageal tube is too short to occupy the entire length from the sixth cervical to the tenth thoracic vertebra (see page 35), the stomach is pulled cranially so as to come into such close contact with the diaphragm that part of the organ may pass through the hiatus and become enclosed in the thoracic cavity (see page 158). The esophagus in such conditions usually terminates at the level of the seventh thoracic vertebra. The junction of the esophagus and the stomach can be recognized by the change of the epithelial lining when examined esophagoscopically. At the point of transition, no narrowing or stricture coarctation is necessarily present, but sometimes a stenosis is found, which, when causing functional disturbances, will require dilation. The chief disadvantage of a congenital short esophagus rests with the lack of an adequate sphincter mechanism (see pages 148 and 158).

The normal, irregular, wavy demarcation line ("Z-Z" line) between esophageal and gastric mucosa, as described earlier (see page 38), is subject to many variations. Thus, *e.g.,* the extensions of the gastric mucosa, usually only a few millimeters long, may protrude in fingerlike fashion upward for 1 or 2 cm. into the distal portion of the esophagus. These striplike projections, between which one can recognize the flattened, paler, squamous epithelium of the esophagus, marking a displacement of gastric structures, have been called *"heterotopia"*, in contrast to the appearance of some small, discrete islands of gastric mucosa, as they are found quite frequently in the more proximal parts of the stomach. The latter, having little, if any, clinical and pathologic significance, should be differentiated from the aberrant extensions of the gastric mucosa near the gastro-esophageal junction and, therefore, have been designated as ectopic gastric epithelium (*ectopia*).

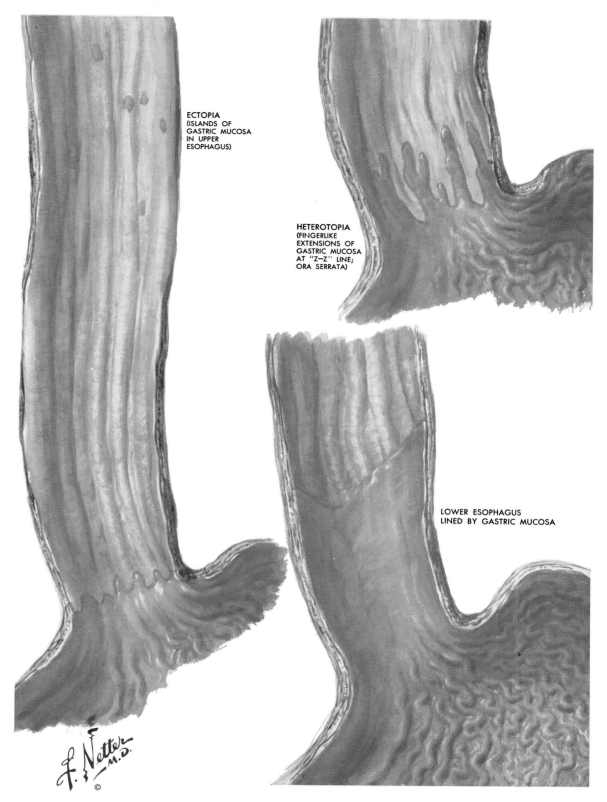

ECTOPIA (ISLANDS OF GASTRIC MUCOSA IN UPPER ESOPHAGUS)

HETEROTOPIA (FINGERLIKE EXTENSIONS OF GASTRIC MUCOSA AT "Z-Z" LINE; ORA SERRATA)

LOWER ESOPHAGUS LINED BY GASTRIC MUCOSA

The heterotopic gastric mucosa in the fingerlike extensions and still more so the strongly exaggerated form of mucosal displacement, for which the term *"gastric-lined esophagus"* has been introduced (Allison, *et al.,* Barrett), give cause to the development of peptic ulcers (see page 148), particularly in the presence of an acquired sliding hernia (see page 158), with sphincter incompetence. This condition, in which the most distal part of the esophageal lumen may be covered with typical gastric mucosa up to 3 or 4 cm. high, is doubtless a congenital anomaly, in spite of the fact that its clinical consequence may become evident only much later in life. The designation "short esophagus" for the "gastric-lined esophagus" is somewhat misleading, because the structure, shape and position of both the stomach and the esophagus, except for the mucosa of the latter in its distal parts, differ in no way from those seen in normal individuals, although one may, of course, consider the esophagus "short" with respect to the length of its own mucosa. The pathogenesis of peptic ulcers in "gastric-lined esophagus" and their diagnosis are discussed elsewhere (see page 148). The recognition of the gastric nature of the lining in the distal esophagus when no ulcer is present may be difficult, not only because this condition may cause no symptoms for a long period of time (if ever) but also because the rugae, typical of the gastric mucosa, may be absent or invisible on endoscopy or even on macroscopic examination.

DISPLACEMENT

Normally, the esophagus shows deviations from a straight downward course as described on pages 34 and 35. More pronounced digressions, along a line marking the shortest distance between pharynx and stomach, are produced by pressure from neoplasms or *thoracic tumor masses* along the entire course of the esophagus. They may cause indentations and displacements of the esophagus as well as actual invasion of the esophageal wall by malignant growth. In the neck the esophagus is often displaced by a large, colloid tumor of the thyroid. The posterior extension of the thyroid tumor may encroach upon the esophagus and compress its lumen. This is especially prone to happen in papillary adenocarcinoma of the thyroid. Metastatic tumors of the neck likewise displace the esophagus and interfere with its physiologic functions. The lymphomas, especially Hodgkin's disease and lymphosarcoma, starting in the neck and extending into the mediastinum, are excellent examples in this respect. On the other hand, thymomas and dermoid cysts of the mediastinum are usually located anteriorly and do not encroach upon the esophagus. The slow-growing carotid body tumors, although commencing high in the neck at the level of the bifurcation of the common carotid artery, may descend into the lower neck and dislocate the esophagus.

Pulsion diverticulum of the esophagus (see page 143), when large enough, may displace the esophageal lumen to the opposite side.

Aneurysms of the aorta can produce both compression and displacement of the esophagus. If the aneurysm involves the arch of the aorta, the esophagus is displaced posteriorly. On the other hand,

DISPLACEMENT OF ESOPHAGUS BY ENLARGED HEART

DISPLACEMENT OF ESOPHAGUS BY ANEURYSM OF AORTA

if the dilatation of the aorta occurs in its descending portion, then the esophagus may be displaced anteriorly, and the compression may be sufficient to cause marked dysphagia. The displacements incident to a double aortic arch and a right subclavian artery, originating in the left descending aorta, are referred to on page 141. One of the most common causes of posterior displacement of the lower esophagus is a dilated left auricle, associated with mitral disease. A swallow of barium will in most cases demonstrate the displacement of the esophagus posteriorly by the enlarged left auricle. In the posterior mediastinum neoplasms such as neuromas and bronchiolar cysts may displace the esophagus medially. Carcinoma of the bronchus with mediastinal lymph nodes not only displaces the esophagus but may actually invade it and produce dysphagia.

Paracardial hernia (see page 159), accompanied by a protrusion of a good portion of the stomach into the thoracic cage, may displace the esophagus to the opposite side while maintaining the normal relationship between the termination of the esophagus and the stomach proper. A large epiphrenic diverticulum (see page 143) may frequently displace the esophagus and produce dysphagia. Similarly, traction may be exerted by the shrinkage of tuberculous mediastinal lymph nodes.

Regular examination of the course of the esophagus will usually demonstrate the location of the displacement and the actual invasion of the esophageal wall in cases of malignancy. Therapy is directed toward the specific etiologic cause of the tumor masses displacing or invading the esophageal musculature. In lymphomas radiotherapy will usually produce prompt palliation but will not result in complete alleviation of symptoms.

ESOPHAGUS
RIGHT COMMON CAROTID ARTERY
RIGHT SUBCLAVIAN ARTERY
LEFT COMMON CAROTID ARTERY
LEFT SUBCLAVIAN ARTERY

DOUBLE AORTIC ARCH
DISTORTING ESOPHAGUS

RIGHT COMMON
CAROTID ARTERY
LEFT COMMON
CAROTID ARTERY
LEFT SUBCLAVIAN
ARTERY

ANOMALOUS RIGHT
SUBCLAVIAN ARTERY

TRACHEA

ANOMALOUS RIGHT
SUBCLAVIAN ARTERY
DISTORTING ESOPHAGUS

X-RAY:
DYSPHAGIA LUSORIA
(ANOMALOUS RIGHT
SUBCLAVIAN ARTERY)

Double Aortic Arch, Dysphagia Lusoria

The aortic arch develops from the fourth of the original six aortic arches in early fetal life. Many combinations of defects can result from anomalies of the various arches, either from their persistence or from their failure to develop. The most common anomalies to occur are the *double aortic arch* with the right arch passing posteriorly around the esophagus to join a small left arch, which, in turn, proceeds into the descending left aorta. The left arch may be greater, and the descending aorta may be on the right side rather than on the left. Other congenital anomalies of the heart are rarely combined with this disorder. The double aortic arch forms a vascular ring which, if not too tight around the trachea and esophagus, may remain symptom-free and the anomaly may be unnoticed until death. Usually, however, respiratory difficulty is evident from the moment the child is born. Flexion of the neck increases the stridor by producing tension on the posterior arch, and extension improves the breathing by relieving this pressure. A barium swallow yields much diagnostic information such as narrowing of the esophagus from both sides and posteriorly. On lateral projection a pulsating mass, displacing both trachea and esophagus anteriorly, may be visible on the posterior esophageal aspect. Angiography will demonstrate the anomaly and show which of the arches is larger, thereby indicating the best approach for surgical division. Other causes of respiratory stri-

dor in early life, especially in infants under 3 months of age, must be excluded, namely, laryngismus stridulus, congenital web of the larynx, tetany, foreign bodies and choanal atresia. The treatment is surgical and the approach is from the left chest in almost all instances. When the vascular ring is very tight, death may occur early in life before institution of treatment. When the posterior arch is replaced by the ligamentum arteriosum, symptoms may not become manifest until later in life. Even after surgery some deformity may persist in the trachea, but ultimately the tracheal lumen will expand owing to the release of pressure incident to the surgery.

An *anomalous right subclavian artery* arising from the left descending aorta may produce dysphagia, so-called "dysphagia lusoria". The right subclavian artery normally takes its origin from the fourth branch of the fetal aortic arch, but in this anomaly it arises

from the descending aorta and pursues a course posterior to the esophagus to reach the right arm. This condition is often associated with progressive dysphagia, so that the patients can swallow only liquids or, at most, a soft diet. The diagnosis is confirmed by a barium swallow, which shows a small indentation on the posterior wall of the esophagus ordinarily at the level of the fourth thoracic vertebra. On esophagoscopy a pulsating transverse linear ridge can be seen on the posterior wall. If this anomaly is entertained, then pressure with the esophagoscopic tube on this pulsating ridge will obliterate the pulse in the right arm and confirm the diagnosis of dysphagia lusoria. Respiratory symptoms are not seen with this anomaly. Therapy consists of ligation and division of the anomalous subclavian artery from the descending aorta. Collateral circulation will promptly establish itself spontaneously.

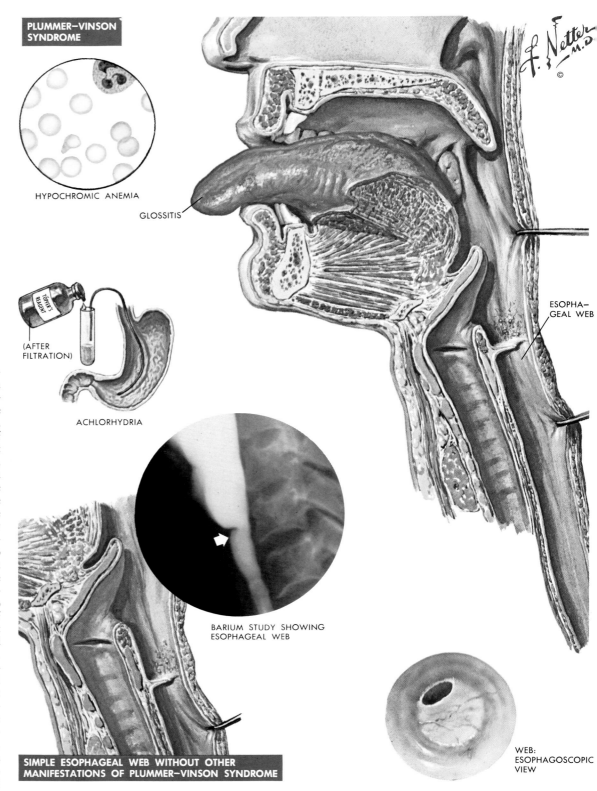

PLUMMER-VINSON SYNDROME

HYPOCHROMIC ANEMIA

GLOSSITIS

(AFTER FILTRATION)

ACHLORHYDRIA

BARIUM STUDY SHOWING ESOPHAGEAL WEB

ESOPHAGEAL WEB

WEB: ESOPHAGOSCOPIC VIEW

SIMPLE ESOPHAGEAL WEB WITHOUT OTHER MANIFESTATIONS OF PLUMMER–VINSON SYNDROME

PLUMMER-VINSON SYNDROME

The chief characteristic of the Plummer-Vinson syndrome is dysphagia which is often accompanied by *hypochromic anemia*. The syndrome may be associated with *achlorhydria, glossitis,* stomatitis, brittle nails and stricture of the mouth of the esophagus; it is most frequently encountered in edentulous, premenopausal, married women. Only a few instances have been reported in the male. The patients are usually in the fourth and fifth decades of life. The patient's chief complaints are invariably difficulty in swallowing, usually accompanied by generalized weakness due to anemia, and dryness of the mouth with burning of the tongue. The syndrome develops gradually over a period of several months or even years and leads to a sensation of obstruction in the back of the throat and neck. Fluids are in almost all cases well tolerated, while solid food may be rejected or impossible to swallow.

Atrophic glossitis and a dry, pharyngeal and buccal mucosa, with painful cracks at the angles of the mouth, present themselves regularly in all patients suffering from this syndrome. The atrophic mucosa may extend into the hypopharynx and into the mouth of the esophagus. Less regular are the brittle fingernails and other evidences of multiple avitaminosis. Splenomegaly has been observed in about 30 per cent of the cases. Although anemia does not invariably occur, when present it is of the iron-deficiency type, being hypochromic and microcytic. The hemoglobin level may be as low as 50 per cent of normal. Achlorhydria is encountered in the great majority of patients.

Formerly, dysphagia was attributed to the presence of an esophageal web found on X-ray examination and/or by esophagoscopy. More recent studies indicate that these webs are often asymptomatic and that the dysphagia of Plummer-Vinson syndrome frequently occurs in the absence of such findings. If a web is present, it is often found in the course of an X-ray examination in which the patient is given a small amount of barium

suspension. On the X-ray film, the web is apparent as a *filling defect* in the wall of the esophagus just below the border of the cricoid cartilage. Such a filling defect may occasionally concern the entire circumference of the upper esophagus, with the barium column being arrested above it and spilling over into the larynx and trachea. Such a stricture, which these roentgen findings obviously indicate, is caused, as can readily be *demonstrated on esophagoscopy,* by the formation of a *weblike structure* usually originating from a site on the anterior wall of the cervical esophagus, somewhere between the hypopharynx and 1 or 2 cm. below the cricopharyngeal region. The web, a few millimeters thick at its root, becomes thinner as it protrudes into the esophageal tube and may be paper-thin at its periphery, where it usually leaves an eccentrically situated lumen between its border and the anterior wall. The mucosa surrounding the inser-

tion of the web is atrophic and shiny, and chronic inflammatory changes and degenerative manifestations of the epithelium in the vicinity have been described, but the true causes leading to the formation of the web remain obscure. It is, however, of interest and certainly of practical significance that in a fairly large percentage of patients with this syndrome the development of a postcricoid carcinoma has been observed.

Only very little pressure is needed to rupture the web while introducing the esophagoscope and to re-establish thereby normal passage through the esophagus. As a result of this procedure, the dysphagia and inflammation of the hypopharynx and esophagus may disappear. Proper alimentation, supported by intake of vitamins and iron preparations, will restore the general status of the patient, including her blood-forming capacity.

PHARYNGO—ESOPHAGEAL
DIVERTICULUM
(ESOPHAGOSCOPIC VIEW)

TRACTION
DIVERTICULUM
(ESOPHAGOSCOPIC
VIEW)

PHARYNGO—ESOPHAGEAL
DIVERTICULUM
(ZENKER'S)

AZYGOS VEIN

PERICARDIUM

DIAPHRAGM

STOMACH

TRACTION
DIVERTICULUM
(MIDTHORACIC)

EPIPHRENIC
DIVERTICULUM
(VIEWED FROM
RIGHT SIDE)

DIVERTICULA

The extrathoracic or *pharyngo-esopha-geal diverticulum,* commonly referred to as Zenker's diverticulum, is of the pulsion variety and is the commonest type of esophageal diverticulum. It usually arises in the posterior midline of the hypopharynx at the pharyngeal dimple in the area bounded above by the horizontal fibers of the inferior constrictor muscle and below by the cricopharyngeal muscle, where a herniation of the mucosa and submucosa of the hypopharynx occurs between the sparse musculature of the inferior constrictor muscles (see pages 21, 36 and 37). The wall of the sac is made up of mucosa, submucosa and fibrous tissue of varying thicknesses and is covered by a rather incomplete muscular coat. These diverticula become more and more enlarged as a result of repeated distention by swallowed food. The sac of mucosa presents posteriorly behind the esophagus and in front of the prevertebral fascia and, eventually, projects to the left of the esophagus. Males (of an average age of 50 years) account for 80 to 90 per cent of the cases. The earliest clinical symptoms are throat irritation, with excessive production of mucus and a sensation of a foreign body on swallowing. Dysphagia is insidious but may rapidly become severe. The patients complain of an irritative type of cough or croaking noise upon the act of swallowing liquids, of regurgitation of undigested food and mucus several hours after ingestion, especially in the supine position, of a distaste for food, nausea and accompanying bad odor in the mouth. Obstruction of the esophagus may become almost complete, with the resultant sequelae of marked weight loss and emaciation. Some asymmetry of the neck, with fullness beneath the lower part of the sternocleidomastoid muscle, may be felt, and an audible, gurgling sound, as a sign of regurgitation, may be produced by pressing the side of the neck. The exact location of the diverticulum, the degree of distention and the size of the pouch are ascertained by X-ray examination. On esophagoscopy the mouth of this pouch is easily entered,

and the mucosa can be seen to end blindly at the distal portion of the pouch. The normal opening of the esophagus is displaced anteriorly and kinked by the diverticulum. The treatment of choice is surgical extirpation by lateral cervical approach.

The *epibronchial diverticulum* is of the traction type. It may or may not be detected endoscopically as an outpocketing of the esophageal mucosa, but roentgen examination reveals that the outpouching of the wall includes all esophageal layers. This condition is invariably associated with inflammatory changes incident to a long-standing tuberculosis.

An *epiphrenic diverticulum* — a combination of pulsion and traction types — is more often found on the right side than on the left, and almost exclusively in males. The majority of cases are associated with achalasia (see page 145), and it might be difficult to decide whether the symptoms (substernal or epigas-

tric pain, regurgitations, vomiting after meals, hiccough, mild dyspepsia and, sometimes, loss of weight or dysphagia) are the result of a cardiospasm or the diverticulum. Precordial pain and cardiographic evidence of coronary insufficiency are probably the result of reflex vagal spasm to direct pressure. At times, differentiation between a large, lower esophageal peptic ulcer, hiatal hernia or an epidiaphragmatic diverticulum may also present problems. Radiographically, the diverticulum exhibits the form of a spherical pouch, with some narrowing at the neck. On esophagoscopy one encounters a vertical partition on one side of which the tube enters the blindly ending pouch, while on the other the tube can be made to enter the esophageal lumen and the stomach. The infected contents of pouches may lead to ulceration of the walls and to perforation, resulting in bronchopulmonary complications.

INFERIOR ESOPHAGEAL RING FORMATION

In many patients with *small, sliding hiatus hernias*, a *circumferential dia-phragmlike intrusion on the lumen* may be seen roentgenologically at the esopha-gogastric junction. When the region is distended by fluid barium, this striking feature becomes manifest along the contours of the segment by sharply demarcated, almost rectangular, toothlike notches projecting into the column and usually connected by a faintly visible, lucent band. Considering that the cali-ber of the "vestibule" (see page 76) is larger than the remainder of the esopha-gus, the over-all diameter at the site of the ring is not remarkably narrowed, though in some cases the maximal dis-tensibility may be distinctly limited. A typical clinical syndrome develops (Schatzki and Gary) in which the lumen cannot be distended beyond a diameter of about 13 mm. The patients, who on the average are over 50 years of age, experience sudden dramatic episodes of pain or discomfort when trying to swal-low solid food that has been insufficiently masticated, because the bolus cannot pass and produces a complete obstruction at the site of the ring.

Though the location and nature of the *lower esophageal ring* are still contro-versial, presently available evidence indi-cates that this ring is static in nature rather than a manifestation of spasms, and that it should be differentiated from contractions of the inferior esophageal sphincter, which are transient and located 2 to 3 cm. above the esophagogastric junction, having an hourglass configura-tion. Sphincteric contractions are seen in patients with small, sliding hiatus hernias, but the contractions disappear, usually, on distention. A thin ring may persist at the level of the sphincter even after distention; it is then, however, clearly situated at the junction of the tubular esophagus and the bell-shaped vestibule rather than at the cardia, and is never as discrete as a lower esopha-geal ring.

Histologically, as demonstrated re-cently (MacMahon, Schatzki and Gary), it is the undersurface of the projecting ridge of tissue where the transition from the squamous esophageal epithelium to the cylindrical gastric epithelium takes place. In this demonstration the core of the ring consisted, for the most part, of areolar connective tissue, with some bun-dles of smooth muscle fibers belonging to the muscularis mucosae. The muscu-

TUBULAR ESOPHAGUS

LOCATION OF INFERIOR ESOPHAGEAL SPHINCTER

VESTIBULE

BARIUM RETAINED IN VESTIBULE AND HERNIAL SAC; DISTAL TUBULAR ESOPHAGUS AND INFERIOR ESOPHAGEAL SPHINCTER REGION CONTRACTED; LOWER ESOPHAGEAL RING INDICATED BY NOTCHES

LOWER ESOPHAGEAL RING

SLIDING HERNIA

PERITONEUM

DIAPHRAGM

PHRENO-ESOPHAGEAL LIGAMENT

PHRENO-ESOPHAGEAL LIGAMENT

TUBULAR ESOPHAGUS

LOCATION OF INFERIOR ESOPHAGEAL SPHINCTER

VESTIBULE

LOWER ESOPHAGEAL RING

SLIDING HERNIA

PERITONEUM

DIAPHRAGM

CONTINUOUS SWALLOWING: LOWER ESOPHAGEAL RING (LOWER ARROW); ALSO FAINT RING AT LEVEL OF INFERIOR ESOPHAGEAL SPHINCTER (UPPER ARROW)

laris propria was not involved in the process, nor could any sign of inflammatory process be seen.

The genesis of the lower esophageal ring is unknown, though in some instances which conform with most, if not all, of the features of the classic description of the ring, a localized peptic esophagitis may have played an etiologic rôle. But the question as to whether esophagitis is the cause in all cases must remain open.

Roentgenologically, the lower esophageal ring can serve as a remarkably useful landmark to identify the level of the esophagogastric junction, and in some cases it is the only finding that permits the recogni-tion of a small, sliding hiatus hernia. Ring formation, notches or incompletely distensible diaphragmlike intrusion have so far never been observed when the junction was located in its normal position. The lower esophageal ring is rarely visible esophagoscopically,

probably because the limited diameter of the instru-ment restricts observation of the area during complete distention.

The lower esophageal ring must be differentiated from a congenital web, which usually becomes evi-dent in early life and is not located at the esophago-gastric junction. Strictures, spasms resulting from peptic esophagitis and carcinoma almost never pre-sent a problem of differential diagnosis.

Obstruction by a poorly masticated bolus at the level of the ring may be relieved by a proteolytic enzyme preparation but, in many instances, requires mechanical help under the esophagoscope. When the lumen in the region of the ring formation is markedly narrowed, and when recurrent episodes of obstruction cannot be prevented by careful masti-cation, operative removal or a plastic procedure must be performed.

CARDIOSPASM

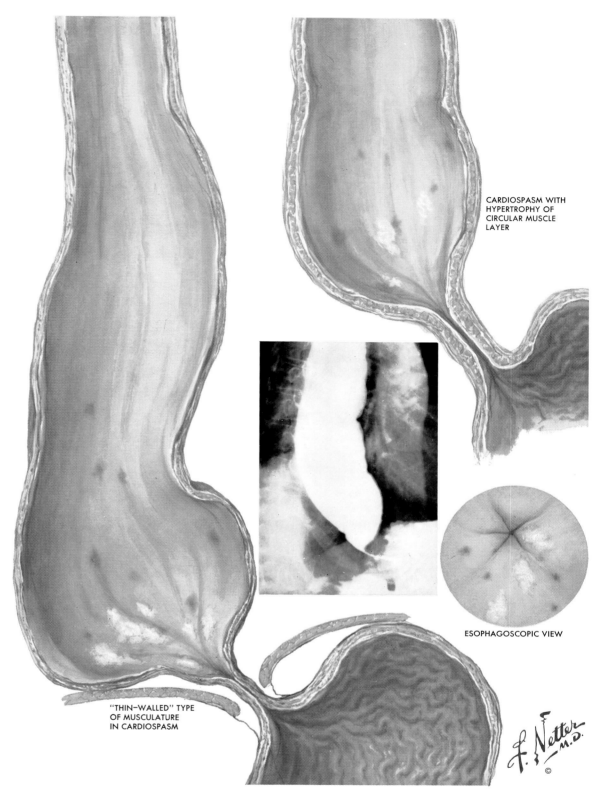

CARDIOSPASM WITH HYPERTROPHY OF CIRCULAR MUSCLE LAYER

ESOPHAGOSCOPIC VIEW

"THIN-WALLED" TYPE OF MUSCULATURE IN CARDIOSPASM

Cardiospasm, or achalasia cardiae, is a motoric disturbance of the distal part of the esophagus characterized by a non-relaxing, obstructing segment at the esophagogastric junction and a dilatation which may involve the entire length of the esophagus. The exact cause of cardiospasm is unknown, but a great number of explanatory theories have been proposed (see also pages 46 and 98). Studying pressure changes with the balloon technique, it has been shown that, in patients with cardiospasm, irregular, low phasic contractions occur simultaneously at all levels, with none of the progressive co-ordinated movements observed with the peristalsis of the normal esophagus (see pages 76 and 77). The esophagus also responds with increased activity to parasympathomimetic agents (see page 98).

In the early stages the patients complain of a feeling of heaviness in the chest or a sensation of constriction in the lower posterior chest when under stress. Food intake causes at first only slight distress, but, eventually, signs of true obstruction become evident. The patient may regurgitate food eaten the day before, dysphagia and substernal pain increase, and a fear of eating develops. Nutritional disturbances may appear, though, remarkably, the vast majority of these patients maintain their nutrition with little weight loss. As a result of the aspiration of regurgitated food particles, recurrent bouts of pneumonia may occur, especially in elderly, advanced cases.

The narrowing of the esophagus at its most distal end is confined to a segment 1 to 2 cm. long. A markedly dilated proximal portion, varying in length but directly evolving from the obstructed part, is the characteristic feature seen upon X-ray examination. One may also observe irregular fluoroscopically spasmodic movements of the entire esophagus, working in an attempt to empty itself without any evidence of success. In time, dilatation, elongation and tortuosity of the esophagus increase, and a typical S-shaped deformity develops. Combining the experience obtained with radiologic studies and at the operating table, two different types of achalasia cardiae have been differentiated. Typical of Type I (75 per cent of the cases) are the very marked dilatation, the lack of peristaltic activity and an amazingly small (in diameter) terminal segment with an abnormally thin muscular layer, which is in contrast to the thick-walled and dilated portion above it. Patients of Type II (25 per cent of the cases) at an early phase of the disease experience pain resulting from esophageal spasms. The dilatation here never assumes the enormous proportions of Type I. Erratic movements and, sometimes, antiperistaltic waves are observed, and at operation the circular musculature of the lower esophagus, including the obstructing segment, is found to be hypertrophied.

The findings on esophagoscopy vary also with the stage of the disease. The amount of retained food particles may be small in the early phases, whereas the dilated lumen in the later stages may be distended by pints of undigested material, necessitating esophageal lavage before esophagoscopy can be adequately performed. Inspissated food particles can often be seen adherent to a thickened mucosa, surrounded by areas of leukoplakia. Measuring the distance from the upper incisor teeth to the cardiac sphincter, the esophagus will, in most cases, be found to be elongated. As a matter of fact, in early cases of cardiospasm its elongation may be more prominent than the dilatation. Esophagoscopy should always be performed at least once in any suspected case of cardiospasm; the tube should always be inserted beyond the sphincter to the point where gastric juice can be readily obtained and gastric rugae can be recognized, in order to rule out a carcinoma of the cardiac end of the stomach.

ESOPHAGITIS, ESOPHAGEAL ULCERS

Peptic Esophagitis

Acute esophagitis may develop owing to a great variety of causes, among which, regrettably, the swallowing of caustic, acid or household cleansing solutions by children figures high in incidence. Other etiologic factors include vomiting, frequent introduction of feeding or suction tubes and some acute infectious diseases, which have the tendency to affect the mucosa of the gastro-intestinal tract without specific preference for the esophagus. Retrosternal pain of varying degree, but sometimes rather severe and radiating to neck and shoulders, and difficulty with deglutition are the dominant clinical manifestations. Aside from emergency treatment with dilute acids and bicarbonates, respectively, when a child has sipped or taken a mouthful of alkaline or acid fluid, therapy is essentially symptomatic (diet and analgesics).

Far more frequent than acute esophagitis, and also more frequent than is generally assumed, is chronic esophagitis, which may be a sequel to an acute esophagitis but is more often an inflammatory reaction of the esophageal mucosa with *erosions and ulcer formation due to the regurgitation* of hydrochloric acid gastric juice with pepsin over a prolonged period of time. For some time the confused state with regard to the terminology has hampered the understanding of the various forms of peptic esophagitis and peptic ulceration. Peptic esophagitis as a clinical entity was first described only a little more than 2 decades ago (Winkelstein) and is characterized as a condition with diffuse inflammatory changes in the distal esophagus which are accompanied by gastric or duodenal ulcers or by a sliding hernia. Pathogenetically, it is, no doubt, the regurgitation of gastric juice which causes, first, the irritation and then the digestion of the esophageal epithelium. Persistent vomiting and prolonged use of an indwelling nasal-gastric feeding tube have been observed to be etiologic factors. Cases have been described in which a peptic esophagitis developed after a protracted coma, during which gastric content entered the esophagus. Depending upon the duration of the disease, one encounters edema and congestion of the mucosa, multiple small superficial ulcerations or larger flat ulcers extending longitudinally. These appear as patches of different sizes covered by coagulated exudation. The lumen of the affected portions of the esophagus is narrow in the early stages as a consequence of the edema and/or spasms, and, later, owing to the development of fibrous tissue, may lead slowly to stricture formation. The proximal section above the contracted part is dilated. These macroscopic findings correspond microscopically to necrosis of the epithelium, erosions, hyalinization of the mucosa, small cell infiltration, hypertrophy of the muscle fibers in the mucosa and connective tissue proliferation, respectively, according to the stage and extent of the inflammatory process. The characteristic site of peptic esophagitis may extend from the gastro-intestinal junction over an area about 10 cm. proximal to it.

The symptoms are essentially the same as those for all esophageal disorders. The patients complain of heartburn, an acid taste with belching, retrosternal pain, discomfort while eating, dysphagia and inability completely to swallow solid food. The narrow segment of the terminal esophagus and the distention of its lumen proximal to the constricted region can be readily recognized by X-ray examination. A small sliding hernia may accompany these

(Continued on page 147)

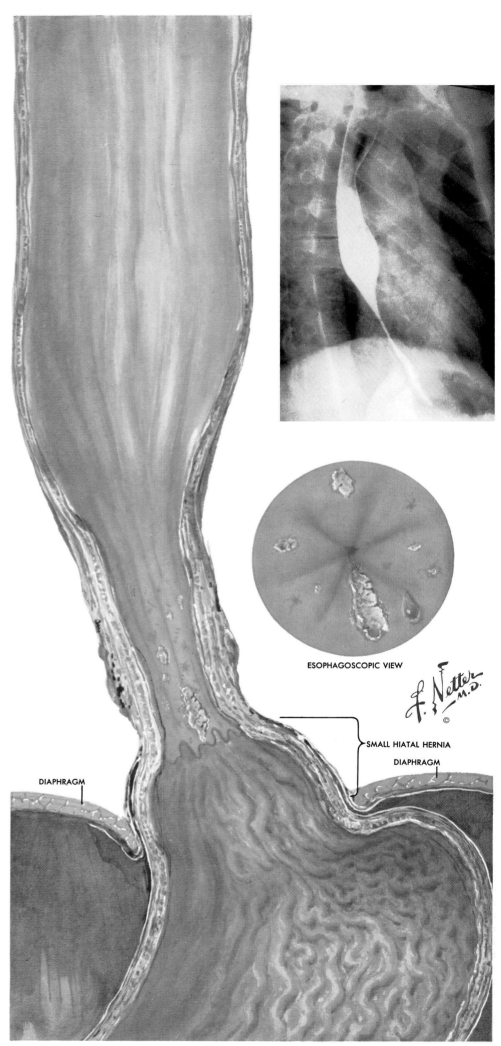

ESOPHAGOSCOPIC VIEW

DIAPHRAGM

SMALL HIATAL HERNIA

DIAPHRAGM

ESOPHAGITIS, ESOPHAGEAL ULCERS
Peptic Esophagitis
(Continued from page 146)

findings. Endoscopy reveals an intense congestion of the lower segment, with a color from the normal pale pink hue to a marked redness, and multiple superficial erosions and pinpoint hemorrhages. The narrow portion may offer some resistance to the esophagoscope, which can usually be overcome by the passage of the rigid 12-cm. instrument. Larger ulcerations become visible the closer the esophagoscope approaches the gastro-esophageal junction.

In the majority of cases, healing occurs, but occasionally a smooth fibrotic stenosis results.

Marginal Ulceration with Hiatal Hernia

Most patients with a short esophagus and *uncomplicated hiatal hernia* (see page 158) are usually symptom-free and show little evidence of esophagitis clinically, as well as by endoscopic examination, when the latter is performed merely as a safeguard after a hiatal hernia has been detected on the roentgen screen. Some patients with hiatal hernia, however, complain of heartburn and other symptoms of regurgitation, and in these, as a rule, esophagitis, localized in the terminal portion of the esophagus with a discrete marginal ulceration, is encountered endoscopically. In such instances unequivocal signs of gastric regurgitation will also be observed. Whereas, normally, no gastric juice is seen with the esophagoscope until the stomach is entered, one meets in these cases with marginal ulceration lesser or greater amounts of gastric fluid welling up from the gastro-esophageal juncture. It even happens that the regurgitated contents of the stomach must be aspirated in order to make visible the inflammatory changes, the erosions and ulcerations in the lowest part of the esophagus. The *ulcer* appears *sharply separated from the surrounding mucosa* and is *covered by a yellowish-gray membrane*, which may readily be removed by suction or forceps without causing much bleeding. The ulcer crater is covered by exuberant granulation tissue, and its edges may sometimes be undermined. Necrosis is seldom found. The lesion is usually elongated, with the proximal edges less distinct than those bordering the mucosa of the thoracic part of the stomach. Islands of heterotopic gastric mucosa will often be found in the region of the ulcer, though it may be impossible to recognize them macroscopically. They can be diagnosed from a biopsy specimen, which should be obtained anyway to exclude the possibility of a tumor.

Proximal to the ulcer the mucosa usually manifests all signs of esophagitis of varying degree (localized inflammation, congestion, edema, spotty and superficial erosions) and, at the site of these inflammatory reactions, the lumen is invariably narrowed as a result of segmental spasms. The proximal portion appears somewhat widened, so that the X-ray picture offers an appearance often described as "butterflylike". Though roentgenologic evidence of an ulceration is not as outspoken and characteristic as with a peptic ulcer of the stomach or duodenum, at the marginal ulceration a small niche of collected barium may occasionally become visible. More often, it is some rigidity or fixation of one side of the terminal esophagus which may arouse the suspicion of the presence of an ulcer.

The healing of discrete ulcerations with hiatal hernia is apt to be accompanied by fibrosis, which leads — and far

(Continued on page 148)

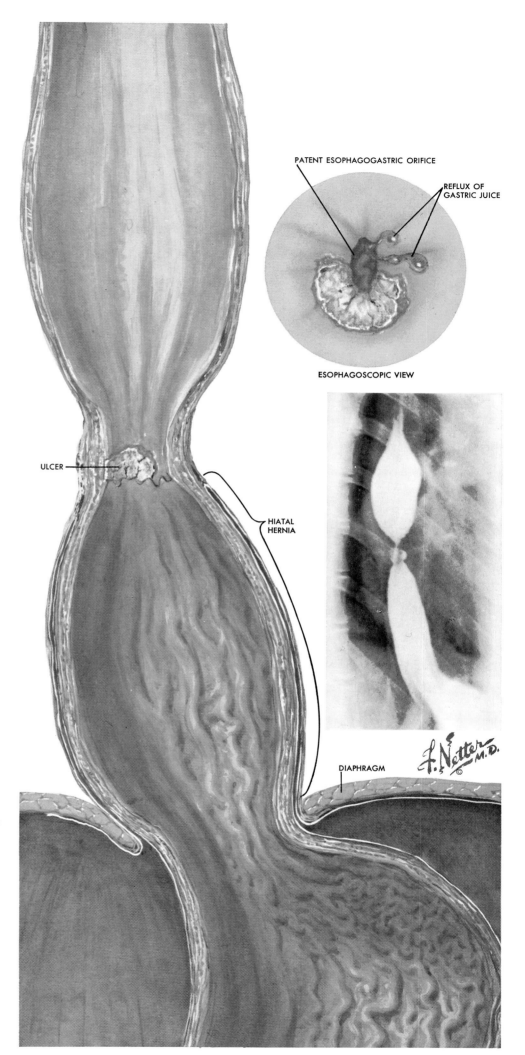

PATENT ESOPHAGOGASTRIC ORIFICE

REFLUX OF GASTRIC JUICE

ESOPHAGOSCOPIC VIEW

ULCER

HIATAL HERNIA

DIAPHRAGM

ESOPHAGITIS, ESOPHAGEAL ULCERS

Peptic Esophagitis

(Continued from page 147)

more often than is the case with ulcers in peptic esophagitis (see above) — to varying degrees of stenosis. In advanced cases the lumen may be restricted to 2 to 3 mm., as measured by the caliber of the bougie which can be accommodated and correlated with the roentgenologic findings. The fact that this condition is more prone to end up with a true stenosis of the distal esophagus explains in part also the more disturbing symptoms such as continuous heartburn, marked retrosternal pain, a severe degree of dysphagia and hematemesis.

Attempts to correct the hiatal hernia are often difficult and unsuccessful because of the presence of periesophagitis and fixation of the esophagus by adhesions. Resection of the lower esophagus and the upper half of the stomach might become inevitable in patients with far-progressed stenosis. In less-advanced cases the lumen might be widened by frequent bougienage to relieve the symptoms. Therapy with antacids and anticholinergics is, of course, indicated but will have no effect on the incompetence of the sphincter mechanism and the free regurgitation of gastric juice, which are the most important factors in this condition.

Gastric Peptic Ulcer in Gastric-Lined Esophagus

An ulcer of a type different from those discussed above may develop in a region which, topographically, belongs to the esophagus when the lumen of the distal part of this organ, instead of being covered with stratified, squamous epithelium (see page 40), is lined with columnar gastric epithelium. Such extension of an atypical gastric mucosa over the esophageal wall has been termed heterotopic gastric epithelium. Since it is a mucosal coat continuous with that of the stomach spreading over (sometimes several centimeters high), it should not be confused with some small, isolated islands of ectopic gastric epithelium, which quite frequently are to be found in the esophagus and rather more often in the proximal than in the distal parts. These ectopic tissue islands rarely, if ever, cause pathologic changes or symptoms. On the other hand, since the heterotopic mucosa in the esophagus seems to be just as susceptible to peptic digestion as the normal esophageal epithelium, the "gastric-lined" part of the terminal gullet may become the site of a *"true" peptic ulcer,* which has all the properties of a peptic gastric

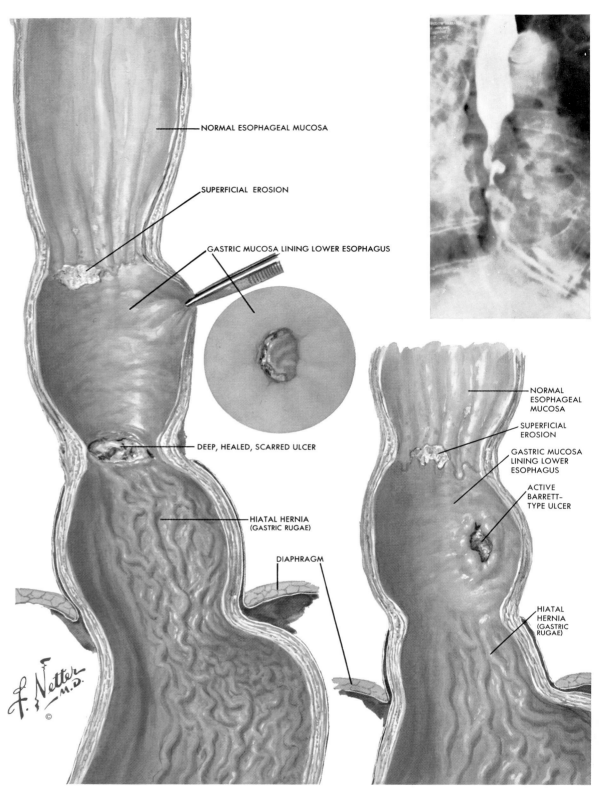

NORMAL ESOPHAGEAL MUCOSA

SUPERFICIAL EROSION

GASTRIC MUCOSA LINING LOWER ESOPHAGUS

DEEP, HEALED, SCARRED ULCER

HIATAL HERNIA (GASTRIC RUGAE)

DIAPHRAGM

NORMAL ESOPHAGEAL MUCOSA

SUPERFICIAL EROSION

GASTRIC MUCOSA LINING LOWER ESOPHAGUS

ACTIVE BARRETT-TYPE ULCER

HIATAL HERNIA (GASTRIC RUGAE)

or duodenal ulcer. In contrast to other peptic ulcers of the esophagus which remain superficial, this "true" peptic ulcer is usually circular and not elongated, possesses a raised edge, extends to the submucosa and even penetrates the deeper layers to the point that severe bleeding and perforation may occur. With these facts in mind, the significance of differentiating the various ulcer types in the esophagus becomes understandable. The heterotopic mucosa is most probably a congenital anomaly (see page 139) in an otherwise absolutely normal esophagus, although the peptic ulcer in the gastric-lined region does not develop until late in life, and it is likely that other factors, such as the acquisition of a hiatal hernia leading to an incompetence of the gastro-esophageal sphincter mechanism with reflux of gastric acid, are necessary to instigate the production of an ulcer.

The diagnosis of this condition rests upon the X-ray

and endoscopic findings. The roentgen picture may be suggestive, if it shows an unusually big ulcer, located relatively high, with a narrowing beginning 2 to 3 cm. above the niche and a second stenotic portion distal to the ulcer and above a hiatal hernia. With esophagoscopy one often encounters a superficial erosion of the squamous esophageal mucosa and, more distally in the readily recognizable region covered with the gastric mucosa, the bed of the "true" peptic or *"Barrett-type" ulcer.* Biopsies taken from the surrounding tissue will establish the diagnosis of a "true" peptic ulcer in a gastric-lined esophagus. The tendency to fibrotic stenosis is great and cases have been reported in which the lumen was restricted to a diameter of not more than 2 to 3 mm.

Resection of the gastric-lined segment, together with the cardia, seems presently to be the most rational therapeutic approach.

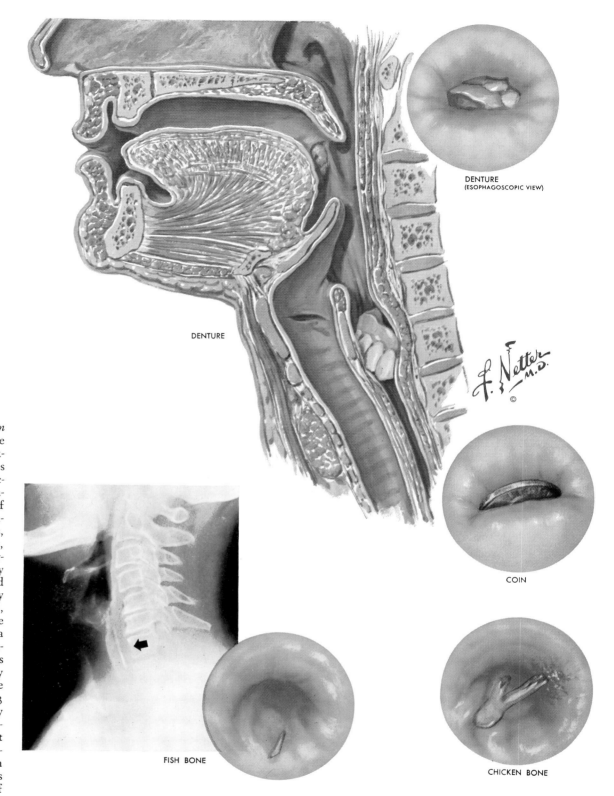

DENTURE

DENTURE
(ESOPHAGOSCOPIC VIEW)

COIN

FISH BONE

CHICKEN BONE

FOREIGN BODIES

The ingestion and arrest of *foreign bodies* in the esophagus is usually the result of carelessness from eating, cooking, playing, putting inedible substances in the mouth or not attending to defective dentures. The loss of palatal sensation owing to the coverage of the roof of the mouth by dentures is often responsible for the swallowing of foreign bodies, such as chicken bones or fish bones, which would otherwise be reflexly regurgitated. Strictures of the esophagus may arrest common foods, such as seeds and peas, which ordinarily would pass freely into the stomach. *Bones* may be lodged, or a bolus too large to pass through the lumen may get stuck in the gullet as a consequence of hasty eating and insufficient mastication. Small objects, such as *coins,* buttons, nuts and hard candy (neither of the latter two should be offered to children under the age of 3 years, unless ground), and even safety pins may become impacted in the esophagus of infants and young children. But foreign bodies are encountered as frequently in adults as in children, and a great number of such accidental events may be traced to the deplorable habit of holding tacks, pins and other pointed objects between the lips, which, in a moment of inattention, may be swallowed to attach themselves in the esophageal wall.

The symptoms of a foreign body in the esophagus depend essentially on its size, shape and consistency. A sensation of choking or gagging usually occurs with the swallowing of too large an object, shortly thereafter followed by dysphagia, drooling of saliva and substernal and/or interscapular pain. Partly because of their inability to express their discomfort and to locate the sensation of pain and partly because of the vagueness of symptoms, diagnosis in children may be difficult and may be supported only by the history of retching, when trying to swallow, and localized cervical tenderness. Radiopaque substances, such as any metallic object, chicken bones and certain fish bones or clumps of meat can readily be recognized on the roentgen film. Nonradiopaque material, to which certain cartilaginous and thin fish bones belong, can be found only by *esophagoscopy,* except when a small amount of barium adheres to the edge of the foreign body, thus permitting recognition by X-ray. In view of the possible serious consequences of a foreign body in the esophagus (perforation, mediastinitis), exploratory esophagoscopy is always warranted, all the more because extraction from the esophagus is also best performed by this technique. Food masses, often accumulating above the engulfed object, must be removed by forceps. Maximal dilation of the esophageal wall prevents foreign bodies from being hidden in the esophageal folds. Sharp or pointed pieces (nails, slivers of tin cans, bristles, etc.) may become embedded within the wall, leaving visible only the point of entrance, at times with utmost difficulty, necessitating swabbing of the mucosa with Acriviolet®, which will adhere to an ulcerated but not to the intact mucosa. The foreign body is extracted by introducing a forceps at the site where the dye has concentrated. A Berman magnet may occasionally be helpful to localize a metallic foreign body and to bring it into a position from which the endoscopist can remove it.

If the esophagus has been perforated, a cervical mediastinotomy is advisable for adequate drainage in case of infection. Search for a foreign body by approach through an external incision is often futile. Pressure of a large mass in the esophagus against the trachea may result in asphyxia which, particularly in children, requires a tracheotomy before removal of the body by endoscopy.

STRICTURE

Strictures of the esophagus are not rare and have a multifarious pathogenetic background. Those of congenital nature (atresia) and those caused by web or ring formation have been illustrated and discussed elsewhere (see pages 138, 142 and 144, respectively).

Cicatricial stenosis of the esophagus is most frequently the result of accidental or suicidal swallowing of caustics ("lye stricture"), which destroy the mucosa. The latter, in turn, is replaced by redundant fibrotic tissue, which contracts the wall and narrows the lumen. Ulcers produced by foreign bodies, and peptic ulcerations also, heal or attempt to heal by proliferation of connective tissue, leaving a fibrotic scar ("peptic stenosis") which may constrict the lumen. Stenosis at the suture line of esophagocardiomyotomies (Heller type of operation for achalasia) or of other esophagogastrostomies has occasionally also been observed, here again developing as a result of an ulcer produced by reflux of gastric juice, unavoidable after by-passing or resection of the cardia.

All patients with strictures of any kind complain about dysphagia, and, depending upon the site of the stenosis, retrosternal or epigastric pain, present themselves usually in poor nutritional states. The patient's past history, as a rule, leads to a conjectural diagnosis which is easily confirmed by X-ray examination or esophagoscopy, or both. Roentgen films show the persistent narrowing of the esophagus in the thoracic region, particularly several centimeters above the diaphragmatic hiatus at the site where marginal ulcers (see page 147) are most frequently located. The proximal portion of the esophagus is dilated and may appear slightly fixed or rigid on the lateral or anterior wall. A conical narrowing of the esophagus presents itself on endoscopic observation, which establishes the diagnosis fairly well, especially if, proximal to the stenosis, signs of superficial inflammatory processes can be seen. The constricted wall offers a definite resist-

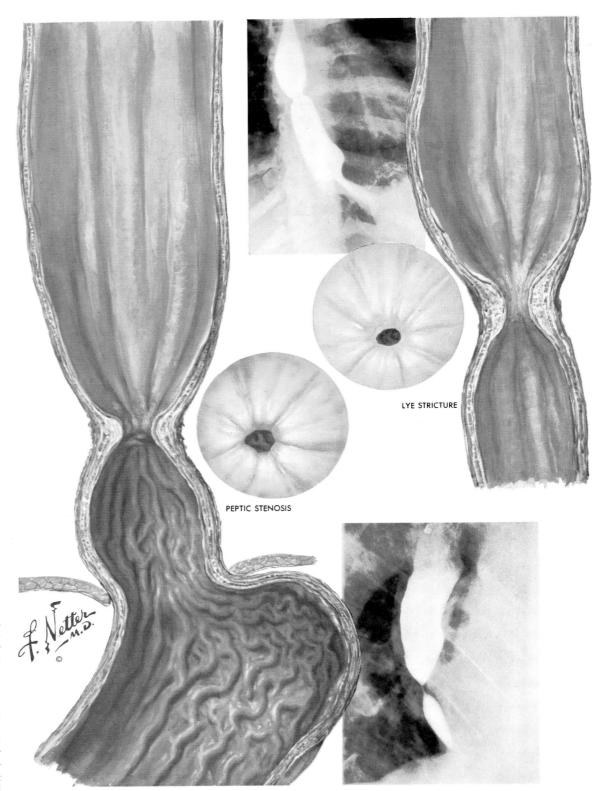

PEPTIC STENOSIS

LYE STRICTURE

ance to the advancing esophagoscope, a resistance which cannot be overcome without applying pressure through a dilating bougie. This fact always indicates the presence of fibrotic tissue. When the stricture has arisen from a marginal ulcer accompanied by a hiatal hernia and parts of the stomach lying above the diaphragm, a constant reflux of the gastric juice above the level of the stenosis may be noticed.

With these types of stricture, relief may be obtained by frequent, regular bougienage. Surgical correction requires an extensive procedure, which often leaves the patient in a deplorable condition as far as alimentation is concerned.

The degree of fibrosis after destruction of the mucosa by caustics is generally greater than that seen following peptic ulcers or ulcers produced by foreign bodies, but here also the depth and width of the original lesion are the deciding factors. The cicatricial

area may be larger, and its color, as seen endoscopically, is paler than in the case of other strictures. The earlier patients who have swallowed a tissue-destroying solution are treated, the better is the final outcome. Extensive cicatrization may be prevented by immediate efforts to neutralize chemically the corrosive material which may have remained in the esophagus and by early passage of graduated Hurst (mercury-weighted) tubes. Administration of anti-inflammatory corticosteroids has been said to decrease the formation of granulations and, thereby, subsequent fibrosis and cicatrization. Once stenosis is fully developed, dilation of the stricture with bougies is the treatment of choice. When the stricture is in the most distal parts of the esophagus, surgical correction is usually inevitable. The substitution of a segment of the colon to re-establish the continuity between esophagus and stomach has recently yielded promising results.

AIR IN
INTERFASCIAL
SPACES DUE TO
PERFORATION
OF CERVICAL
ESOPHAGUS

CAROTID SHEATH
PREVERTEBRAL FASCIA
AIR SPACE
RENT IN ESOPHAGUS
THYROID GLAND
PURULENT EXUDATE

Rupture and Perforation

ESOPHAGOSCOPIC VIEW

TRAUMATIC PERFORATION
OF CERVICAL ESOPHAGUS

AIR IN MEDIASTINUM DUE
TO SPONTANEOUS RUPTURE
OF LOWER ESOPHAGUS

SPONTANEOUS
RUPTURE
OF LOWER
ESOPHAGUS

Spontaneous rupture of the esophagus, though an extremely rare event, occurs when the esophageal wall, presumably owing to a pre-existing weakness, gives way to a sudden increase of intra-esophageal pressure during violent coughing or excessive vomiting, to which alcoholics are particularly prone. It is usually the lower third of the posterolateral wall which ruptures linearly (2 to 3 cm.) into the left pleural space. The patients complain of sudden excruciating pain in the epigastrium, which lasts and radiates to the chest, to the back or to both. Dyspnea, cyanosis and shock soon set in and dominate the clinical picture. Emphysema and pneumo- or hydropneumothorax, especially in the left mediastinum, develop and may become visible radiologically. This serious condition has been encountered in men who previously were healthy and seemingly strong and vigorous but who, in most cases, had a history of a gastro-intestinal disease such as duodenal or gastric ulcer. A possible association of spontaneous rupture of the esophagus with brain tumors, especially following cerebral surgery, has recently been reported (Fincher and Swanson).

Having eliminated other conditions that may cause a similar clinical picture (such as perforation of peptic ulcer, acute pancreatitis, spontaneous pneumothorax, intra-abdominal thrombosis, etc.), thoracotomy and other emergency measures (chemotherapy, parenteral fluids) are urgently indicated and can save about 2 out of 3 patients, all of whom would have died before the advent of modern thoracic surgery and a series of auxiliary measures.

Perforations of the esophagus caused by trauma, including penetration of the wall by a foreign body (see page 149),

or by the ingestion of a corrosive liquid or by a peptic ulcer, together are somewhat more frequent than is spontaneous rupture. The symptoms and signs of a perforation in the thoracic esophagus are, in general, the same as those outlined above, as is the need for immediate surgical interference.

Perforation of the cervical esophagus, e.g., in the hypopharyngeal region, results most often from the introduction of an instrument, particularly from an attempt to pass the esophagoscopic tube. In most cases the esophagoscopist is immediately aware of having produced a tear or false passage. Bleeding and the loss of normal landmarks should arouse suspicion of a perforation. Immediate withdrawal of the endoscopic tube is indicated. The administration of large doses of antibiotic therapy is mandatory, as well as sedation and parenteral feeding. After a short interval the classical syndrome of fever, dysphagia, crepitation

and severe interscapular pain will ensue. The X-ray evidence of subcutaneous emphysema, with the demonstration of air in the prevertebral fascia and the subcutaneous tissues of the skin, will establish the diagnosis.

Experience has proved that conservative therapy, including administration of antibiotics and parenteral feeding, will prevent further complications in the great majority of cases. Occasionally, cervical drainage of a localized periesophageal abscess will be required. Further esophagoscopic manipulation is contraindicated. On rare occasions the signs of perforation and periesophageal infection may not become manifest until several days after esophagoscopy. This is especially prone to happen in elderly patients with cervical dorsal kyphosis or where the patient is unable to open the mouth widely because of fixed bridgework or muscular contraction, as found in scleroderma.

VARICOSIS

The cardinal symptoms of esophageal varicosities are recurrent severe hematemesis and melena. The immediate cause of the bleeding is not yet fully understood. It is probable that acid regurgitation from the stomach plays a rôle in the mucosal erosion necessary to produce bleeding. On the other hand, the mechanisms by which the esophageal veins become distended have been fairly well established as a consequence of the anatomic relationships between the venous drainage of the supramesocolonic organs (see pages 42 and 62) and the intrahepatic structural changes leading to portal hypertension (see CIBA COLLECTION, Vol. 3/III, pages 68, 69 and 72). The varices are most frequent in the lower third of the esophagus but may extend throughout the entire length of this organ.

On *endoscopy* the varices appear as isolated, bluish spheres surrounded by congested mucosa or as bluish-red tortuosities protruding into the lumen, if they have clustered, as they often do, in the most distal parts, particularly around the gastro-esophageal juncture. The varicosities are easily compressible and offer no resistance to the passage of the esophagoscope. Erosion of the superficial mucosa, with an adherent blood clot, signifies the site of a recent hemorrhage. When the presence of esophageal varices is established, a search should also be made for gastric varicosities, since the surgical treatment may have to be modified by the knowledge of their existence. The use of esophagoscopy is recommended in any patient with unexplained hemorrhage from the upper gastro-intestinal tract in order to exclude esophageal varices or to corroborate their clinical and X-ray evidence in patients with recurrent hematemesis. Provided adequate care is exercised by experienced esophagoscopists, the risk of initiating bleeding from the varices is negligible. If, with the inserted esophagoscope and after aspiration of the contents of the esophagus, no signs of varicosities are encountered, it may be concluded that the bleeding is not esophageal in origin and that a gastric lesion, most likely a peptic ulcer, exists.

Roentgen examination will not always reveal the presence of esophageal varices; as a matter of fact, only about 40 per cent

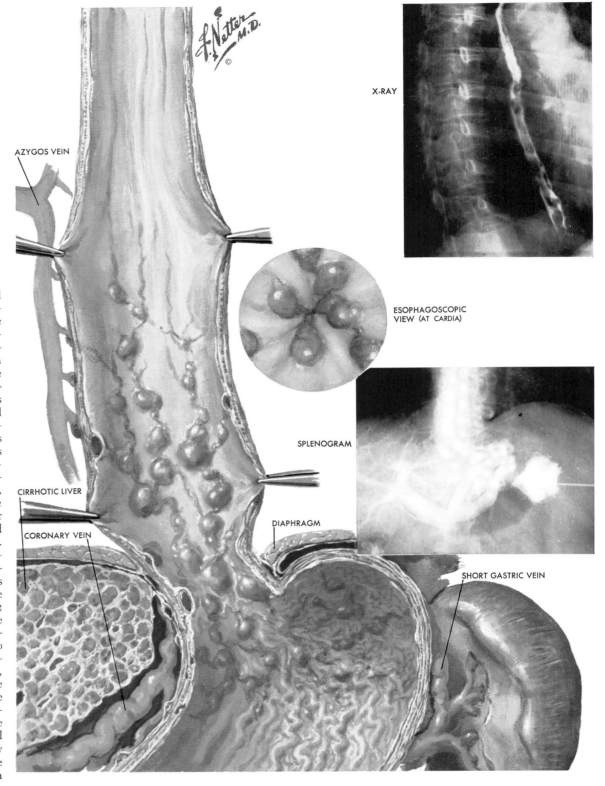

AZYGOS VEIN

X-RAY

ESOPHAGOSCOPIC VIEW (AT CARDIA)

CIRRHOTIC LIVER

SPLENOGRAM

CORONARY VEIN

DIAPHRAGM

SHORT GASTRIC VEIN

of true cases of varicosities are demonstrable by *X-ray photography*. A typical picture shows a honeycombed appearance produced by the thin layer of barium which surrounds the venous protrusions but does not distend or constrict the lumen of the esophagus. Varicose distention and distortion of the gastric veins may also be demonstrated occasionally. Radiologic studies with simultaneous injection of contrast medium into the spleen may also be helpful to clarify the basic process responsible for the development of the varices. With such a *"splenogram"* or "portal venogram" (see CIBA COLLECTION, Vol. 3/III, page 54), the increase in portal hypertension may be demonstrated, or thrombosis of the splenic vein (see CIBA COLLECTION, Vol. 3/III, page 72) may be diagnosed.

Varices of the esophagus are accountable for only a small portion of upper gastro-intestinal hemorrhages, but, in view of their inclination toward serious hemor-

rhage, their presence constitutes an ever-impending danger for the life of the patient. It has been estimated (Blakemore) that only 50 per cent of patients with liver cirrhosis and varices can be expected to live 1 year following the first hemorrhage if surgical therapy is not instituted. The elevation of the blood urea in hemorrhages stemming from varicose veins of the esophagus as a result of liver cirrhosis has recently been shown to be a valuable diagnostic aid.

During the acute phase of a hemorrhage, tamponade with the Sengstaken balloon is indicated as emergency treatment. Present thinking, however, points in the direction of surgical relief (see CIBA COLLECTION, Vol. 3/III, page 73) of portal hypertension and venous congestion in the esophagus, spleen, stomach, etc., as soon as the patient's condition permits it, or as soon as the diagnosis of varices has been made.

BENIGN TUMORS

Benign tumors of the esophagus, though relatively rare, are being recognized (and treated successfully) with increasing frequency. The great majority of these tumors are nonepithelial in origin. From the clinical point of view, they are best classified as (1) mucosal (intraluminal) and (2) mural (muscle-wall) tumors, the former including essentially *lipomas,* fibrolipomas and fibromyxomas, whereas the latter comprise chiefly the various types of leiomyomas. Unless of fairly large size and filling the lumen, as pedunculated or polypoid growth, the tumors arising from the mucosa are asymptomatic. Occasionally, they may bleed as a result of surface ulceration produced by the passing of food particles, and this is apt to occur with tumors of angiomatous structure. The usual *pedunculated type of tumor* may cause dysphagia and mild substernal distress, and the patient may be bothered by cough when esophageal secretions overflow into the tracheobronchial tree. The stalk or pedicle of such an intraluminal mass may become progressively stretched and elongated by the propulsive force of deglutition or eructation, and that has led, on rare occasions, to an aspiration of a *highly attached pedunculated tumor* into the pharynx and to suffocation. Fibromyoma, often located in the uppermost part of the esophagus, may reach sizes from 7 to 10 cm. in length and become freely suspended in the lumen. On hypopharyngoscopy a round mass covered with intact mucosa is visible in these instances. The tumor is freely movable, can easily be grasped and, after displacement into the pharynx, can be removed by a diathermy snare under suspension laryngoscopy.

The *intramural leiomyomas*—the largest group of esophageal benign tumors—are most often located in the lower third of the esophagus and, occasionally, may extend into the stomach. They are firm, rubbery, elastic, well-circumscribed, as a rule not pedunculated, but almost invariably encapsulated masses covered by an intact mucosa. In time, these oval or rounded submucosal tumors may encircle the lumen of the esophagus in the form of a U and may become firmly adherent to the surrounding tissue without being invasive. The leiomyoma may take on various forms

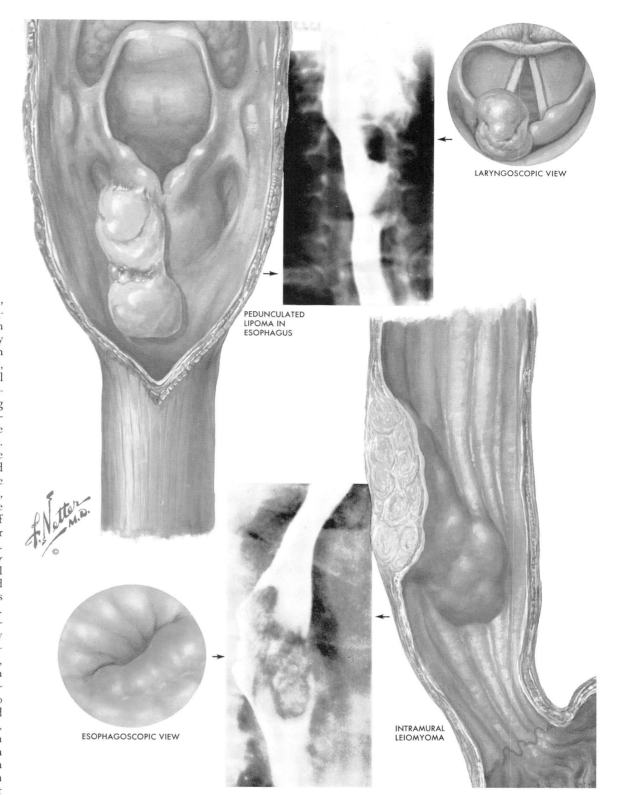

LARYNGOSCOPIC VIEW

PEDUNCULATED LIPOMA IN ESOPHAGUS

ESOPHAGOSCOPIC VIEW

INTRAMURAL LEIOMYOMA

(simple or nodular or lobulated) and may be a single tumor or may appear in multiples. The symptoms are essentially the same as with the intraluminal tumors discussed above, except that bleeding from a mural tumor is most unusual. Pain, if existing, is felt substernally or in the epigastrium and may radiate to the back or shoulder and, most often, at the time of deglutition. Even large tumors may be asymptomatic, owing to the fact that the lumen is usually not narrowed enough to interfere with the passage of the bolus, although the esophagoscopist may observe a more or less marked prominence of the esophageal wall, which creates the impression that an extra-esophageal mass compresses the lumen. It may even happen that the tube cannot be passed beyond the proximal bulge of the tumor.

Polypoid and endoluminal tumors are visible in *X-ray pictures* as smooth, round or oval filling defects,

and the pedicle, if not seen directly, may be surmised by noting the degree of the tumor's motility. Smooth indentations of the esophageal contour or changes in the configuration of the mucosal folds point to the presence of an intramural tumor, but it should be kept in mind that the pressure exerted, *e.g.,* by large mediastinal lymph nodes, may elicit similar radiologic findings. On rare occasions a dilatation of the esophagus proximal to a very large, lobulated leiomyoma situated in the lower third may have developed.

If both roentgenologist and endoscopist suspect the presence of an intramural leiomyoma, a biopsy of the mass should not be undertaken, because, to be useful, it must be made by ulcerating the mucosa, and this will complicate a subsequent surgical enucleation. On the other hand, should an ulceration be detected on esophagoscopy, a biopsy becomes mandatory because of the likelihood of a malignancy or leiomyosarcoma.

MALIGNANT TUMORS I
Upper Part of Esophagus

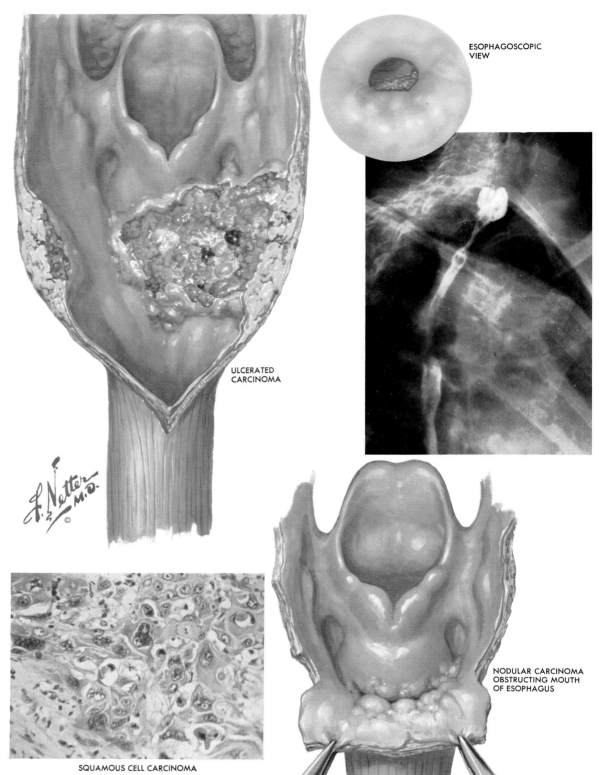

ESOPHAGOSCOPIC VIEW

ULCERATED CARCINOMA

SQUAMOUS CELL CARCINOMA

NODULAR CARCINOMA OBSTRUCTING MOUTH OF ESOPHAGUS

Over 80 per cent of carcinoma in the alimentary tract occurs in men. Only the carcinomas of the upper third of the esophagus make an exception, being more often encountered in women, but, of all esophageal tumor sites, the upper third is also the least frequent. An etiologic relationship between a carcinoma of the mouth of the esophagus and a chronic hypopharyngitis seems to exist, and the incidence of such malignant tumors in women suffering from the Plummer-Vinson syndrome (see page 142) is also suggestive of some sort of pathogenic association. Pathohistologically, the tumors of this region are squamous and of the anaplastic, immature type.

The patients' chief complaints are dysphagia, hoarseness, otalgia and frequent regurgitations of food into the trachea. The hoarseness must be attributed to the involvement of the recurrent laryngeal nerves. The difficulty in swallowing is, in most cases, the first and sometimes the only symptom and, whenever present, should be cause for a most careful examination, including endoscopy and X-ray studies, either to diagnose a postcricoid or upper esophageal malignant growth or to exclude it. Roentgen examination may or may not uncover a constant filling defect in the upper esophagus. With mirror laryngoscopy, the most proximal end of a tumor in the piriform fossa of the hypopharynx may occasionally be detected, and with direct hypopharyngoscopy the upper part of the lesion can often be visualized as a granulomatous ulceration. In such instances biopsy is indicated and will almost invariably reveal an anaplastic immature carcinoma. Exploring further with the esophago-

scope, one can visualize an ulcerating funduslike growth obstructing the lumen of the mouth of the esophagus and its extension into one or the other piriform fossa. To determine the distal extent of the lesion in order to appraise the chances and possible complications of surgical removal, roentgenography may be helpful, especially using the Trendelenburg position. If this fails, the insertion of a Jackson bougie can establish how far down the lesion has grown. The bougie can be inserted beyond the stenotic region and then withdrawn, so that the extent of the constricted part of the esophagus can be measured in relation to its distance from the upper incisor teeth. Knowing, as a result of direct visualization by laryngoscopy, the upper end of the tumor and assuming that its terminal end coincides with the site at which the bougie meets resistance on withdrawal, the area of the growth can be reasonably well established.

Unfortunately, radiation therapy of these malignancies has been disappointing. The recognized and most hopeful approach is surgical extirpation of the laryngo-esophagus and its primary reconstruction by a skin graft. In most cases, since the posterior half of the larynx and cricoid cartilage are so often involved, the larynx must be sacrificed, and a radical dissection of the lymph nodes in the neck and the superior mediastinum must be performed. Usually, the anterior portions of the larynx and trachea are not involved by the lesion and may be preserved and then used to form the anterior wall of the new pharyngo-esophagus, the posterior wall of which can be constructed with a skin graft. (Operation described by Som.)

Photomicrograph kindly provided by Sadao Otani, M.D., Department of Pathology, The Mount Sinai Hospital, New York.

Malignant Tumors II
Midportion of Esophagus

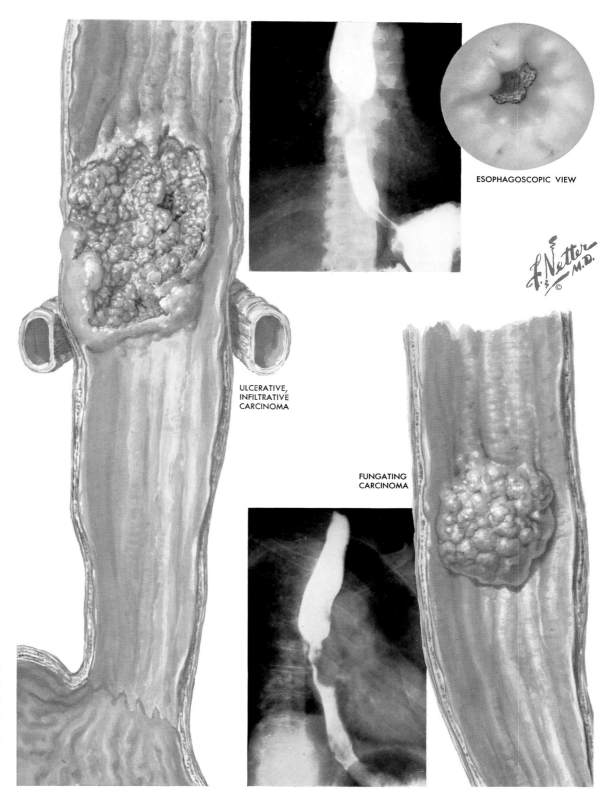

ESOPHAGOSCOPIC VIEW

ULCERATIVE, INFILTRATIVE CARCINOMA

FUNGATING CARCINOMA

Of all esophageal carcinomas, about 37 per cent are found in the middle third of the organ, meaning that this region is the second most frequent site. Two types of cancer predominate here — first, the *exophytic or proliferative type of lesion,* and, second, the ulcerating or infiltrating and stenosing mode of growth. The latter, though it also starts as a small mucosal lesion, which causes only few or no symptoms and is therefore detected only in very rare cases, is the most treacherous and dangerous. The neoplasm may convert the greater part of the esophagus into a rigid, constricted tube, fixing the organ to the adjacent structures. It may expand directly to the pericardium, the pleura, the mediastinum and into the tracheobronchial tree, causing a tracheo-esophageal fistula. With the exophytic type of growth, dysphagia may appear only relatively late in the disease, after the tumor has grown to a large size.

Concerning the causal factors of these esophageal lesions, we know as little as we do about the appearance of carcinoma in other places of the body, but the consumption of hot food and drinks, the excessive use of alcoholic beverages and poor dental hygiene have been regarded as possible etiologic factors.

The dominant clinical features are dysphagia, pain, regurgitation of food into the trachea, and cachexia. Radiating pain into the interscapular region is a frequent complaint even in only moderately progressed cases of the infiltrating type. The diagnosis may be suspected by X-ray examination, but it must be confirmed by esophagoscopy. It is important to observe, on roentgenography, a constant, irregular margin of the filling defect to exclude stenosis on the basis of some benign lesion. On endoscopy, the exophytic tumor type presents a polypoid growth, which should be biopsied for pathohistologic diagnosis. In the annular or infiltrative type, the stenosis may be very pronounced, so that the forceps, in order to get an adequate biopsy specimen, must be introduced beyond the stenotic area. The mucosa of the dilated esophagus proximal to the tumor often shows signs of inflammatory changes which, when submitted to the pathologist as a biopsy specimen, may not reveal the carcinoma. Bronchoscopy should also be performed to exclude the existence of a broncho-esophageal or tracheo-esophageal fistula, which would render the case inoperable.

The therapeutic approach is essentially surgical, but, with pain in the interscapular region or with involvement of the recurrent nerve, a total extirpation of the tumor may be impossible. Palliative surgery for alimentation is of questionable value. In inoperable cases with marked obstruction, the insertion of a nasogastric feeding tube to improve the patient's nutritional status is indicated. Radiotherapy, preferably with radioactive cobalt, may be palliative, to the extent that the obstruction may be relieved for many months. In the absence of the mentioned contraindications, surgical extirpation, with a high gastro-esophageal anastomosis or using a tube introduced by Gavrilow, may be tried in spite of the fact that the 5-year cure rate still remains at a disappointingly low level.

MALIGNANT TUMORS III

Lower End of Esophagus

The most frequent site of an esophageal carcinoma is the lower third of this organ (43 per cent). The tumors are usually of the scirrhous, infiltrating or of the proliferative, exophytic type. Both types eventually give rise to obstruction, producing dysphagia, progressive dyspepsia and discomfort after eating. In the scirrhous type the esophageal lumen may appear, on the roentgen film, eccentric and angulated, and the passage of a barium bolus is delayed because of a stenosed, rigid segment due to extension of the tumor. This may be an important observation for the differentiation from benign lesions such as cardiospasm or peptic esophagitis, in which the esophageal wall above the stenosis remains distensible. In time, dilatation of the esophagus proximal to the obstructing tumor increases and may reach magnitudes such as are seen in cardiospasm, although complete obstruction by a carcinoma is a rare finding. Irregular, mostly multiple and ulcerated masses are characteristic of the exophytic type of tumor. They produce soft tissue shadows in the X-ray picture, easy to differentiate from the thin, uniform barium column in the lumen, which occasionally takes a bizarre course. Squamous cell carcinoma of the lower third of the esophagus can be very extensive, occasionally almost reaching the cervical portion of the organ.

In many instances the *tumor of the lower esophagus* presents an *extension from a carcinoma of the gastric cardia* and fundus, which may have grown insidiously until it invades the terminal esophagus, causing there an obstruction by submucosal infiltration. If that has happened, the stenotic area may appear, endoscopically, quite smooth, with findings indistinguishable from cardiospasm.

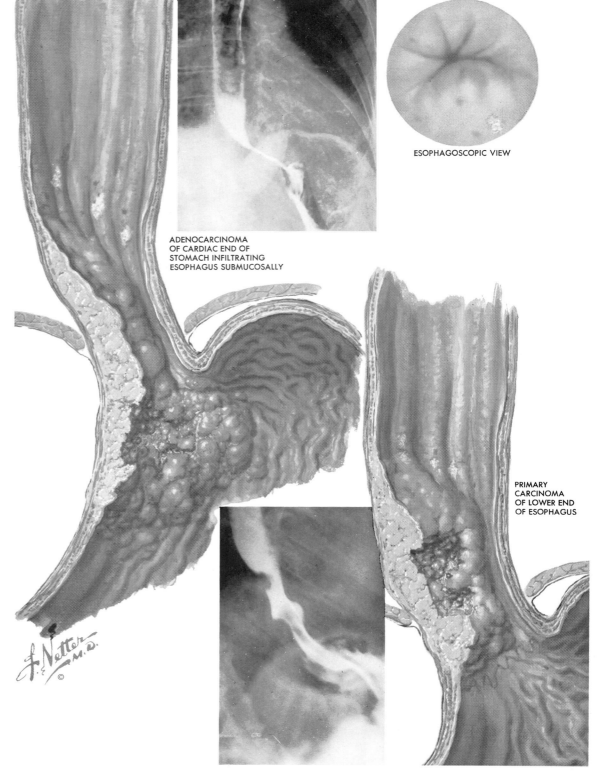

ADENOCARCINOMA
OF CARDIAC END OF
STOMACH INFILTRATING
ESOPHAGUS SUBMUCOSALLY

ESOPHAGOSCOPIC VIEW

PRIMARY
CARCINOMA
OF LOWER END
OF ESOPHAGUS

The differential diagnosis rests, in such cases, on the study of the peristalsis by X-ray examination. In the presence of cancer, the peristaltic activity of the esophagus is usually maintained, and stands in contrast to the repetitive secondary and tertiary contractions which distort the peristalsis in achalasia. The roentgenologist is in a more favorable position to determine the extension of an esophageal tumor. The endoscopist can usually see only its proximal portion, except when polypoid tumors permit the esophagoscope to pass the distal end of the neoplasm until normal esophageal mucosa can again be recognized.

In some cases the differential diagnosis between carcinoma and benign lesions, such as cicatricial strictures, peptic ulcers, cardiospasm and hiatal hernia may be decided only by an adequate biopsy specimen taken distal to the point of stenosis.

Primary adenocarcinoma of the esophagus, prob-ably arising from cardiac glands in the esophageal wall, is a very rare finding, but adenocarcinoma of the cardia extends, quite frequently, proximally to the lower esophagus, usually by submucosal infiltration. The primary esophageal adenocarcinoma is surrounded by a smooth and normal esophageal mucosa. If the microscopist reports adenocarcinoma in a biopsy specimen excised deeply from the submucosa, one may confidently assume the existence of a neoplasm of the cardia. The mucosa overlying an infiltrating cardiac adenocarcinoma appears puckered or nodular, and the lumen is conically narrowed, with the tapered end toward the stomach.

The therapy promising the greatest hope is surgical extirpation at an early stage. In inoperable cases, passage of a nasogastric feeding tube for alimentation is essential before ionizing radiation (supervoltage or radioactive cobalt) is tried.

Section VII

DISEASES OF THE STOMACH AND DUODENUM

by

FRANK H. NETTER, M.D.

in collaboration with

PROF. RUDOLF NISSEN, M.D.

THORACIC STOMACH I

Short Esophagus, Sliding Hernia

Protrusion of any abdominal viscera or parts thereof into the thoracic cavity through a congenital or acquired opening in the diaphragm is termed a diaphragmatic hernia. To those diaphragmatic hernias which involve the stomach belong the relatively rare cases in which this organ enters the chest through a gap in the side of the diaphragm posteriorly which failed to fuse at an early stage in the very complex development of the diaphragm.

A second congenital condition, in which part of the stomach is found above the diaphragm, and one which has received increasing attention in recent years, is attributable to innate *shortness of the esophagus* (brachyesophagus, see also page 139). From the pathologic-anatomic point of view, this condition does not represent a true hernia because of the lack of a hernial sac. The gastric cardia and part of the fundus have been pulled cranially and hang bell-like at the end of an esophagus which has not descended sufficiently or was not adequately elongated. The cause or causes (they may be manifold) of such thoracic position of parts of the stomach have not been definitely clarified, but, as operative experience shows, the shortness of the esophagus may be only spurious, and the elasticity and recoiling of the esophageal tube may permit the stomach to be drawn and fixed in its normal position. The thoracic stomach resulting from a short esophagus (the clinical consequences of which are discussed on page 147) is not to be confused with the state of what has become known as "gastric-lined esophagus" (see pages 38 and 148).

An acquired form of short esophagus, the so-called "pseudobrachyesophagus", may develop on the basis of a chronic esophagitis with reflux manifestations and a periesophagitis and subsequent shrinkage. This may be considered as the terminal stage of a long-standing sliding hernia, leading to a thoracic fixation of the prolapsed fundus.

Of all diaphragmatic herniae the *sliding* or "rolling" *esophageal hernia* is the

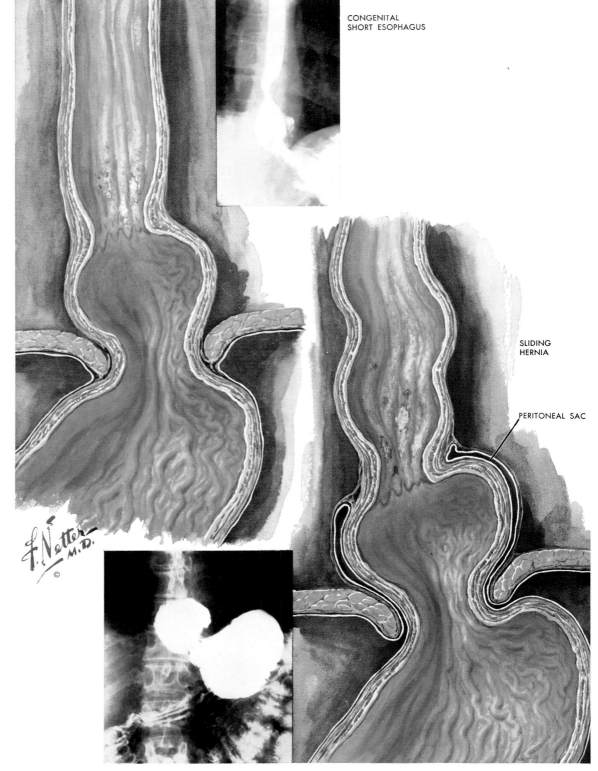

CONGENITAL SHORT ESOPHAGUS

SLIDING HERNIA

PERITONEAL SAC

one most frequently encountered. It develops mostly in women of middle and more advanced ages, as a result of a progressive slackness of the phreno-esophageal ligament (see page 38), from which a dilatation of the esophageal hiatus ensues, permitting the cardia and fundus to glide into the thoracic cavity either with a change of body position or following the suction effect of each inspiratory movement. In the early stages the stomach moves down- and upward, according to the respiratory phase, position or state of gastric filling (reversible hiatus hernia). Later on, adhesions may form between the hernial sac and pleura and fix the hernia. The mobility of the cardia and the formation of a hernial sac by the duplication of the peritoneum are the characteristic pathologic signs. The disease may remain symptomless for many years and may be discovered only accidentally during the search for the cause of a variety of epigastric symptoms, usually those produced by the accompanying reflux esophagitis (see pages 146-148). The diagnosis is readily established by adequate X-ray examination and endoscopy, which, in particular, is able to confirm the reflux phenomenon.

The striking X-ray findings of a sliding esophageal hernia, however, should not cause one, as often happens, to overlook other diseases such as peptic ulcer or cholelithiasis, which are primarily responsible for the patient's symptoms, while the sliding hernia still has no true clinical significance. It should also be kept in mind that a sliding esophageal hernia may simulate some symptoms of coronary disease or, conversely, that such a vascular ailment may be accompanied by a clinically insignificant hernia. Mild cases of esophageal hernia can be helped with antacids and spasmolytics. Persistent and moderate-to-severe symptoms are indications for surgical repair of the hernia.

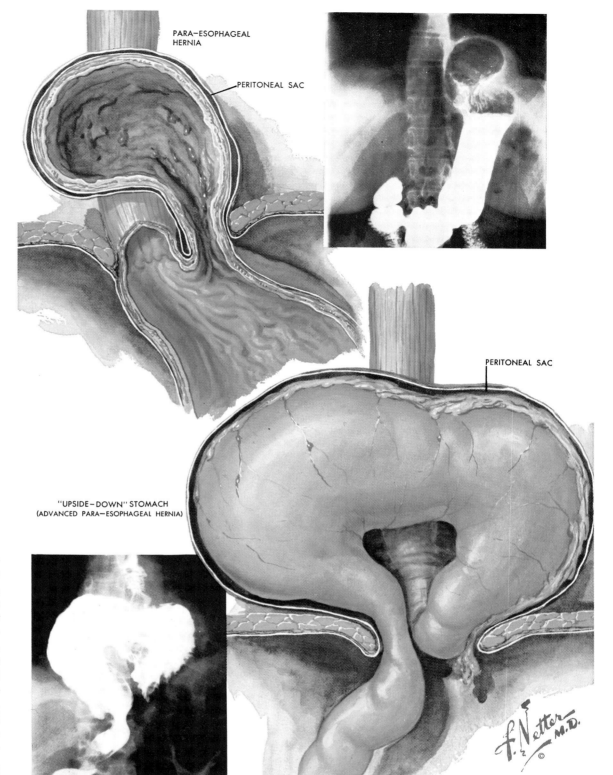

PARA—ESOPHAGEAL HERNIA

PERITONEAL SAC

Thoracic Stomach II
Paracardial Hernia

"UPSIDE—DOWN" STOMACH
(ADVANCED PARA—ESOPHAGEAL HERNIA)

PERITONEAL SAC

A paracardial or *para-esophageal hernia,* which is seen far less frequently than is a sliding diaphragmatic hernia, is characterized by the protrusion of a sometimes rather large, sometimes smaller part of the gastric fundus into the intrathoracic space alongside the esophagus, which is of normal length and in the usual and fixed position. The cardia and its attachment by the gastrophrenic ligament also have usually remained intact. The fundus (or parts of it) has slipped through a fibromuscular aperture directly to the left or right of the gastro-esophageal junction. The parietal peritoneum, which normally covers the abdominal surface of the diaphragm, has prolapsed and serves as the outer wall of the *hernial sac.* These anatomic relations explain why, with a para-esophageal hernia, there is no insufficiency of the esophagocardial sphincter mechanism, and hence no peptic esophagitis occurs.

The hiatus between the terminal portion of the esophagus and the diaphragmatic crus (or the phreno-esophageal ligament) (see page 38) is, as a rule, so narrow that it may interfere with the circulation of the prolapsed portion of the fundus, which will consequently become congested. The venous congestion leads to inflammatory reactions of the mucosa, which tends then to erode

or bleed, particularly in the area of the hiatal aperture. The resulting blood loss, in some cases, may be of such magnitude as to produce a chronic and recurrent anemia, which may be the first and only clinical sign of the disease. The para-esophageal hernia, however, assumes its clinical significance essentially by the potential danger of strangulation of the herniated parts. The predominant symptoms with this type of hernia are epigastric and substernal pain, nausea and, but only rarely, dysphagia. An increase of the intermittent attacks of pain, the appearance of hematemesis and a tendency toward cardiovascular collapse should always arouse the suspicion of a possible strangulation. Meticulous roentgen examination reveals the herniated gastric fundus adjacent to the normally placed esophagus with normal topo-

graphic relations of the gastro-esophageal junction.

An extreme variant of the para-esophageal hernia has been quite pertinently called the *"upside-down" stomach.* In such instances a markedly widened hiatus in the diaphragm has permitted the entire stomach to enter the thorax and to lie within the herniated sac. The stomach is rotated around its longitudinal axis, and the more movable major curvature thus becomes the dome of the prolapse. The cardia and pylorus are in close apposition to each other, and lie, with such a complete herniation of the organ, at the same level.

Once the diagnosis of a para-esophageal hernia has been established, its surgical repair is definitely indicated, not only because of the symptoms and signs (epigastric pain and anemia) but more so because of the always imminent danger of incarceration.

HYPERTROPHIC PYLORIC STENOSIS

Hypertrophic pyloric stenosis is a neonatal disorder. Its etiology and pathogenesis have been debated for many decades and still remain unsettled. The majority of authors, at least in the United States, seem to favor the concept that it is a congenital disease. Other observers, impressed by the facts (1) that symptoms never occur before the tenth day of life and (2) that medical treatment with parasympatholytics and appropriate nursing may yield in many hospitals (and even in private homes) as good or even better results than the best surgical therapy, stress the significance of environmental and nervous factors, neuromuscular dysfunction and other postnatal processes. They believe that the basic defect is not a primary (congenital) excessive development of the pyloric muscular mass but that the latter comes into existence, admittedly with astounding rapidity, secondarily as the result of spasms.

From the pathologic point of view, the designation of this condition is a misnomer, in so far as the microscopic findings indicate, for it is not a hypertrophy but a hyperplasia of the smooth muscle layers of the prepyloric region, particularly of the circular layer. The increase in muscular mass greatly *diminishes the size of the lumen,* thus causing obstruction. Depending upon the degree of the obstruction and its duration, the stomach may be enormously dilated. The *pylorus* is *pale or grayish from its serosal aspect,* as well as on its cut surface; its *contour* is smooth, though it bulges forward like a tumor, which terminates abruptly at the beginning of the duodenum at one end and, on the average, about 2 cm. proximally at the other end. The consistency of the pylorus in this condition is remarkably firm, sometimes almost as hard as that of cartilage. The mucosa of the pyloric region may appear normal but, at times, may show signs of irritation and inflammation. The condition occurs from five to seven times more frequently in boys than in girls.

Vomiting is always the first symptom and may appear between the second and sixth weeks of life. It increases in frequency and severity and early assumes the character of vomiting carried out sud-

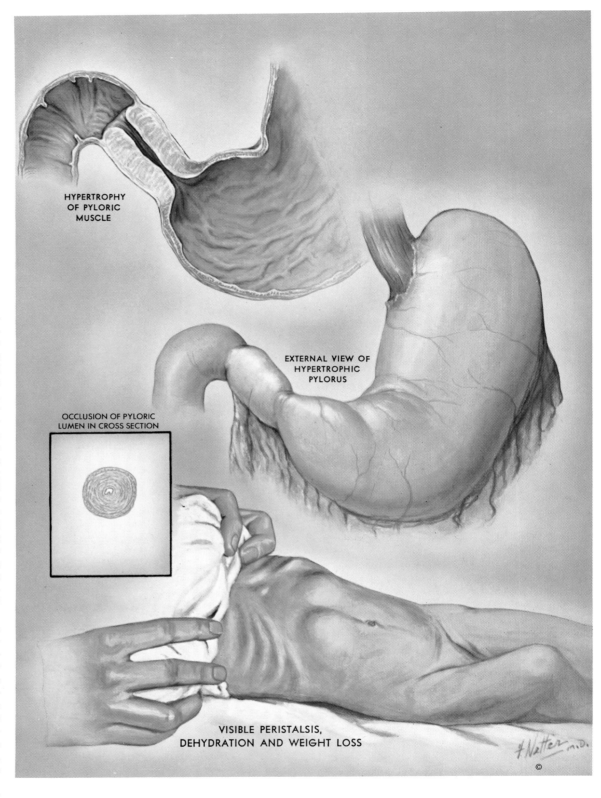

HYPERTROPHY OF PYLORIC MUSCLE

EXTERNAL VIEW OF HYPERTROPHIC PYLORUS

OCCLUSION OF PYLORIC LUMEN IN CROSS SECTION

VISIBLE PERISTALSIS, DEHYDRATION AND WEIGHT LOSS

denly and with great force (projectile type of vomiting). The infants, the vast majority of whom are males, cry, indicating hunger and willingness to take food. With less and less food or fluid passing through the obstructed pylorus, the *patients* lose weight and become *dehydrated.* In this stage a metabolic alkalosis may present a serious problem. The pylorus may be palpated, and strong peristaltic movements of the stomach may be observed on simple inspection of the abdominal wall. Diagnosis can be made in almost every case based on the history and physical examination alone. X-ray examination is rarely necessary and is considered not desirable by some clinicians. It can, however, be performed without the use of a barium suspension. The abnormally large, dilated stomach will be outlined by the air in it. When barium is administered, the increased size of the stomach becomes clearly visible, and no contrast

medium will appear in the duodenum until from ½ to 2 hours have passed after the instillation.

Opinions as to the treatment of hypertrophic pyloric stenosis are divided in line with those concerning its pathogenesis. Pylorotomy (Fredet-Ramstedt's operation) seems to be widely accepted in many countries; however, it should be performed not as an emergency operation but only after adequate preparation and regulation of the electrolyte and fluid situation and the state of nourishment. With such medical treatment, including the use of parasympatholytics, the improvement may be such that an operation becomes unnecessary. With a team available, who are experienced in pediatric surgery, anesthesia and postoperative care, the mortality rate of pylorotomy nowadays is less than 1 per cent or, as claimed by some authors, zero. The resulting cure is permanent, leaving no tendency to diseases of the upper gastro-intestinal tract.

DIVERTICULUM OF STOMACH, GASTRODUODENAL PROLAPSE

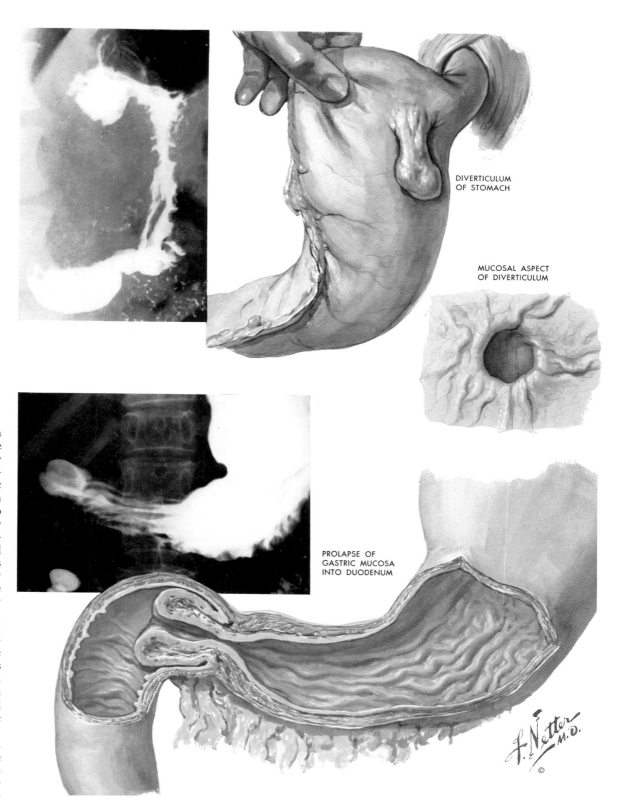

DIVERTICULUM
OF STOMACH

MUCOSAL ASPECT
OF DIVERTICULUM

PROLAPSE OF
GASTRIC MUCOSA
INTO DUODENUM

A *diverticulum of the stomach* is a rare occurrence and, therefore, of little practical significance, but occasions may arise which make it worth while to consider it in differential diagnosis. Gastric diverticula are practically all located on the posterior wall of the cardia and to the left of the esophagus. Whether they develop in postnatal life or originate during the fetal period cannot be decided upon with certainty. Small sacculations of the posterior wall have occasionally been observed in the stomach of the human fetus, and even more frequently in that of the hog and other animals. These facts favor a congenital etiology. On the other hand, the structural weakness of the longitudinal muscles on the posterior surface (see page 53) points also to the possibility that the diverticula may be acquired during lifetime by a pulsion mechanism. Both theories could explain the site of predilection and the rare occurrence of diverticula.

As a rule, all layers of the stomach participate in forming the pouch of the gastric diverticula, but, occasionally, one or the other layer may be absent totally or in part. The diverticula are usually 2 to 3 cm. long and from 1 to 2 cm. in diameter. The opening of the diverticulum is, in most cases, wide enough to allow free communication between the pouch and the stomach, and these patients have no complaints. Occasionally, the ingesta may become impacted and then cause inflammation. The danger of a perforation seems relatively small. *Roentgenologically,* a diverticulum of the stomach may be demonstrated as a saccular structure which fills with barium when the patient is asked to lie down and, a few minutes later, to stand up. The pouch on the posterior wall may be seen within the cardiac air bubble at some distance to the left of the esophageal entrance. Overdistention of the stomach with barium may obscure the

deformity. Sometimes it may be necessary to turn the patient obliquely, with his right side against the screen or film. The diverticulum will then appear to extend from the lesser curvature. A penetrating ulcer in the upper regions of the stomach may produce X-ray pictures quite similar to those of a diverticulum, and, if the clinical manifestations are very pronounced, it is preferable to assume the presence of an ulcer.

Diverticula located at the pyloric end of the stomach or on the anterior wall of the cardia have been reported only in a few isolated cases.

A *prolapse of the gastric mucosa into the duodenum* probably develops because of an extreme movability of the antral mucosa and submucosa, which, for one reason or another, adhere only loosely to the external layers of the wall. The mucosa of the antrum, which normally is thicker than the mucosa of other parts of the stomach and sometimes assumes a cush-

ionlike quality, is pushed through the pyloric ring to lie like a turned-back cuff of a sleeve within the duodenum. A fully developed prolapse is rare, but partial ones are quite frequent, though they have little or no clinical significance. In the X-ray picture the bulb of the duodenum appears as if it were filled with a tuberous mass, which has irregular contours owing to the fact that the contrast medium lies only on top of the mucosal folds and is absent in the pits. The diagnosis is, thanks to the typical configuration, easy, and in only a few special cases is it difficult to differentiate such a prolapse from a polyp or an acute ulcer with a marked mucosal edema of its surroundings.

Strangulation of the prolapsed segment and extreme swelling of the mucosa, with subsequent signs of a pyloric stenosis or hemorrhages from congested mucosal blood vessels, are rare occurrences.

DIVERTICULA OF DUODENUM

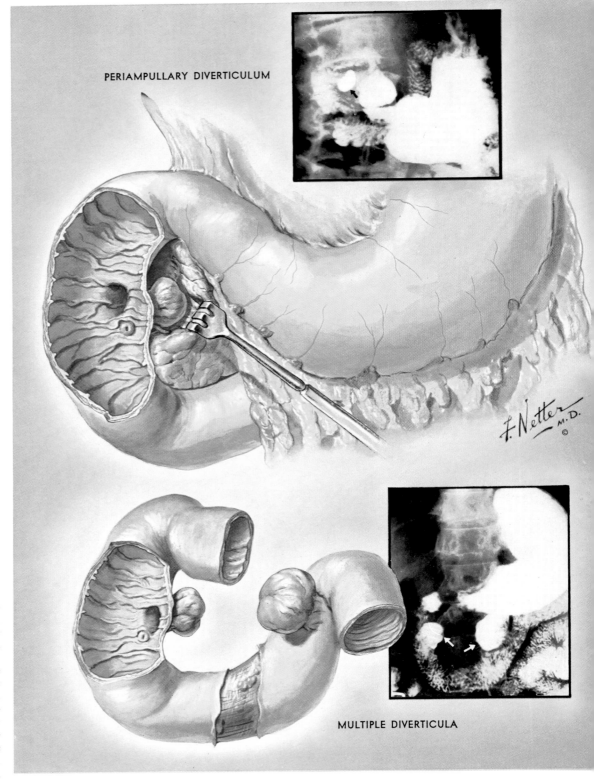

PERIAMPULLARY DIVERTICULUM

MULTIPLE DIVERTICULA

A comparatively common abnormality of the duodenum is a diverticulum. This is a saccular structure originating from any part of the duodenal curve, though a true diverticulum originating from the first portion of the duodenum must be extremely rare if, indeed, it ever occurs, since many experienced observers have never been able to find a case of this kind. This, of course, excludes the pre-stenotic type of diverticulum described on page 171, which develops second-arily to the narrowing associated with a duodenal ulcer.

As a rule, diverticula are single. The site of predilection is the *region of the ampulla of Vater*. Development of a diverticulum in this region is probably related to an area of diminished resistance to intraduodenal pressure. Some evidence, however, is available to indicate that such anomalies may be congenital. In addition to the periampullary region, diverticula may also occur in other parts of the duodenal curve beyond the bulb. In rare instances *diverticula* may be *multiple,* as many as five being present at one time. Usually, the diverticula origi-nate from the inner or concave border of the duodenal curve. In rare instances, however, they have arisen from the outer border or from the posterior wall.

The diagnosis is ordinarily made dur-ing routine radiologic study, since duo-denal diverticula are rarely responsible for clinical symptoms. Abdominal dis-comfort, however, may result when a diverticulum becomes inflamed, particu-larly as a consequence of prolonged retention of duodenal content for hours or even days after the stomach has been emptied. Occasionally, secondary inflam-mation of the pancreatic head has been encountered, resulting from an expansion of a duodenal diverticu-litis. In some cases of obstructive jaundice, the only pathologic finding may be a diverticulum originating from the region of the papilla of Vater. Removal of such a diverticulum has relieved the jaundice, so that it may be rightly assumed that either direct pres-sure of the diverticulum or a secondary inflamma-tion indirectly connected with it was responsible for the manifestations of an obstruction.

On *radiologic* examination the diverticulum appears to have a *circular contour* with a neck com-municating with the duodenum itself. Strands of mucosa may be noted within the neck but none within the diverticulum. As stated, the clinical sig-nificance of such a finding must not be overempha-sized, and the cause of the abdominal symptoms must, as a rule, be sought for elsewhere. With the patient in the erect position, a duodenal diverticulum may show a fluid level capped by gas. It may so overlap the pyloric region of the stomach as to simulate the niche of an ulcer in this region. Moreover, the diver-ticulum may overlap the lesser curvature of the mid-portion of the stomach and simulate a niche. Careful fluoroscopic observation with manual palpation so as to separate overlapping parts, as well as observation through various angles of obliquity, will eliminate this possible error of interpretation. As long as a diverticulum, usually an accidental roentgenologic finding, produces no signs of inflammation, obstruc-tion, hemorrhage or perforation, it is best left alone. In case of complications, as indicated, surgical removal is the best treatment, though the operation may at times be rather difficult. Palliative procedures (gastrojejunostomy or gastroduodenal resection) are useless.

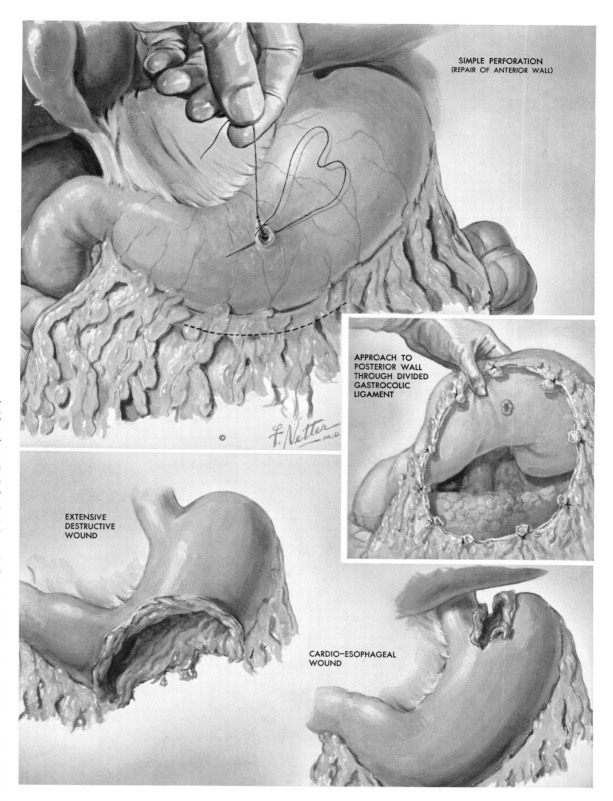

SIMPLE PERFORATION
(REPAIR OF ANTERIOR WALL)

APPROACH TO POSTERIOR WALL THROUGH DIVIDED GASTROCOLIC LIGAMENT

EXTENSIVE DESTRUCTIVE WOUND

CARDIO-ESOPHAGEAL WOUND

F. Netter

TRAUMA OF STOMACH

Injuries of the stomach occur relatively frequently with any penetrating or perforating wound of the abdomen. According to statistical data of war surgery, about 8 per cent of all abdominal wounds involve the stomach, and in approximately 5 per cent the stomach alone is injured. With blunt trauma to the upper abdominal region, the stomach may become lacerated, or it may even rupture if the organ is filled and distended at the moment of impact.

The type of gastric wound produced by a bullet or sharp instrument depends upon the size, shape, course and velocity of the wounding agent. Bullets which enter from the front, taking an anteroposterior course, often cause only small perforations of the wall. Larger shell fragments, on the other hand, can produce rather *extensive jagged lacerations,* which may completely sever the stomach from the duodenum, particularly if they include the gastric antrum. *Wounds of the cardia* often involve the lower end of the *esophagus* and mediastinum.

The clinical manifestations of any perforating injury of the stomach are, as a rule, very dramatic. Depending upon the size of the wound, the loss of blood, and the presence or absence of concomitant injuries, either shock or signs of peritonitis dominate the clinical picture. Small perforations, causing little shock, may first cause localized and then diffuse pain, which is soon followed by rigidity of the abdominal wall, nausea and vomiting of bloody material. The entry of air into the abdominal cavity can be demonstrated roentgenologically.

It may be added that small *perforating injuries of the cardia* produce, in the beginning, very few or no clinical symptoms. In most cases only a left shoulder pain due to inflammatory reaction of the diaphragmatic peritoneum is present.

The prognosis of any gastric wound depends nowadays upon the promptness of the appropriate surgical intervention rather than upon the type and degree

of the injury. In World War I the mortality rate of all gastric wounds ranged between 50 and 60 per cent, owing to the frequency of hemorrhagic shock and peritoneal infection, and from 25 to 50 per cent of those cases in which the wound was not complicated and was restricted to the stomach. The progress made in the meantime in treating shock and infections, as well as the improved military organization for the transport of battle victims, has tremendously reduced these figures in later conflicts.

The only treatment for injuries of the stomach is surgical, and that at the earliest possible time. With both gunshot and stab wounds, the *posterior* as well as the anterior *wall* may be *injured* simultaneously, so that it becomes obligatory to explore the posterior wall in every instance by adequately detaching the gastrocolic ligament and pulling the stomach upward. Cases in which the anterior gastric wall has remained

intact, while the posterior wall alone was perforated, even though the shot or puncturing instrument entered through the anterior abdominal wall, have been reported. This can happen if, at the time of the accident, the stomach was so tightly filled that the greater curvature, rotating around the longitudinal axis of the stomach, has turned forward and upward. In this position the inferior aspect of the posterior wall approaches the anterior abdominal wall.

Extensive destructive wounds, with major defects of the stomach, cannot be repaired and make a typical gastrectomy or removal of large parts of the stomach inevitable.

If the cardia has been injured, a left thoracotomy becomes necessary in order to assure a sufficient view and also freedom of action to perform a gastroesophageal resection in those instances in which the esophagus also is found to be involved.

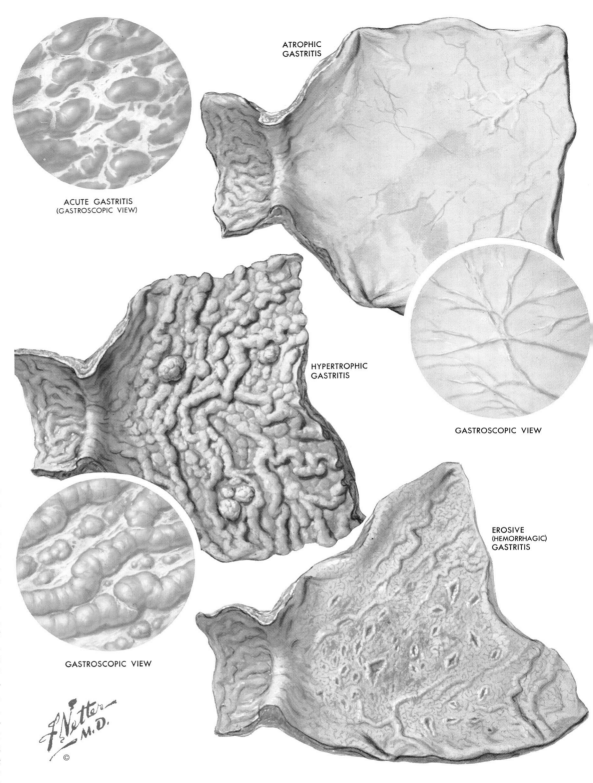

ATROPHIC GASTRITIS

ACUTE GASTRITIS
(GASTROSCOPIC VIEW)

HYPERTROPHIC GASTRITIS

GASTROSCOPIC VIEW

EROSIVE (HEMORRHAGIC) GASTRITIS

GASTROSCOPIC VIEW

GASTRITIS

Irritation from dietary indiscretions (excessive food intake, insufficiently masticated or spoiled or strongly seasoned food), from abuse of alcohol, coffee and tobacco and, last but not least, from chemicals used as drugs is the main cause of *acute gastritis*, but it may develop also as a concomitant symptom with many febrile infections (typhoid, pneumonia, diphtheria, etc.). The mucous membrane in acute gastritis (Beaumont in his classical work, 1833) is erythematous, with livid, sometimes sanguineous areas, and covered with a thick, ropy mucus. The most common symptoms are epigastric distress, nausea, belching, disagreeable taste and vomiting, all of which vary in intensity.

A corrosive type of gastritis, originating from the intake of strong chemicals, such as lye, can lead to a localized or diffuse necrosis and permanent scarring. *Chronic atrophic gastritis* may be an aftermath of an acute gastritis, but many other possible etiologic factors of exogenous or endogenous origin have been considered, all with some justification. Its relation and association with malignancies are not definitely clarified, but its close relationship to pernicious anemia is firmly established. The characteristic gross pathologic features gastroscopically are the disappearance of the folds and the thinness of the gray-colored mucosa through which shines the vascular net, both arterial and venous. Microscopically, the chief and parietal cells are considerably reduced in size and number; the epithelial cells are transformed to a great extent into goblet cells, or undergo metaplastic changes. The clinical manifestations, subjective and objective, are rather nonspecific and rarely permit adequate differentiation from any of the other diseases of the stomach and gastro-intestinal tract. Even gastric analysis is unreliable, since only in less than one third of the patients with atrophic gastritis are values found that indicate anacidity or hypacidity. X-ray examination is usually of little help, and only gastroscopy is able to establish the diagnosis beyond doubt.

With chronic *hypertrophic gastritis* the situation is clinically much the same, except that hyperacidity is present in most cases, and the distribution of the rugae and the "cobblestone" appearance of the mucosal surface, seen roentgenographically, provide more often the right clue for the diagnosis which can, however, only be made unequivocally by gastroscopy. The rugae are strikingly thickened and, even at autopsy, do not flatten out when the wall is stretched.

Erosive hemorrhagic gastritis is characterized by multiple, diffuse erosions in an inflamed mucosa, and it acquires a special clinical significance through its tendency to severe, often life-endangering hemorrhages. Larger arteries extend quite frequently as far up as the epithelium and may become involved in some of the many small, but by no means superficial, erosions. Whenever the origin of gastro-intestinal bleeding cannot be identified, the possibility of an erosive, hemorrhagic gastritis must be seriously considered. X-ray examination is of little or no avail, and gastroscopy during an episode of acute bleeding is not without danger. At laparotomy the diagnosis may still be difficult, because, even when viewing the mucosa directly after gastrotomy, the small erosions, *i.e.*, the source of the bleeding, may not be seen macroscopically.

A similar type of hemorrhagic gastritis (see page 188) has been observed after partial resection of the stomach or after gastro-enterostomy or ulcer. This should be kept in mind if the suspicion of a bleeding peptic "anastomotic ulcer" cannot be confirmed unequivocally by X-ray studies or at laparotomy. Under such circumstances vagotomy seems to be the best procedure to stop the bleeding. It has helped in many cases and, in any event, is preferable to an additional resection.

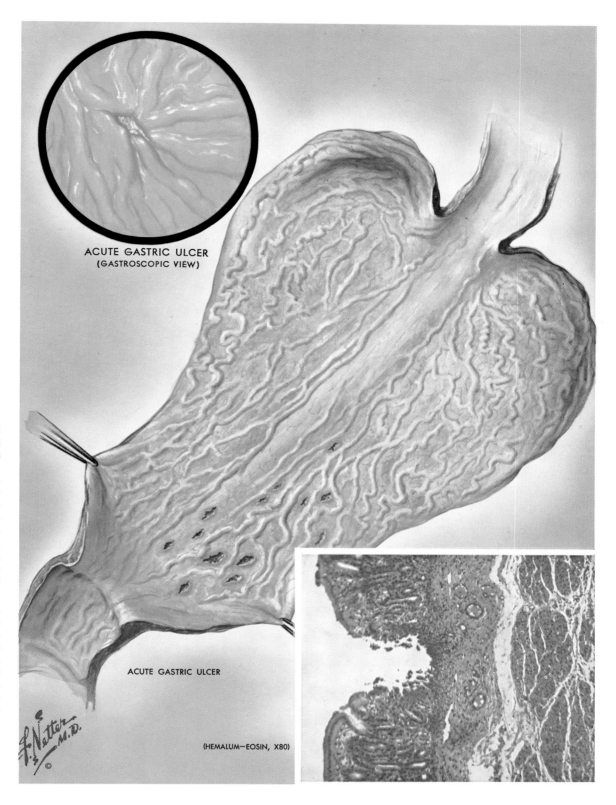

ACUTE GASTRIC ULCER
(GASTROSCOPIC VIEW)

ACUTE GASTRIC ULCER

(HEMALUM—EOSIN, X80)

PEPTIC ULCER I

Acute Gastric Ulcer

The etiology of gastric or duodenal peptic ulcers has been a matter of debate during several decades and still remains unsettled.

Small superficial erosions of the gastric mucosa, even those with a tendency to bleed (see page 164), may cause few or no symptoms, though in the past they were noted quite often by the pathologist at autopsy or, more recently, by the gastroscopist. *Acute ulcers* are said to be characterized by a somewhat greater defect of the mucosa and sometimes of the uppermost stratum of the submucosa. Their size varies considerably between the extremes of a few millimeters to 3 to 4 cm. The very small ones may sometimes be seen only when the mucous membrane is stretched. Acute ulcers are usually multiple, and, the greater their number, the smaller is their size. Single acute ulcers are rare. The site of predilection for acute ulcers is in the prepyloric region, but occasionally very small ones may arise in the mucosa of the body and along the greater curvature. In contrast, larger acute ulcers are sometimes found along the so-called "Magenstrasse" (see pages 52 and 53).

In its earliest stages an acute ulcer appears as a shallow necrotic region, with a slightly raised soft margin surrounded by tissue which may or may not show a mild inflammatory reaction. The sloughed floor of the ulcer usually appears black, as a consequence of the chemical changes produced by the hydrochloric acid on the blood which oozes from the lesions. At times the bleeding may be more pronounced, or even severe, with a relatively small ulcer. Should the ulcerative process reach the muscularis mucosae, this layer retracts, drawing the edges of the ulcer downward in apposition to each other. The original shape of the acute ulcer is oval, but it assumes a slitlike shape when the stomach wall contracts.

Although it is generally agreed that acute ulcers may become subacute or chronic, as a rule they have a good and relatively rapid healing tendency. The healing process starts with growth of the epithelium from the margins across the area from which the necrotic parts have been sloughed. From the newly formed epithelium the growth is downward. Even the muscularis mucosae, if involved in the process, may be completely restored.

The diagnosis of an acute ulcer is not often made on clinical grounds, except when *gastroscopy* is employed. But the application of this technique, in patients with acute gastric ulcer, is rarely indicated, provided the individual suffers from no other disease. The symptoms, if any, are negligible and certainly less pronounced than with an acute diffuse gastritis.

A special type of acute peptic ulcer of the stomach or duodenum, the so-called "stress ulcer", has been discussed widely, the pathophysiologic relation of which has not yet been completely clarified. It may develop following extensive burns ("Curling's ulcer"), in the course of tetanus, after brain surgery ("Cushing's ulcer") or in the course of therapy with corticotropin and corticosteroids ("steroid ulcer") (see also page 92) or even with pyrazolones. The specific features of this ulcer type are the rapidity with which they come into existence, the lack of any inflammatory reaction around the ulcer, complete painlessness and a pronounced tendency to perforation and bleeding. The frequency of ulcer formation during steroid therapy, however, has been overestimated. Statistical analysis of ulcer incidence has led to the conclusion that the percentage of ulcer development in patients treated with steroids is not greater, but rather somewhat smaller, than in a population that has not undergone this type of therapy.

PEPTIC ULCER II

Subacute Ulcer of Stomach

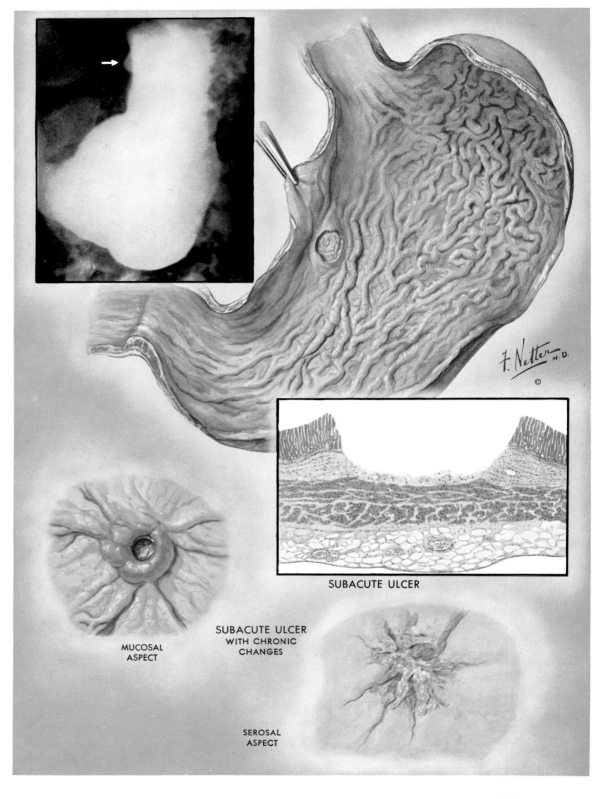

SUBACUTE ULCER

MUCOSAL
ASPECT

SUBACUTE ULCER
WITH CHRONIC
CHANGES

SEROSAL
ASPECT

The transitional stage between an acute and a chronic ulcer has often been termed "subacute ulcer". Morphologically, it differs in degree from an acute ulcer in so far as it is more rounded and has a greater depth. Its walls are thicker and higher, its shape occasionally funnel-like, with irregular contours. The subacute phase of a peptic ulcer has *involved both mucosa and submucosa,* but at times may reach the muscular coat. In any event, the subacute ulcer may present the same potential danger of perforation or profuse bleeding (see page 172) as does an acute or a chronic ulcer. At the *floor of the ulcer,* one finds, as a rule, purulent, grayish-yellow, necrotic material. The grayish-white color on the floor or edges may be due also to proliferating fibroblasts, as token of a healing tendency and the beginning of scar formation.

Usually, the subacute ulcer is single, but, even if multiple ulcers are present, they are larger than the multiple or single acute ulcer, though, as a rule, smaller than a fully developed chronic lesion (see page 172).

The concept of the subacute ulcer is

derived essentially from the observations of the pathologist, and, in view of the enormous variability in size, shape, depth, etc., characteristic of any transitional stage or form of pathologic process, the term, understandably, cannot be sharply defined. Clinically, it is almost impossible to commit oneself definitely to the diagnosis of subacute ulcer, except occasionally, when the duration of the patient's history and the shallowness of the ulcer, if identified radiologically, may justify the diagnostic use of this term. The symptoms of subacute ulcer are the same as those of either an acute or a chronic ulcer, or both. In addition, a subacute ulcer may run a symptom-free course for an indefinite period of time, and its presence may become evident only after a sudden massive hemorrhage or after the dramatic signs of acute perforation or the less dra-

matic ones of a "chronic perforation" (see page 172).

On the X-ray screen or film, a subacute ulcer is usually demonstrable at or near the *lesser curvature.* The *niche* is, as a rule, clearly outlined and sharply delimited from the contour of the curvature. It is a fixed deformity, remaining stationary during the radiologic study, in contrast to the greater part of the lesser curvature, which participates freely in the peristaltic activity. When the wall of the ulcer is edematous, the apparent depth may be exaggerated. But with the diminution or disappearance of the wall or its margins, it is sometimes difficult, if not impossible, to demonstrate the niche of a fairly superficial subacute ulcer, though, in spite of the lack of or vanishing radiologic evidence, the ulcer itself may still be present.

Peptic Ulcer III

Chronic Gastric Ulcer

The chronic gastric ulcer is almost invariably single, although scars of previous ulcers that have healed can be found in association with the sole, active, chronic lesion. Not infrequently, a duodenal ulcer develops simultaneously with a chronic gastric ulcer.

Most benign *chronic gastric ulcers* occur at or *near the lesser curvature* of the stomach in its mid-area and, frequently, on the posterior wall near the lesser curvature. They arise less commonly at the cardiac portion of the stomach or near the pyloric ring. Only rarely does an ulcer on the greater curvature prove to be benign.

Chronic gastric ulcers vary considerably in size, but about 80 per cent of them are less than 1.8 cm. in diameter. The ulcer is usually round, but at times it may be elongated. The margins of a chronic ulcer are raised and, usually, considerably undermined, as a result of the retraction of the muscular strata, whose continuity has, in a chronic ulcer, always been interrupted. Fibrotic tissue, covered, at times, by a fibrinous, purulent exudate, forms the floor of the ulcer. The *penetrating* ulcerative process may also involve the serosa, which subsequently becomes thickened by production of fibrotic tissue ("Narbenpflaster") (see pages 172 and 174).

At times, obliterative endarteritis appears in the blood vessels on the floor of the chronic peptic ulcer. The associated veins sometimes show evidence of thickening. Thrombosis of the veins and arteries may occur, sometimes with endarteritis in the same vessel. The nerves at the floor of the ulcer occasionally display perineural fibrosis.

The dominant and also most characteristic symptom of chronic gastric ulcer is epigastric pain, which the patient locates at some place between the xiphoid process and the umbilicus, or somewhat left of this line toward the left costal margin. The intensity and character of the pain, which the patient may describe as "cutting", "gnawing", "burning", etc., depend upon a variety of factors, such as the location, size and "activity" of the ulcer and the sensitiveness of the individual patient. The pain may radiate to the back, usually to the level of the eighth to the tenth thoracic vertebrae. Rather typical, but by no means absolutely pathognomonic of a chronic ulcer (or sufficiently invariable as to exclude the possibility of a malignant growth),

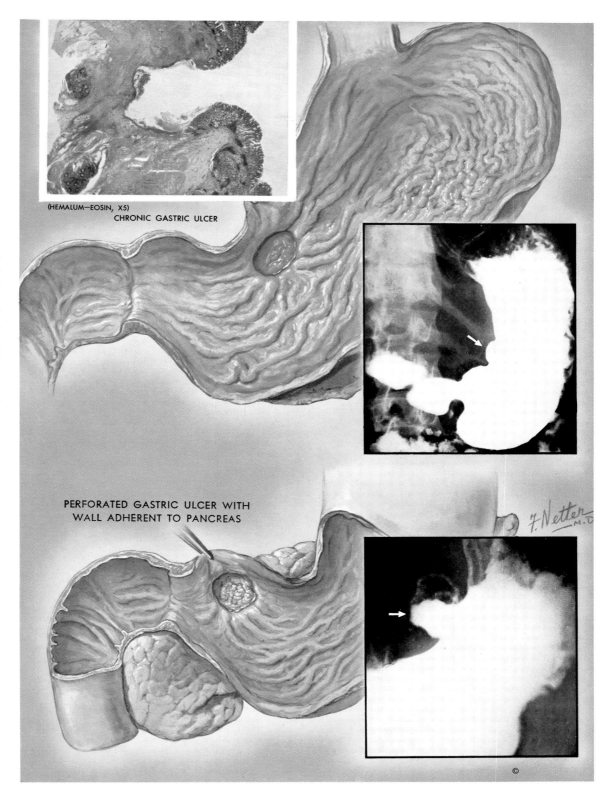

(HEMALUM—EOSIN, X5)
CHRONIC GASTRIC ULCER

PERFORATED GASTRIC ULCER WITH WALL ADHERENT TO PANCREAS

is the rhythmic and periodic recurrence of the pain. Usually shortly after ingestion of food, the pain disappears only to recur ½ to 1 hour after the meal (see also page 88). It may then abate spontaneously before the next intake of food. This "food-comfort-pain" rhythm, as it has been called, may persist or may respond more or less satisfactorily to medical treatment. It may fade gradually and disappear suddenly, failing to reappear for many months, or even years, if the ulcerating, penetrating or accompanying inflammatory processes have slowed to a stop. If, on the other hand, the pain becomes more intense, or loses its periodic rhythm and becomes persistent, this should always be taken as an ominous sign of increasing danger of further complications.

Though the patient's history and complaints, as well as a careful physical examination, will be helpful in diagnosing a gastric ulcer, the final diagnosis can be made only by X-ray studies. Radiologically, the chronic gastric ulcer is characterized by a niche projecting from the barium-filled stomach. As a rule, the niche is deeper than that of a subacute ulcer, though it is not always possible to determine the exact depth of the crater from the size of a niche, owing to the variability in the thickness of the edematous and swollen wall. In spite of the great value of the roentgen examination in diagnosing a peptic ulcer, still 10 to 20 per cent of patients remain with signs of ulcer in whom the benignancy of an ulcerative lesion cannot be definitely ascertained. In line with the opinion of experienced clinicians, these patients, and those whose symptoms do not improve or become more severe after several weeks of medical treatment, or where the size of the niche does not decrease in spite of subjective improvement, should be subjected to prompt surgical exploration.

PEPTIC ULCER IV

Ulcer Near Cardia

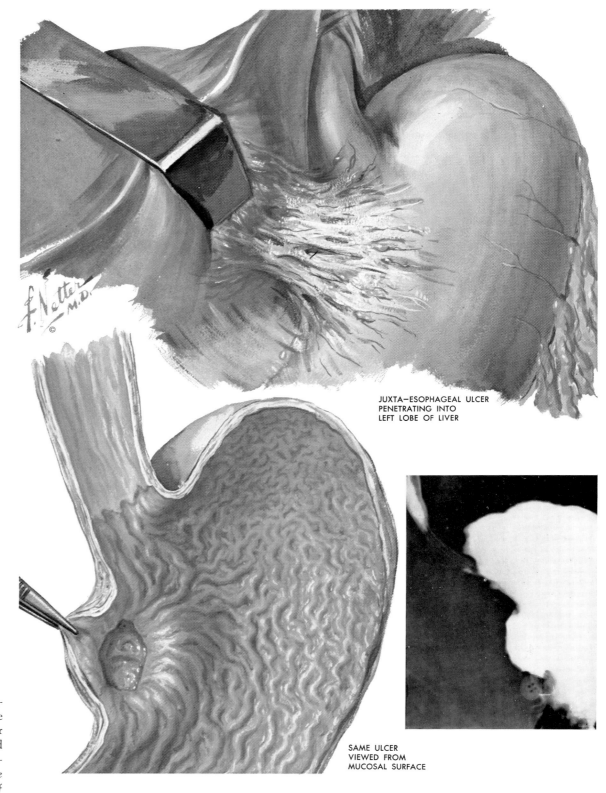

JUXTA-ESOPHAGEAL ULCER
PENETRATING INTO
LEFT LOBE OF LIVER

SAME ULCER
VIEWED FROM
MUCOSAL SURFACE

Approximately 7 per cent of all peptic ulcers (stomach and duodenum) are located within the cardia or at the lesser curvature near the cardia (Portis and Jaffee). These ulcers merit special consideration, because they may *penetrate* and grow *into the adjacent left lobe of the liver*. A marked periulcerous inflammation, with shrinkage of the gastrohepatic ligament (omentum minor), and *broad pannuslike adhesions* are associated with this penetrating process, which may proceed to such a point that the floor of the ulcer is formed by the parenchyma of the liver. Similarly, an ulcer located on the posterior wall of the stomach may infiltrate the body or tail of the pancreas. In such stages the condition is characterized clinically by severe, persistent pain, which, from time to time, may even be punctuated with more severe episodes as a result of irregular intensification of the inflammatory proc-

ess. But, in general, any real freedom from pain and, particularly, its correlation to meals, which is so typical of other ulcer patients, are missing. The patients, once the ulcer has penetrated to the underlying organ, lose appetite and, consequently, weight. In this stage, X-ray examination reveals usually a rather large niche, with a strongly developed wall and some fixation of the surrounding parts.

The differentiation from an ulcerated carcinoma (see page 184) may, under these circumstances, become, clinically as well as roentgenologically, almost impossible, so that surgical intervention must be considered the course of choice.

The localization of the ulcer and the involvement of liver or pancreas present some intricate problems for the surgeon planning resection. An extensive

resection, including the lesser curvature from its beginning at the cardia ("Schlauchresektion"), will, as a rule, permit removal of an ulcer which is still confined to the gastric wall. With one of the rare juxta-esophageal ulcers, however, it will be necessary to perform a transpleural gastro-esophageal resection. If the ulcer has penetrated either the liver or the pancreas, it is more prudent to leave the ulcer itself in situ, after having separated it from the gastric wall, provided, of course, that the absence of a malignancy has been clearly established by a frozen section of a specimen obtained during the operation. In view of the fact that the diagnosis from a frozen section is reliable only in about 80 per cent of the submitted specimens, some surgeons consider it safer to remove the ulcer and the surrounding tissue whenever possible.

Peptic Ulcer V

Giant Ulcer

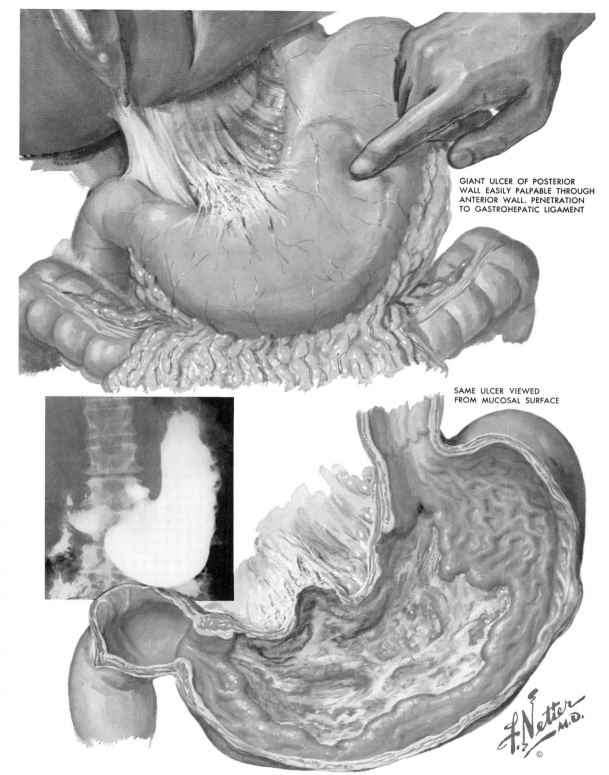

GIANT ULCER OF POSTERIOR WALL EASILY PALPABLE THROUGH ANTERIOR WALL. PENETRATION TO GASTROHEPATIC LIGAMENT

SAME ULCER VIEWED FROM MUCOSAL SURFACE

Ulcers of the stomach measuring over 3 cm. in their least diameter have been thought, until recently, to be rare except in the presence of extensive carcinoma. It is apparent, however, that a group of large, lesser-curvature gastric ulcers exist, particularly in the age group over 35, of which only a small proportion are malignant (5 per cent or less). These ulcers, because of their penetrating and extensive qualities, are serious threats to the health of the patient if not given adequate care, and are not easily amenable to surgery, as, even on the operating table, they give the appearance of a malignant lesion, so that more extensive surgery is performed for them than in many instances is justified. In the overall group of gastric ulceration, they are a rarity. The site of origin is usually *on the posterior wall* and may progressively involve the lesser curvature by extension. They may *penetrate the gastrohepatic ligament* and even involve the liver and pancreas. They are particularly deceptive in that they are of such great extent that there may be *no characteristic niche in the X-ray picture,* because the flattened floor of the ulcer is so extensive that it resembles an atrophic area of gastric mucosa. A very similar pathologic picture can be produced acutely by the corrosive action of acids or alkalis. When due to caustic agents, however, the material puddles in the prepyloric region and on the posterior wall of the stomach if the patient assumes a supine position immediately after the accident of ingestion, and this characteristic distribution, shown either on X-ray or by operative

procedures, should lead to suspicions as to the true agent, which often may have been self-administered.

The true giant benign ulcers usually have a long history of ulcerative disease, and usually ulcerative symptoms are at least 4 to 6 months old. The symptoms may occasionally have been present as long as 30 years. They may even involve the duodenum as well. The great majority of these patients are over the age of 50, although cases have been reported in the third and fourth decades. The patient may have lost much weight and may show advanced stages of malnutrition verging on cachexia. It is probably no coincidence that many of these patients have fairly far-advanced peripheral vascular disease with involvement of the mesenteric arterioles in an arteriosclerotic process, and, perhaps because of this diminished blood supply, the ulcer has proceeded to this striking size. Perforation or massive hemorrhage as a terminal

event is not unusual. Generally, with an ulcer history as long as that indicated above, one is dealing with an unco-operative patient as well.

It is interesting that this type of ulcer, usually 30 years ago thought to have been characteristically a carcinoma, has swung to the position of one of the more benign lesions if properly tended with vigorous medical management. Gastroscopy is usually valueless and may be hazardous. Surgical exploration may lead to more extensive surgery than is proper. It must still be remembered, however, that ulcers of this magnitude, and particularly in the prepyloric region in the absence of a caustic ingestion history, must be considered malignant until proved otherwise by biopsy by the pathologist, and that adenomatous changes of serious malignant import can occur in giant ulcer craters just as they can in the smaller ulcers of the stomach.

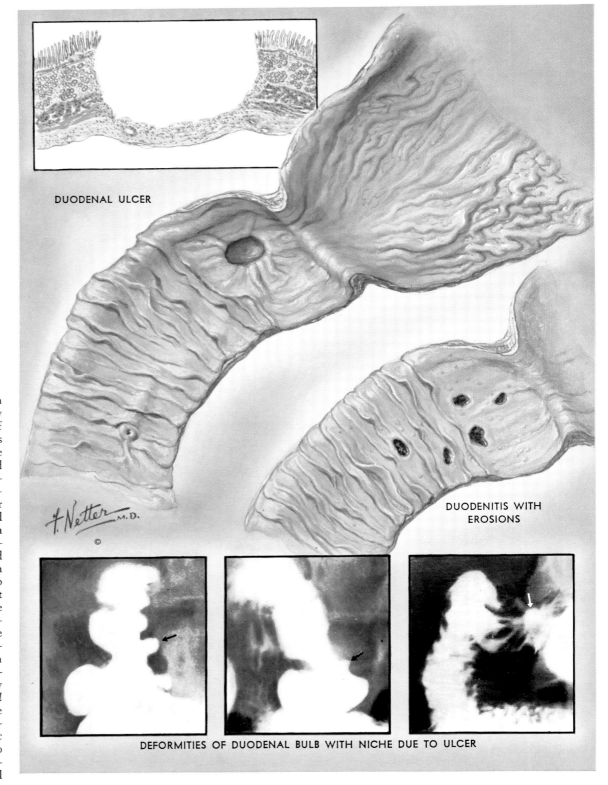

DUODENAL ULCER

DUODENITIS WITH EROSIONS

DEFORMITIES OF DUODENAL BULB WITH NICHE DUE TO ULCER

Peptic Ulcer VI

Duodenitis and Ulcer of Duodenal Bulb

If, as happens not infrequently in medical practice, the most careful X-ray examination fails to find any evidence of a duodenal ulcer in a patient who has typical ulcer symptoms, and if a disease of the gastric mucosa can be excluded after gastroscopy, the most probable diagnosis is that of *duodenitis, i.e.,* an inflammation of the mucosa in the bulbar region. The diagnosis may be supported when, in the roentgen film, the mucosa of the most proximal part of the duodenum appears somewhat mottled and when, fluoroscopically, spasms and an increased motility of the duodenal cap can be observed. It has been said that emotional disturbances play a rôle in the pathogenesis of this disease, but its etiology has remained otherwise obscure. The inflamed duodenal mucosa has a relatively strong tendency to bleed, even in the absence of an actual ulcerative process. At times, however, duodenitis may be associated with *multiple superficial erosions*. On the other hand, diffuse duodenitis may also be present in association with a characteristic chronic peptic ulcer. Duodenitis is usually confined to the most proximal parts of the duodenum, but, occasionally, the antral mucosa as well may participate in the inflammatory reaction. Since, in most instances, the diagnosis can be made only per exclusionem, continued observation and treatment of the patient are of paramount importance. Medical treatment for duodenitis is the same as that for peptic ulcer. Massive hemorrhages from duodenitis with erosion may, in rare cases, make exploration necessary, although, as a matter of general principle, surgical intervention is not recommended unless the source of the bleeding has been determined (see page 175).

More common, and clinically more important, is the *chronic duodenal ulcer*. With rare exceptions (see page 171) this lesion is seated within the duodenal bulb. It develops with essentially the same frequency on the anterior or posterior wall. The average size of a duodenal ulcer is 0.5 cm., but the ulcers on the posterior wall are usually larger than those on the anterior wall, mainly because the former, walled off by the pancreas lying below the ulcer, can increase in size without free perforation (see also page 173).

The duodenal peptic ulcer is usually round and has a punched-out appearance, but as a small ulcer it may sometimes be slitlike, crescent-shaped or triangular. The chronic ulcer, in contrast to an acute ulcer which stops at the submucosa, involves all layers. It penetrates to the muscular coat and deeper. An ulcer on the anterior wall may show a moderate amount of proliferation, whereas that on the posterior wall will give evidence of considerable edema and fibrosis. Healing may proceed just as it does with a gastric ulcer (see page 176), with disappearance of the crater and bridging of the gap by formation of fibrous tissue covered by new mucous membrane, but healing becomes more difficult once the destruction of the muscular layer has gone too far.

The symptoms of a chronic ulcer are, as a rule, typical and are characterized by periodic episodes of gnawing pain (see also page 88), usually located in the epigastrium. The pain occurs 1 to 2 hours after meals and may be relieved by food.

Roentgen examination reveals the classic features of deformity: (1) a niche corresponding to the actual ulcer crater, (2) a shortening of the upper curvature of the bulb and (3) contraction of the opposite side, which probably is the result of spasms of the circular muscle fibers in the plane of the ulcer or of edema and cicatrization. Radiating folds due to puckering from scar formation are sometimes demonstrable at the edge of the niche.

PEPTIC ULCER VII

Duodenal Ulcers Distal to
Duodenal Cap, Multiple
Ulcers, Prestenotic
Pseudodiverticula

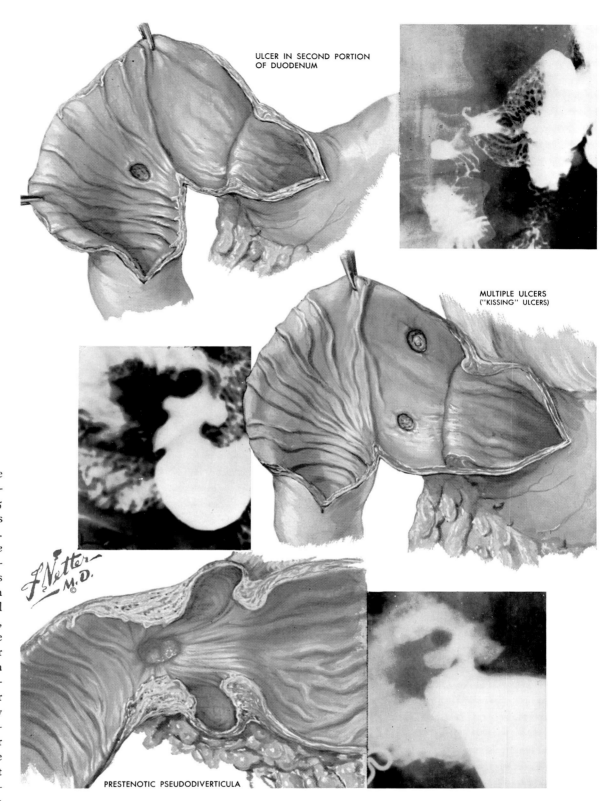

ULCER IN SECOND PORTION OF DUODENUM

MULTIPLE ULCERS ("KISSING" ULCERS)

PRESTENOTIC PSEUDODIVERTICULA

Peptic ulcers in a region distal to the duodenal bulb are rare, and their frequency, altogether probably less than 5 per cent of all duodenal ulcers, decreases with their distance from the pylorus. *Ulcers in the second portion of the duodenum* give rise to the same symptoms and are beset with the same dangers and complications as is the case with ulcers of the bulb. The acute clinical picture and later significance, however, may be far more complex because of the functional and anatomic implications for the adjoining structures. By the edema of its margin and surroundings, by penetration or by shrinkage, such an ulcer may cause obstruction and eventually stenosis of any one of the following structures: the papilla of Vater, the lower part of the common bile duct and one or both of the pancreatic ducts, so that chronic pancreatitis and/or biliary obstruction with jaundice may result. Deep penetration may give rise to choledocho-duodenal fistula.

Multiple chronic ulcers of the duodenum are fairly common. Their frequency, according to statistical data obtained from cases coming to autopsy, ranges between 11 and 45 per cent. As a rule, the number is restricted to two, and only in rare instances have more than two been found. When ulcers develop on both the anterior and posterior walls, they are referred to as "kissing" ulcers. Only a very small percentage of patients with an active duodenal ulcer have also an active gastric ulcer. Roentgenologic demonstration of more than one ulcer requires

a more detailed study, including visualization of the mucosal relief with a thin layer of barium and compression of the duodenum, to bring out the niche on the posterior wall. Serial "spot-film" comparisons of the fluoroscopic findings may also be necessary.

A great variety of anatomic changes and roentgen deformities of the duodenum can be associated with an ulcer or can develop during the course of its extension or involution. One of the most typical duodenal deformities occurring with the ulcerative process is the *prestenotic pseudodiverticulum.* Seen from the lumen, it represents a relatively flat, sinuslike indentation, located usually between the pylorus and the site of the ulcer or proximal to a duodenal stricture resulting from a cicatricial remnant of an ulcer.

Although all layers of the duodenal wall partici-

pate in the formation of such a pouch, they differ from a true duodenal diverticulum (see page 162), in that the mucosa has not evaginated through a small muscular gap. The pseudodiverticula need not cause any clinical symptoms, but they produce quite characteristic X-ray pictures, which have been described as a "typical bulbus deformity" in cases of chronic peptic ulcer (Akerlund), though, at times, their differentiation from an active duodenal ulcer niche may be difficult. Although the prestenotic diverticulum is usually single, the development of multiple pouches is not rare. Often two pseudodiverticula may appear symmetrically in the upper and lower parts of the duodenal bulb, and a third one may deform the bulb into what has been called roentgenologically the "clover-leaf bulbus" ("Kleeblattbulbus").

PEPTIC ULCER VIII

Complications of Gastric and Duodenal Ulcers

Perforation (Rupture)

The two most serious complications of gastric or duodenal peptic ulcers are perforation and hemorrhage. Their incidence cannot be judged, because of the large number of ulcer patients who escape statistical calculations. The frequency of acute perforations in patients hospitalized for peptic ulcer varies from 2 to 25 per cent. It can, however, be stated that perforation occurs with far greater frequency in men than in women. It is also recognized that peptic ulcer tends to perforate more often in individuals between the ages of 25 and 50 years than in younger or older persons.

The previous duration of an ulcer, of either the stomach or the duodenum, seems to have no influence on the speed with which the ulcerative and inflammatory processes penetrate the muscular coat and the serous layer. An acute peptic ulcer may rapidly permeate the gastric or intestinal wall, so that, in some instances, the patients even FAIL TO GIVE ANY HISTORY OF TYPICAL ULCER SYMPTOMS. Many chronic ulcers, on the other hand, may exist for years without progressing so far in depth as to implicate the serosa, although no chronic ulcers with severe and persistent symptoms or recurrent or calloused ulcers are ever exempt from the potential danger of a perforation. The rapidity with which the digestive effect of the strongly acid gastric juice destroys the layers of the wall and approaches the serosa cannot be anticipated.

Once perforation has taken place, the location of the ulcer plays a dominant rôle as to the subsequent development of the disease. *Ulcers of the anterior wall* of both the stomach and the duodenum have a greater access to the "free" peritoneal cavity than do those on the posterior wall. From the posterior aspects the ulcer may proceed to penetrate the underlying organs such as the left lobe of the liver (see page 168), the pancreas (see page 173) or the gastrohepatic ligament (see page 169). These may block off the ulcer and prevent the entry of gastric or duodenal contents into the peritoneal cavity. This blocked perforation, in which a new floor for the ulcer has been organized outside the visceral wall, has been called "chronic perforation" or "penetration", whereas the term "subacute perforation" has been reserved for certain tiny ruptures in the serosa, which occur only with a relatively slowly advancing penetration of a chronic gastric ulcer. In such instances fibrinous adhesions to contiguous parenchymal organs or peri-

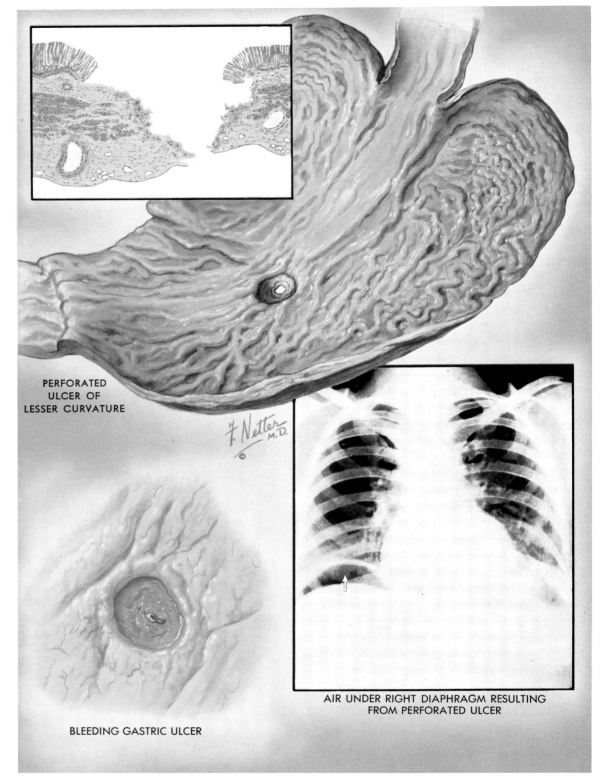

PERFORATED ULCER OF LESSER CURVATURE

BLEEDING GASTRIC ULCER

AIR UNDER RIGHT DIAPHRAGM RESULTING FROM PERFORATED ULCER

toneal attachments have come into existence, as a result of peri-inflammatory tissue reactions, long before the ulcer has permeated to the serosal layer. The adhesions intercept the small amount of gastric content which might escape through what are usually very small apertures, thus enveloping the fluid, which may lead to the development of localized abscesses.

A "free perforation" occurs most frequently with ulcers of the anterior wall of the duodenal bulb (as illustrated on page 173). The hole resulting from an acute perforation is usually round, varying in diameter from 2 to 4 mm. One of the characteristic features of these holes is their sharp edge, which makes them appear to have been punched out. The surrounding tissue may fail to show any signs of chronic induration, edema or inflammation.

The clinical picture of an acute and free perforation, whether it occurs in the stomach or in the duodenum, is one of the most dramatic episodes a physician may encounter. At the moment of perforation, the patient is seized by a sudden, excruciating, explosive pain, which is of a severity "almost beyond description" (Moynihan). It is felt all over the abdomen and may radiate to the chest and shoulder. The patient is pale, his haggard face is covered with cold perspiration and his suffering is expressed in every feature of his countenance. In an effort to reduce the abdominal pain, he flexes the thighs toward the abdomen, which is extremely rigid and tender ("doubling up"). During this early phase, which may last from 10 minutes to a few hours, in part depending on the amount and type of gastro-intestinal content released into the peritoneal cavity, the body temperature is subnormal, while pulse and blood pressure remain within the normal range (or the rate of the pulse may

(Continued on page 173)

PEPTIC ULCER VIII

Complications of Gastric and
Duodenal Ulcers

(Continued from page 172)

even be rather slow), though respiration may assume a superficial and panting character. Within a short time, in some instances introduced by a period of apparent subjective improvement, all the typical signs (nausea, vomiting, dry tongue, rapid pulse, fever, leukocytosis, etc.) of a severe, acute, diffuse peritonitis appear. The tenderness, in the early phase confined mostly to the upper part of the abdomen, has spread, as a rule, over the total abdominal area. It may be excessive in the lower right quadrant if, with a perforation of a duodenal ulcer, the intestinal material is dissipated in the right lumbar gutter along the ascending colon.

The differential diagnosis between a perforated gastric or duodenal ulcer and pancreatitis or a mesenteric thrombosis may be rather difficult in some cases, but such difficulties are seldom encountered with a ruptured appendix. Other conditions, such as an ectopic pregnancy, ruptured diverticulum, renal colic, acute episodes of biliary tract diseases (see, *e.g.,* CIBA COLLECTION, Vol. 3/III, page 131), acute intestinal obstruction or volvulus and, in some instances, coronary thrombosis must also be considered.

The sign which is most helpful in confirming the suspected diagnosis of ulcer perforation is the *presence of free air* in the peritoneal cavity, particularly *in the subphrenic space,* demonstrable by upright X-ray examination. If it is possible for the patient to sit or stand, the air will accumulate under the diaphragm. Escaped air is present, in rare cases, under the left diaphragm only; not infrequently air may be detected under both diaphragmatic leaves and, more usually, under the right only.

With the finding of air, operation is indicated without further delay. The prognosis of a perforated gastric or duodenal ulcer is better the earlier an operation is performed. The mortality rate increases relentlessly when the operation is performed more than 6 hours after perforation. The operation of choice is a subtotal gastric resection in younger individuals who are in good general condition. This is true if the surgeon is permitted to work within the first 6 hours after the ulcer has perforated, under optimal hospital conditions, with carefully supervised anesthesia, with every auxiliary necessary to combat successfully the vascular collapse and infection. Under suboptimal facilities, and with the patient in poor general condition, efforts to treat conservatively with suction through an indwelling catheter in the stomach, massive antibiotics and supportive therapy entail a greater risk and are less success-

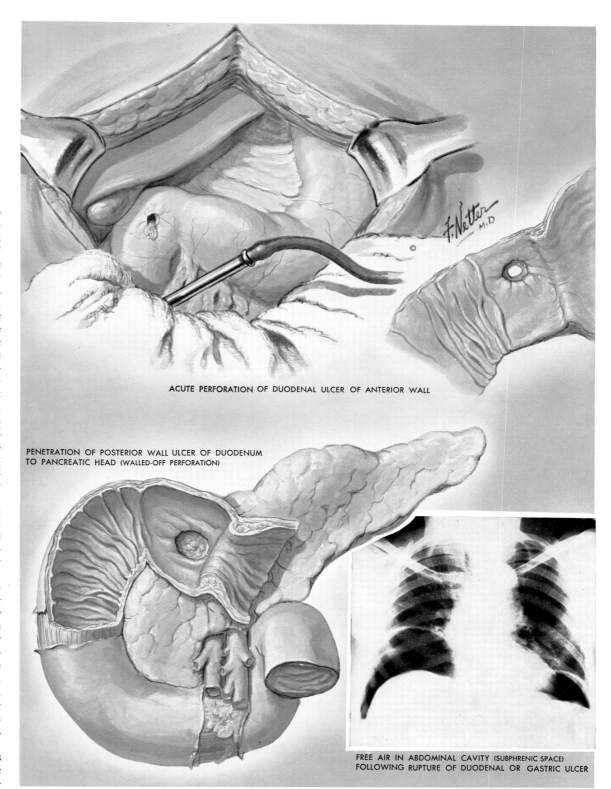

ACUTE PERFORATION OF DUODENAL ULCER OF ANTERIOR WALL

PENETRATION OF POSTERIOR WALL ULCER OF DUODENUM TO PANCREATIC HEAD (WALLED-OFF PERFORATION)

FREE AIR IN ABDOMINAL CAVITY (SUBPHRENIC SPACE) FOLLOWING RUPTURE OF DUODENAL OR GASTRIC ULCER

ful than is surgical treatment, although in some isolated instances the life of the patient so treated has been saved. The simple closure of the perforation, postponing the more definitive surgery, if necessary, until such time as the patient may be in a more favorable condition, should be reserved for cases that come to the surgeon's attention later than 6 hours after the onset of the acute illness, or for elderly patients (over 60 years of age), when the shock tends to be massive, or when the cardiopulmonary situation requires an operation of the shortest possible duration. In approximately 60 per cent of those cases in which the perforation is closed by simple suture, the more radical operation becomes inevitable at a later time.

The symptomatology of a spontaneously closing ulcer perforation (so-called "subacute perforation", see above) lacks the dramatic accents of an "acute" or free perforation. The majority of these patients

may not feel more than some intensification of their usual ulcer pains. It has, indeed, happened, not infrequently, that anamnestically the tissue into which the ulcer had penetrated could not be detected, and the perforation has been established only at operation for medically intractable ulcer. In other instances the patient, as well as the physician, may have been well aware of the acute event, but the signs pointing to a perforation (sharp epigastric pain, abdominal rigidity, elevated temperature and pulse rate, etc.) disappeared within such a short period of time that operation was deferred as not critical. Sooner or later, however, most of these patients must be operated upon because of a localized peritonitis, an abscess which may form in the subphrenic or subhepatic regions or, later, a partial gastric or duodenal obstruction by the massive scar formation.

(Continued on page 174)

Peptic Ulcer VIII

Complications of Gastric and Duodenal Ulcers

(Continued from page 173)

The erosion of the serosal layer by a chronic peptic ulcer on the posterior walls of the stomach and duodenum and its penetration into a contiguous organ is such a slow process that the actual perforation is rarely detected by the patient. The typical ulcer pains and their relation to and relief as a result of food intake gradually give place to continuous, gnawing, boring pain, which no longer responds to the ingestion of food. The pain may radiate to the back, shoulder, clavicular areas or umbilicus, or downward to the lumbar vertebrae and the pubic or inguinal regions. Considering the peripheral distribution of pain pathways and their origin in a spinal segment (see page 85 and Ciba Collection, Vol. 3/III, pages 21 and 31), the site where the patient allocates the radiating pain or the detection of a hyperesthesia in a certain region of the skin may give a clue to determining the organ involved. A classic example of a *"chronic perforation"* is the *ulcer of the posterior wall of the duodenal bulb,* penetrating into and walled off by the pancreas (see page 173). In operating for this condition and attempting to remove the entire ulcer with its floor in the pancreatic tissue, one runs the risk of producing a pancreatic lesion which may open accessory pancreatic ducts. It is, therefore, advisable in these cases to leave the ulcer floor untouched after careful dissection of the ulcer from the duodenal wall.

Ulcers located in the upper parts of the *posterior duodenal wall* have a great tendency to *penetrate the hepatoduodenal ligament* (see page 49). This process is usually accompanied by the development of extensive, fibrous and thickened adhesions, to which the greater omentum may contribute. The supra- and retroduodenal portions of the common bile duct, taking its course within the leaves of the ligament (see page 50), may become compromised in these adhesions. As a result of a constriction or distortion of the common duct, a mild obstructive icterus may confuse the clinical picture. Fortunately, perforation into the duct, with a subsequent cholangitis, is a rare event. In the surgical approach to an ulcer of that kind, the anatomic relations of the common bile duct must be kept acutely in mind, whether or not signs of duct involvement are present. Disastrous lesions can be avoided by a preliminary exposure of the duct and by the introduction of a T tube, which serves as a good guide in disentangling the adhesions and exposing the duodenal wall and the ulcer. Very seldom does an acute perforated ulcer of the

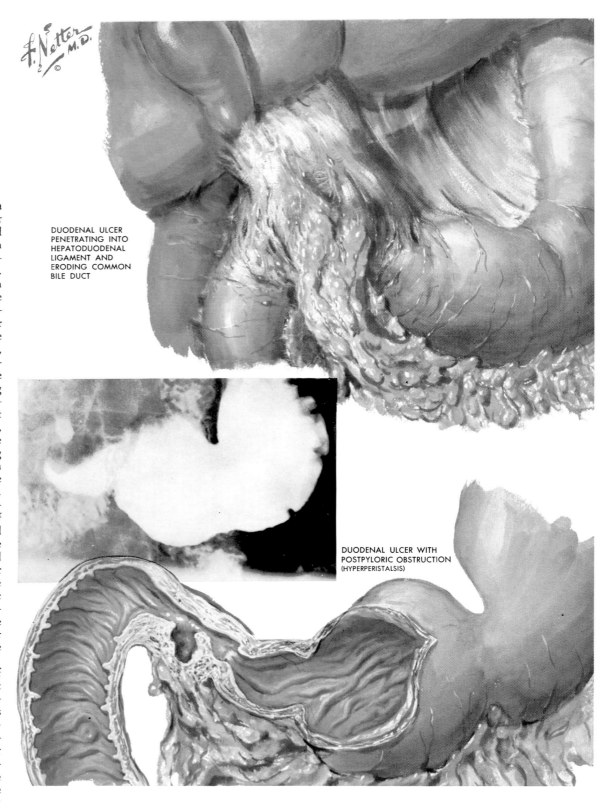

DUODENAL ULCER PENETRATING INTO HEPATODUODENAL LIGAMENT AND ERODING COMMON BILE DUCT

DUODENAL ULCER WITH POSTPYLORIC OBSTRUCTION (HYPERPERISTALSIS)

posterior gastric wall release chyme into the bursa omentalis, producing only signs of localized peritonitis without free air in the abdominal cavity.

Pyloric Stenosis

Another typical complication of the chronic relapsing duodenal or juxtapyloric ulcer is *stenosis of the pylorus,* which develops gradually as the result of the little-by-little thickening of the duodenal wall and the progressive fibrotic narrowing of the lumen. The incidence of complete pyloric stenosis as a sequel to an ulcer has decreased in recent decades, apparently because of improved medical management of this type of ulcer and prompt recognition of its initial phases. When the pyloric lumen begins to narrow, the stomach tries to overcome the impediment by increased peristalsis (see page 89), and its muscular

wall becomes hypertrophic. This is the stage that has been called "compensated pyloric stenosis", because, with these adaptation phenomena, the stomach succeeds in expelling its contents with only mild degrees of gastric retention. Later, when the lumen is appreciably narrowed, the expulsive efforts of the stomach fail, and the clinical picture will be dominated by incessant vomiting and by distress, owing to a progressive dilatation of the stomach, which, at times, may become massive. This condition of "decompensated pyloric stenosis", which results in the retention of ingested material and the products of gastric secretion, is, as a rule, irreversible and is an unequivocal indication for surgical intervention. The operation of choice is a subtotal gastrectomy, but, in view of the characteristically poor general condition of the patient, the surgeon may sometimes have to resort

(Continued on page 175)

Peptic Ulcer VIII

Complications of Gastric and Duodenal Ulcers

(Continued from page 174)

to less radical procedures, such as a gastrojejunostomy. In the presence of a still-active ulcer, those operations which reroute the gastric content around the duodenum in the most simple fashion should be supplemented by a bilateral vagotomy.

Hemorrhage

Minor bleeding occurs in the majority of patients with acute or chronic peptic ulcer. "Occult" blood can be found with fair regularity in the stools or gastric juice of the majority of ulcer patients. This is the result of the oozing characteristic of every ulcerative lesion. Massive hemorrhage, which, together with perforation, typifies the most dangerous of all ulcer complications, is fortunately far less frequent. Reliable figures of its incidence are not available, but it has been estimated that, of all massive hemorrhages of the gastro-intestinal tract, 60 to 75 per cent stem from a peptic ulcer. Obliterative endarteritis or thrombosis of the mucosal and submucosal vessels in the ulcerated tissue proves to be a natural protection against bleeding from the more superficial ulcers. As a rule, the hemorrhage is caused by erosion into a large vessel, though excessive bleeding occasionally also derives from smaller arteries or veins whose drainage is impaired. A decisive factor for the degree of bleeding is the location of the ulcer. Gastric ulcers (see page 172) have often caused excessive blood loss, but the most frequent origin of a *massive hemorrhage* is the *ulcer of the posterior portion of the duodenal bulb*, because here the ulcer can penetrate into the walls of the gastroduodenal and retroduodenal (posterior and superior pancreaticoduodenal) arteries, which course just behind the first portion of the duodenum (see pages 56 and 57).

The essential clinical signs of a duodenal ulcer perforated into an artery are massive melena and acute vascular collapse. The shock may appear suddenly and very shortly after the opening of an artery, or it may be delayed for several hours. In striking contrast to the hemorrhages due to gastric ulcer and esophageal ulcers or varices, hematemesis is rare with bleeding from a duodenal ulcer, because the blood, originating from beyond the spastic pylorus, is propelled into the small intestine and does not regurgitate to the stomach. In some cases sudden bleeding comes as a complete surprise to patients who have had no previous complaints or signs pointing to

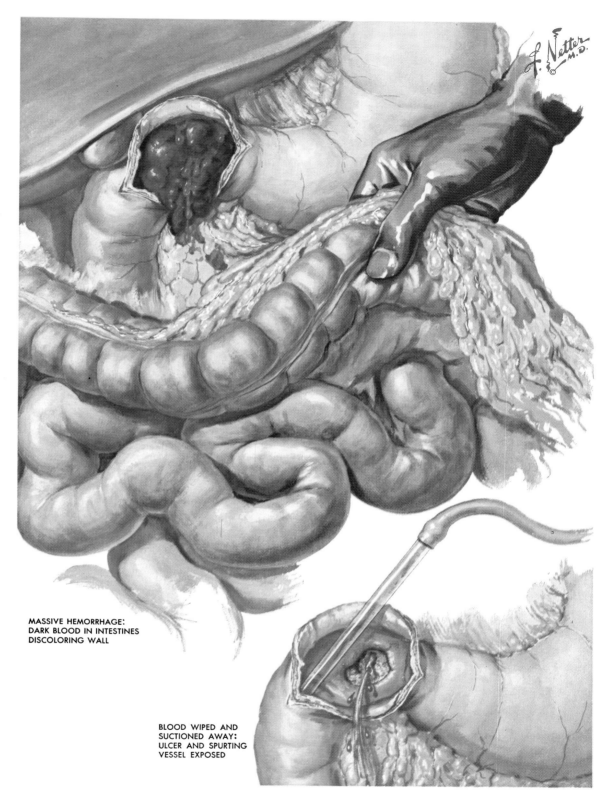

MASSIVE HEMORRHAGE: DARK BLOOD IN INTESTINES DISCOLORING WALL

BLOOD WIPED AND SUCTIONED AWAY: ULCER AND SPURTING VESSEL EXPOSED

the presence of an ulcer, and this may be the first event to indicate the existence of a "silent" ulcer. The differential diagnosis of the origin of the bleeding and its localization may, at times, be extremely difficult. X-ray examination, which in the hospital can be performed unhesitatingly, is often of little help, because such a bleeding ulcer may fail to show the usually typical perifocal changes, and because the niche may be filled with blood coagulum. An X-ray may exclude the esophageal origin of the bleeding and thus may aid in reaching a decision concerning treatment and operative approach.

Massive and continuous bleeding from an ulcer should be treated surgically; however, opinions as to the best time for such an operation are not unanimous. The first hemorrhage, showing a tendency to stop, is within the realm of a conservative treatment. Bleeding may often be an isolated episode, which, for

reasons little understood, may end in permanent healing. Repeated hemorrhages are adequate indication for surgical intervention. A rapid major blood loss, the advanced age of the patient and shock not immediately responsive to appropriate measures make operation imperative. On an average, surgical results in these cases are definitely better than are those of conservative therapy.

Even during operation it is often difficult to establish the origin of hemorrhage. A bluish discoloration of the upper jejunal loops permits no more than a suspicion that the bleeding has originated in the gastroduodenal or esophageal area. The ulcer itself cannot always be palpated, and only after duodenotomy may the ulcer crater be found. The bleeding can then be provisionally secured by ligation of the bleeding vessel. The final arrest of the hemorrhage is, however, attained only by a subtotal resection.

Peptic Ulcer IX
Healing of Gastric Ulcer

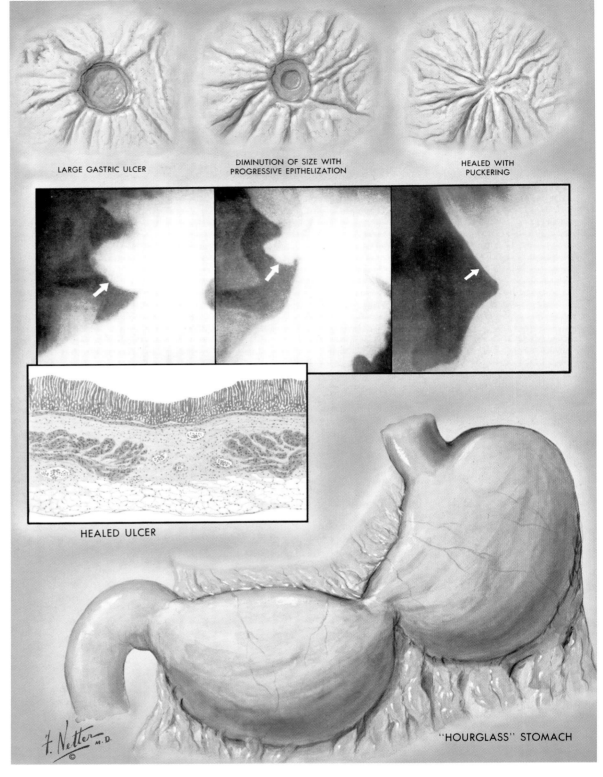

LARGE GASTRIC ULCER

DIMINUTION OF SIZE WITH PROGRESSIVE EPITHELIZATION

HEALED WITH PUCKERING

HEALED ULCER

"HOURGLASS" STOMACH

In many cases the chronic gastric ulcer will heal. Inflammation and edema of the ulcer wall subside. As a result, the wall tends to become flattened. The fibrinopurulent exudate on the floor of the ulcer separates off, is discarded and is replaced by healthy granulation and, subsequently, by fibrous tissue. The size and depth of the ulcer are reduced, chiefly by cicatrization and the contraction of the fibroblasts on the floor and in the wall of the lesion. In addition, the epithelium grows inward from each margin to cover the area of ulceration. From this epithelial layer, projections downward eventually develop, forming simple glands. Finally, the entire area is covered by epithelium. As the contraction of the fibrous tissue progresses, a permanent scar and, in some cases, *radiation of the mucosal folds* develop.

During the healing process the ends of the muscular coat may fuse with the muscularis mucosae. But, although severed ends of the muscular layer approximate one another as a result of the cicatrizing process, restitution of a muscular breach is never complete. This remains as permanent evidence of the original lesion. *Puckering* and radiating streaks on the serosal surface are further evidences of the scar produced in the healing process of the chronic gastric ulcer. The healing of a chronic gastric ulcer sometimes is complete, but not infrequently such ulcers are prone to recur, particularly if the newly formed mucous membrane is thin and its vascular supply deficient. In other cases the recurrence of ulcer symp-

toms is due to an entirely new ulcer, the scar of the original lesion remaining permanent.

The *gradual transition* that occurs *in the healing* process of a chronic gastric ulcer is demonstrable roentgenologically by following the changes in the size of the niche corresponding to the crater of the ulcer. As a result of the healing process, the niche diminishes until it has completely disappeared. At other times, with clinical recurrence of symptoms, the ulcer becomes reactivated, and the niche reappears.

As a result of the healing of a large gastric ulcer, a number of deformities may develop, of which the bilocular or *"hourglass" stomach* is the best known. It is a rare phenomenon but occurs more frequently in the female sex than in the male, in spite of the higher incidence of gastric ulcer in the latter. With

an "hourglass" stomach, the viscus is divided into two cavities connected by a channel with a lumen of varying size. The deformity originates mostly from a large ulcer, located in the corpus of the stomach, which has healed by an extensive contracting scar formation. It rarely causes complete obstruction, but the clinical symptoms are so unspecific, particularly when the original ulcer is still active, that the diagnosis must depend on the results of the X-ray examination, which, in some instances, also may not yield unequivocal answers, because constriction due to a malignant growth, temporary spasms associated with an active gastric ulcer and the formerly rather frequent gastric manifestations of syphilis may simulate the roentgen appearance of an ulcer dependent on "hourglass" stomach.

BENIGN TUMORS OF STOMACH

Benign tumors, compared with carcinoma, are relatively rare, but since many of them remain small and may cause no symptoms, their true incidence may be greater than the reported statistical data indicate. The majority of benign tumors were formerly discovered only at autopsy, but the number of clinically diagnosed neoplasms of this kind has increased in past years, since the advent of gastroscopy.

The etiology of benign tumors is disputed, and it has remained undecided whether they develop from normal constituents of the gastric wall or whether they derive from hamartomas or other structural anomalies. It is possible that environmental, mechanical or inflammatory factors play a rôle. Benign tumors may be located in the mucosa, in the submucosa, within the muscular layers or in the subserosal tissues. Accordingly, the histologic type of the tumor varies. They may be typical epithelial tumors, such as the adenoma, or they may belong to the connective tissue and mixed types, such as the leiomyoma, fibromyoma, hemangioma, neurofibroma, lipoma, etc.

Symptomatologically, as already mentioned, benign tumors may remain silent throughout the patient's lifetime. Sometimes they may be discovered accidentally on the occasion of an X-ray study instigated for quite other reasons. If a benign tumor enlarges sufficiently, or if it happens to be located near the cardiac or pyloric ends, it may interfere with the motor or secretory functions of the stomach, e.g., with the regular progression of peristalsis or with normal emptying. Under such circumstances, signs of stasis or obstruction may become apparent. These tumors may have a tendency to chronic, sometimes profuse bleeding, so that anemia or hematemesis may dominate the clinical picture. The tumors produce pain or epigastric distress only infrequently, and, if they do, the problem arises as to how to differentiate them from a peptic ulcer. In such instances roentgenologic and/or gastroscopic examination may or may not provide the answer.

Clinically, the paramount importance of benign tumors lies in their potential to undergo malignant degeneration. For this reason, and because of the fact that it is often difficult or impossible to differentiate a benign tumor from a carcinoma, even with the aid of X-ray studies and gastroscopy, surgical intervention is indicated whenever a tumor is diagnosed or even seriously suspected. The type of operation to be performed depends upon

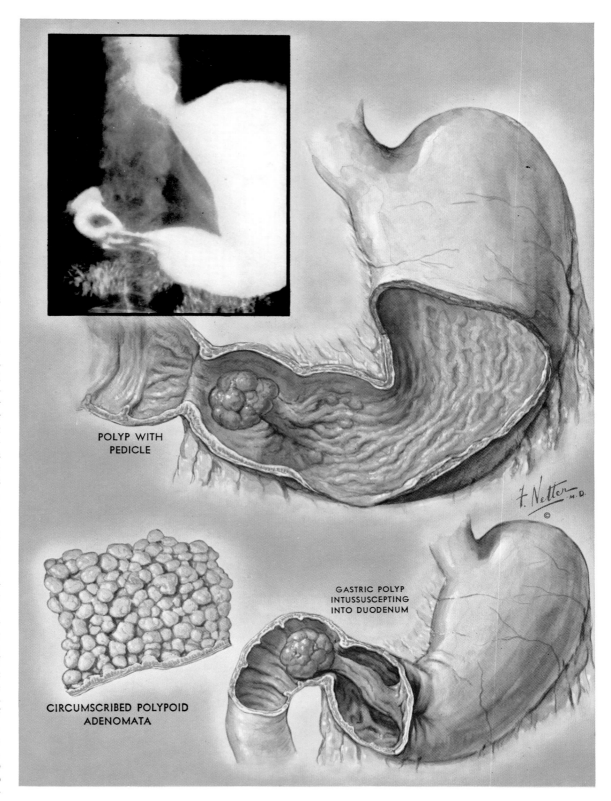

POLYP WITH PEDICLE

CIRCUMSCRIBED POLYPOID ADENOMATA

GASTRIC POLYP INTUSSUSCEPTING INTO DUODENUM

F. Netter M.D.

the location and extension of the tumor. A pedunculated tumor may be removed after ligation of the pedicle, depending upon its anatomic relation to the wall of the stomach. At times the tumor may be enucleated or extirpated with a section of the wall out of which it arises. If these more conservative operations are not possible, because of the size of the tumor or because of its broad invasion into the wall, a gastric resection is necessary.

The most frequent type of benign gastric tumor is the adenoma, represented in the illustration by a *"polyp with pedicle"*, a term that refers to its macroscopic shape rather than to its microscopic structure. The gastric adenoma, sessile or pedunculated, contains more or less regular epithelial tubules embedded in loose connective tissue. The pedicle of such a solitary "polyp" of the stomach usually is broad where it attaches to the gastric wall, but the stalk is

thin and permits free mobility of the tumor proper. Its site of predilection is the corpus or the antrum. In the latter case the tumor is able to move in front of the pylorus or may even be pushed by peristalsis, with the gastric contents, through the pylorus, where it appears in the X-ray picture as a circular, translucent filling defect in the duodenal bulb. Usually, in such cases, the obstruction is only partial and does not seriously affect gastric emptying. The pendulous, to-and-fro movements, however, give rise to irritation and stretching of the tumor's mucosa, which account for the epigastric pain and well-recognized bleeding seen with these tumors. In some cases, recurrent or profuse hematemesis may be the first clinical manifestation.

Adenomas may be single or multiple, and both types, the pedunculated and the sessile, may be pres-

(Continued on page 178)

Benign Tumors of Stomach

(*Continued from page 177*)

ent simultaneously. In rare instances an incalculable number of small, *circumscribed, polypoid adenomas* may lie closely packed together, covering smaller or larger areas and, indeed, sometimes the entire mucosa. This condition has been designated as polyposis gastrica (multiple polyposis, "polyadenomoes polypeux"). The individual tumors are small (2 to 5 mm. in diameter) and have a broad attachment to the gastric wall. They are covered by columnar epithelium and contain glands. Some evidence points to the probability that this condition may evolve from a chronic gastritis and that it expands gradually over the mucosa, starting, as a rule, in the antral region. Because of the great bleeding tendency on the surface of these structures (being more vulnerable than the normal mucosa), most patients with these neoplastic changes suffer from a marked anemia, which may be hypochromic and microcytic but may also assume the character of a pernicious anemia, owing to a gradually increasing atrophy of the gastric glands and subsequent loss of the intrinsic factor. The gastroscopic picture of a polyposis gastrica is unique and permits an unequivocal diagnosis. The X-ray picture may also help, showing the countless number of indentations in the gastric mucosal outline. Opinions as to the danger that these originally benign tumors may undergo malignant transformation are conflicting, and so are ideas about the most appropriate therapy. It seems that radical surgical intervention is justifiable, as long as the extent of the lesion permits a resection with preservation of part of the gastric wall. Total gastrectomy, with its own complications, as a "prophylactic" measure does not seem warranted. X-ray treatment has also been advocated for this condition.

Reports as to the frequency of leiomyoma of the stomach are contradictory. Some believe it to be more, others less, common than adenoma. The *leiomyoma* belongs to the group of smooth muscle tissue tumors, which include such mixed tumors as fibromyoma, adenomyoma, etc. Histologically, the gastric leiomyoma possesses the same characteristics as does myoma elsewhere in the body. It is usually well encapsulated and grayish-white on the cut surface; it originates from the muscular layers and develops below or within the submucosa. In extremely rare cases such a leiomyoma may enlarge through the serosa to form an extragastric tumor. Intragastric tumors may attain

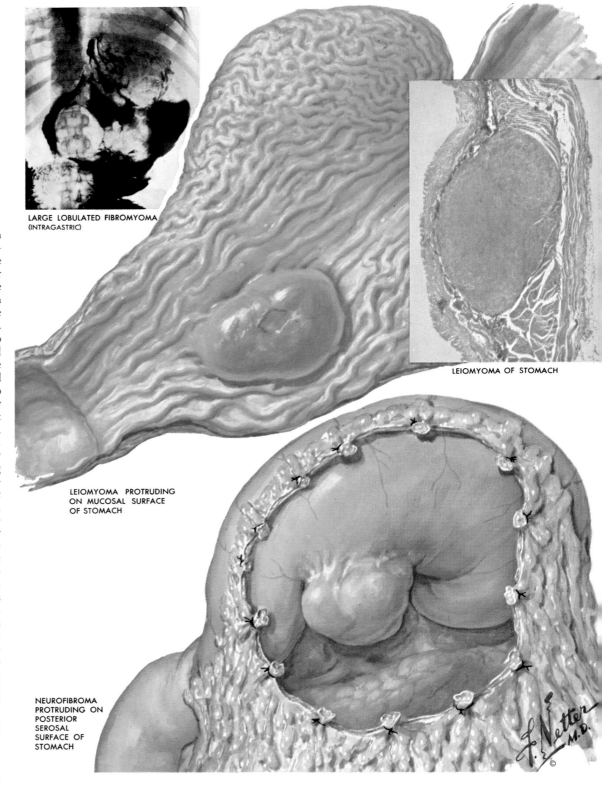

LARGE LOBULATED FIBROMYOMA (INTRAGASTRIC)

LEIOMYOMA OF STOMACH

LEIOMYOMA PROTRUDING ON MUCOSAL SURFACE OF STOMACH

NEUROFIBROMA PROTRUDING ON POSTERIOR SEROSAL SURFACE OF STOMACH

such size as to occupy a large part of the lumen. In such instances they may cause obstruction, or at least serious impairment, of the filling and emptying of the stomach. Smaller tumors, occasionally multiple, usually have no clinical significance. The mucosa above a large leiomyoma is stretched tightly and tends to ulcerate and, subsequently, to bleed profusely. In addition, they may, rarely, undergo sarcomatous degeneration. In the X-ray picture the neoplasm may appear as a circular, at times lobulated but fairly distinct, filling defect. The roentgen film reproduced in the illustration was obtained from a patient previously gastrectomized because of a duodenal ulcer and demonstrates an enormously large fibromyoma of the fundus and a monstrous dilatation of the remainder of the stomach. The treatment of gastric leiomyoma is surgical removal by extirpation or partial resection of the stomach.

Neurofibroma, probably the least frequent type of benign gastric tumor, is a slow-growing neoplasm, usually originating from a nerve sheath coursing along the lesser curvature. The tumor may also occasionally represent part of a generalized neurofibromatosis (von Recklinghausen's disease). A neurofibroma may expand in the direction of the lumen and may produce there a submucosal protrusion, or it may project outward into the peritoneal cavity, in which case it may sometimes become pedunculated. Provided the mucosa is sufficiently stretched, intragastric neurofibroma may also give rise to bleeding, as do other benign tumors. If not, they display little, if any, clinical symptoms. Cystic degeneration of a neurofibroma has been reported.

Another rare benign tumor of the stomach is a hemangioma (not illustrated). Its specific characteristic is the marked tendency to cause bleeding.

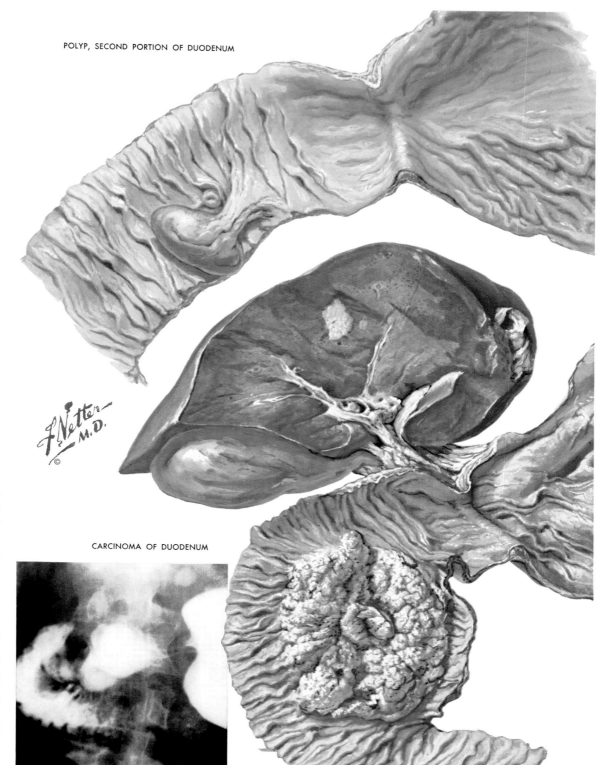

POLYP, SECOND PORTION OF DUODENUM

CARCINOMA OF DUODENUM

TUMORS OF DUODENUM

Tumors of the duodenum are extremely rare. The benign neoplasms, which may be encountered occasionally, include polyp, adenoma originating from Brunner's glands, polypoid adenoma, lipoma, leiomyoma, neurofibroma, hemangioma and aberrant pancreatic rest, all of which, however, reach scarcely more than the size of elevations beneath the mucosa and cannot be considered true tumors. The chief clinical symptom of a benign tumor is bleeding, which, if persistent, may lead to anemia. The bleeding results, as a rule, from erosions and ulcerations of the mucosa lying above the growth. To produce signs of partial obstruction, the tumor must have grown quite large, which is seldom the case. A *polyp, the pedicles* of which may assume a length of several centimeters, may be very mobile, shifting back and forth by peristaltic movements and even passing retrogressively through the pylorus to enter the stomach. In view of their translucency, these polyps may, under such circumstances, produce most confusing X-ray pictures.

The anatomic situation of the duodenum makes it impossible to palpate benign duodenal tumors, and their diagnosis rests with X-ray examination. Depending upon the type, localization and relation to the duodenal wall, the tumors usually reveal themselves by a distinct, either mobile or fixed, filling defect. If the tumors present an obstacle to the free passage of the intestinal contents, that part of the duodenum lying proximally to the neoplasm will be found dilated, with signs of congestion.

Primary carcinoma of the duodenum is likewise relatively rare. Its ratio of incidence, compared with carcinoma of the stomach, is said to be 1:100. The majority of duodenal carcinomas arise from the papilla Vateri and from peripapillary tissues. The early symptoms are vague and unspecific (nausea, dyspepsia, fatigue), and patients seek medical advice in most cases only when they have become icteric and when the tumor has produced the complex clinical picture of an obstruction of the common bile and pancreatic ducts. In the absence of biliary colic and a palpable gallbladder (Courvoisier's law, see CIBA COLLECTION, Vol. 3/III, page 82), it may be possible to differentiate preoperatively the duodenal papillary tumor from cholelithiasis, but it is impossible to separate clinically such a duodenal carcinoma from a tumor of the pancreas head or of the ductus choledochus. Certain clues may be obtained from X-ray examination. The papillary carcinoma of the duodenum may, at times, be recognized as a circular, more or less regular, but distinct filling defect in the medial wall of the second duodenal portion, whereas the carcinoma of the pancreatic head remains usually radiologically invisible, except when it has assumed such a conspicuous size as to displace and change the contours of the duodenal arc (see also CIBA COLLECTION, Vol. 3/III, page 148).

The differentiation of these tumors has a practical significance, because the relatively favorable long-term results of a radical removal of a papillary carcinoma justifies a pancreatoduodenectomy, whereas, in the case of pancreatic carcinoma, the long-term results are so poor that they rarely warrant the risk of such an extensive procedure and make preferable palliative operations such as cholecysto- or choledochojejunostomies (to unburden the biliary tract) or gastrojejunostomies (when the duodenal passages are obstructed).

Other localizations of malignant duodenal growths in the duodenal bulb (or at the duodenojejunal flexure), some of them resulting from degeneration of a polyp or an ulcer, are so rare that they may almost be considered curiosities.

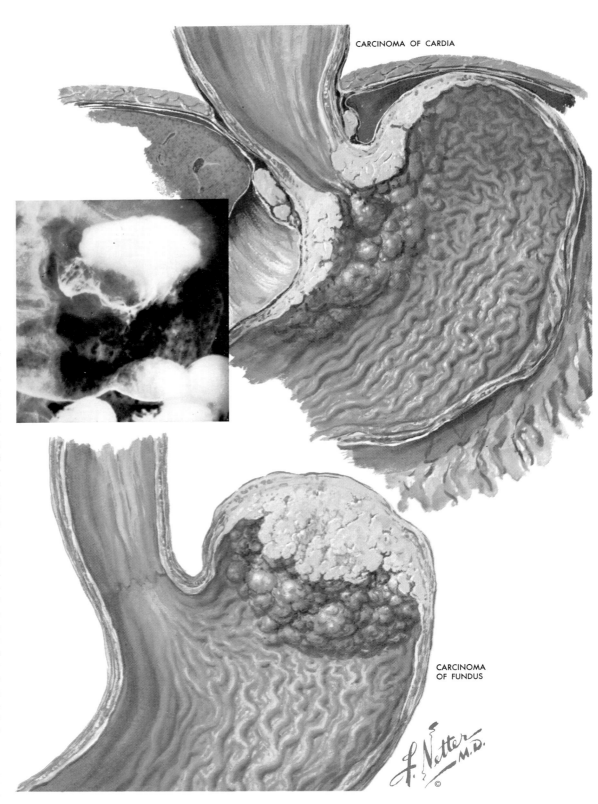

CARCINOMA OF CARDIA

CARCINOMA OF FUNDUS

Carcinoma of Stomach

In mortality statistics the first position was formerly held by cancer of the stomach in that portion of the male population who died of malignant neoplasms. However, in recent decades the incidence of lung carcinoma has begun to increase, so that the figures for gastric cancer, varyingly quoted between 16 and 25 per cent, have slowly decreased. In women, cancers of the uterus and of the breast are more frequent than of the stomach. In general, cancer of the stomach is seen more than twice as often in men as in women. It is essentially a disease of middle and old age, about 85 per cent of the cases arising after the age of 40.

As with all malignant growths, the etiology of gastric carcinoma has so far remained obscure. The significance of several potential contributory factors, however, has been widely discussed. Heredity may well play a part, because not too infrequently gastric cancer has been observed for several generations in members of the same family. However, the available data on the frequency of gastric cancer among relatives of patients with this disease and among families in which no cancer has been detected in several generations are not sufficient to decide whether a genetic component is or is not an etiologic factor.

Atrophic gastritis (see page 164), though by no means invariably leading to cancer, is considered by many a precancerous, or at least a potential precancerous, lesion. Transitional changes from an atrophic mucosa to hyperplastic and papillomatous areas have been demonstrated (Konjetzny). The rôle of chronic peptic ulcer of the stomach (see page 167) as a precursor of carcinoma is firmly established. Its tendency to malignant degeneration, according to a fairly general opinion on the part of pathologists, is between 10 and 20 per cent. This means that about 17 per cent of all gastric cancers arise in ulcers and that approximately 10 per cent of benign ulcers later become malignant (Stewart). Apparently, the location of the ulcer has a little influence on its fate, as ulcers in the region of the pylorus and the angulus ventriculi, or those near the cardia (see page 168), seem to have a greater tend-

ency to become malignant than do those situated in the vertical portion of the minor curvature. It would, however, be tragic to rely on location and the percentage figures quoted in the literature, because a carcinoma of the stomach may develop in any location from or in the presence of a gastric ulcer or an atrophic gastritis. It is always a matter of primary concern for the physician to exclude the possibility of a malignancy by most complete examination and continuous supervision. The suspicion of cancer should never be set aside because of the common difficulty in differentiating, on clinical grounds, the benign chronic ulcer from an ulcerating carcinoma (see page 184).

Applying a variety of parameters, macroscopic or microscopic characteristics, location, infiltrative potency or clinical behavior, several classifications of gastric carcinoma have been proposed, of which that of Borrmann has received the widest attention in

almost all textbooks on gastro-enterology, internal medicine and pathology. In view of the multiform nature of the tumors, however, no one system of classification has proved completely satisfactory, and none permits a clear-cut separation of all the individual varieties of gastric carcinoma.

Carcinoma Near the Cardia and in the Fundus

Though carcinoma of the stomach has no site of predilection and may develop in any part of the organ, it seems justified from the clinical point of view, by reason of the diagnostic, prognostic and operative-technical aspects, to segregate distinctly at least two types of carcinoma in the upper portions of the stomach, namely, those located in the cardia on

(Continued on page 181)

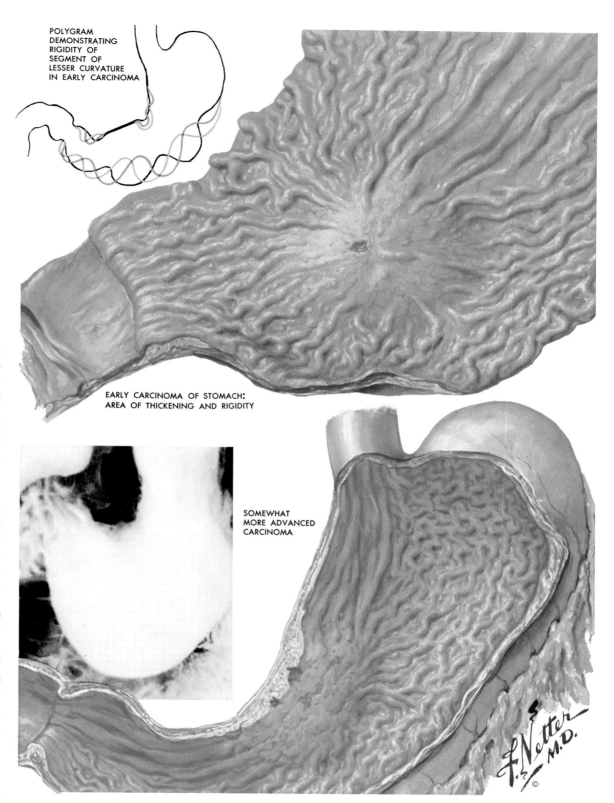

POLYGRAM
DEMONSTRATING
RIGIDITY OF
SEGMENT OF
LESSER CURVATURE
IN EARLY CARCINOMA

EARLY CARCINOMA OF STOMACH:
AREA OF THICKENING AND RIGIDITY

SOMEWHAT
MORE ADVANCED
CARCINOMA

CARCINOMA OF STOMACH

(Continued from page 180)

the side of the lesser curvature, which involve the gastro-esophageal junction, and those which occupy the fundus, infiltrating in the direction of the major curvature. The *cardiac carcinoma*, even in its earlier stages, interferes with the free passage of food, causing marked dysphagia. This fact often permits a relatively early diagnosis. Thus, it is not surprising that it is the operative treatment of these tumors which yields probably the best long-term results of all carcinoma of the stomach. In contrast, the *fundic carcinoma* (see also page 180), as do other neoplasms in the so-called "silent" gastric zones, remains undiscovered usually for a long time. Since they do have a marked tendency to bleed once they have reached a certain size, severe chronic anemia or a sudden hemorrhage may give the first late clue to their existence.

The cardiac carcinoma often exceeds the bounds of the stomach, either by submucosal infiltration or by more superficial extension, and narrows the cardiac orifice or even the most distal portions of the esophagus. In such instances it is difficult, or sometimes impossible, to differentiate roentgenologically, or even on direct macroscopic inspection, a cardiac carcinoma from primary cancer of the distal end of the esophagus. This question may sometimes be decided when the esophagoscopist submits a biopsy specimen to the pathologist (see page 156). Otherwise, the X-ray diagnosis of cancer in the upper part of the stomach is relatively easy, particularly if the growth has altered the anatomic relation of stomach and esophagus. If a stenosis is present, the adjacent portion of the esophagus will be dilated, and entry of the barium meal into the stomach will be delayed. Such findings have rarely more than one possible explanation. When doubts still exist, the age of the patient, his past history and endoscopy may help to exclude achalasia and other benign stenotic lesions (esophagitis, peptic esophageal ulcer, see pages 146 and 147, strictures deriving from corrosion, see page 150). Surgical exploration is always indicated if even the slightest uncertainty or the faintest suspicion remains. If passage through the cardia is not disturbed, the

tumor may be overlooked, particularly if one fails to examine the fundic region with the patient in supine position and with the lower part of the body elevated. Occasionally, a fundic carcinoma may be so flat and infiltration may have proceeded so superficially and broadly that the gastric contour is altered very little.

Surgically, the cardiac carcinoma is best approached by a left thoracotomy or thoraco-abdominal incision, because these approaches guarantee complete freedom of action should an additional resection of the esophagus be necessary. Tumors of the fundus, located at a reasonable distance from the cardiac orifice, can be handled through the abdominal approach, since a subdiaphragmatic transsection of the esophagus seems to fulfill the requirements of a radical removal of the neoplastic tissues. Should doubts arise during operation that the subdiaphragmatic esophageal resection is adequate, the field can be widened

by prolonging the incision into the thoracic wall and the diaphragm, or by continuing the operation by a separate thoracotomy. The distal portion of the stomach should not be removed unless absolutely necessary because of the extension of the tumor. The physiologic significance of preserving a segment of the stomach has been demonstrated experimentally as well as clinically.

Early Carcinoma of Stomach

Some gastric cancers start with a relatively sharply circumscribed area of infiltration, spreading superficially on an almost even level, without polypoid proliferation (see page 182) and showing little, if any, ulceration. Of the numerous pathologic-anatomic forms in which carcinoma of the stomach

(Continued on page 182)

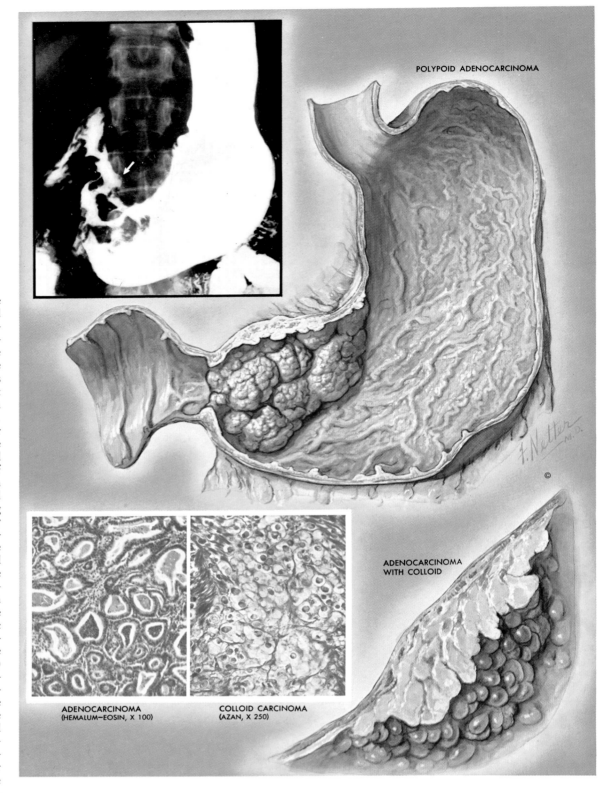

POLYPOID ADENOCARCINOMA

ADENOCARCINOMA
WITH COLLOID

ADENOCARCINOMA
(HEMALUM—EOSIN, X 100)

COLLOID CARCINOMA
(AZAN, X 250)

Carcinoma of Stomach

(Continued from page 181)

can make its appearance, this is the one that most often escapes early clinical recognition, because it leaves the mucosal pattern and the contour of the stomach unchanged for a long time, until the malignant growth has involved a large area. In the early stages this type expands only within the mucosal layer; then it seizes the submucosa and only much later encroaches upon the muscular coat. Its most frequent location is the lesser curvature between the pylorus and the angular incisura. Irregular flattening and breaks in the mucosal folds, distortion of the rugae, particularly where they begin and end, more or less frank epithelial defects and, sometimes, small bleeding areas of erosion are the macroscopically visible characteristics of this slow-growing tumor in its early stages. As time passes, local inflammatory reactions and the extension of the neoplasm in the muscularis takes place. On X-ray examination, first a scarcely noticeable, then increasingly striking stiffening of the region appears. The normal peristaltic waves are interrupted in the rigid segment of the gastric wall. A *polygram* (see upper left corner of plate on page 181) of the peristaltic waves by repeated roentgenography of several phases of a peristaltic movement on one and the same plate may be most informative in these cases. It is, indeed, a most profitable and gratifying task for the radiologist to discover such a tumor early in its development. In view of the fact that the contour of the organ is not changed either by the formation of an ulcer crater or by endophytic growth, only the most careful fluoroscopic examination of the condition of the gastric wall or a series of spot films or a motion picture will permit one to prove the presence of this type of gastric carcinoma.

Adenocarcinoma of Stomach

From the histopathologic point of view, the most frequent malignant growth in the stomach is the adenocarcinoma. Its macroscopic appearance, as the surgeon or the pathologist sees it, depends essentially upon the time or the developmental stage at which it happens to be recognized. It its early stages it may represent a relatively small, cauliflower-like mass only a few centimeters in diameter, which projects into the lumen. Unfortunately, however, it reaches, though still well circumscribed, far larger dimensions before causing local symptoms and before having metastasized to more distant structures. In any event, the size of the tumor alone is not indicative of the spread to neighboring organs. If it grows in the prepyloric area, as do about two thirds of gastric cancers, it may bring about early signs of obstruction, gastric enlargement and disturbances of the motoric function of the stomach, which lead to its discovery. Macroscopically visible invasion of the pylorus proper or of the duodenum by an adenocarcinoma is, however, considered an extreme rarity.

The adenocarcinoma usually arises from a broad base. Less frequently, a papillary adenocarcinoma arises from a polyp or pedunculated adenoma and invades the gastric wall through the stalk. Some adenocarcinomas assume on their surface a *polypoid* or *fungating appearance*, with necrotic and ulcerating foci. On the cut section this "vegetative" type of carcinoma, as it has been called, presents a yellowish, solid mass in a gray fibrillar stroma. The histologic architecture of the adenocarcinoma may sometimes exhibit the typical columnar cell arrangement, with formation of glandular spaces but it is usually more complicated and varies considerably. Atypical tubular glands may replace the normal mucosal pattern, penetrating into the muscularis mucosae or spreading from the submucosa as far as the serosal coat. The nuclei of the tumor cells stain, as a rule, distinctly darker than do those of the normal surrounding glands. At times, the tumor consists only of closely grouped alveoli with cylindrical and cuboidal cells and hyperchromatic nuclei. The cells lining these alveoli may, in some

(Continued on page 183)

CARCINOMA OF STOMACH

(Continued from page 182)

cases, contain substantial amounts of mucus and, occasionally, the entire tumor may be replaced by gelatinous or slimy *colloid material,* in which only a few embedded cancer cells may be found. In such instances the displaced nuclei and overextended, ruptured or disintegrated cells in this mucinous matrix may create a most *complex histologic picture.*

Scirrhous Carcinoma of Stomach

To the diffuse infiltrating variants of the gastric carcinoma belongs the relatively less frequent but highly malignant spheroidal cell carcinoma, which probably originates in the chief cells of the gastric glands. It is a peculiar type of cancer in that it develops in some well-circumscribed areas of the mucosa, which appear elevated, and penetrates rapidly the submucosa and muscularis, metastasizing early to the regional lymph nodes.

Far more common is the other diffuse infiltrating type, the *scirrhous carcinoma* of the stomach. This category produces a diffuse thickening of all layers and involves a large part of or, sometimes, the entire gastric wall, which becomes contracted and rigid. The scirrhous malignant lesion usually begins in the pyloric canal and may, in some cases, remain limited to this region, where it may soon cause signs of obstruction, because the profuse growth of its fibrotic components markedly reduces the lumen. The same phenomenon takes place over the whole gastric cavity, when the scirrhous growth has expanded extensively over the entire lining. The mucosal folds become immobile and inflexible, while simultaneously, as a result of the abundant formation of fibrous tissue, the whole organ shrinks, assuming a shape that has been described as the "leather-bottle" stomach.

Histologically, nests of epithelial cells are scattered in dense fibrous tissue, which leaves nothing of the normal gastric structures. The number of recognizable malignant cells is gradually reduced, and, in the advanced stages, it is difficult to demonstrate their presence except by the most painstaking microscopic study. In some cases the fibrotic reaction has gone so far as to make recognition of the original nature of the process practically

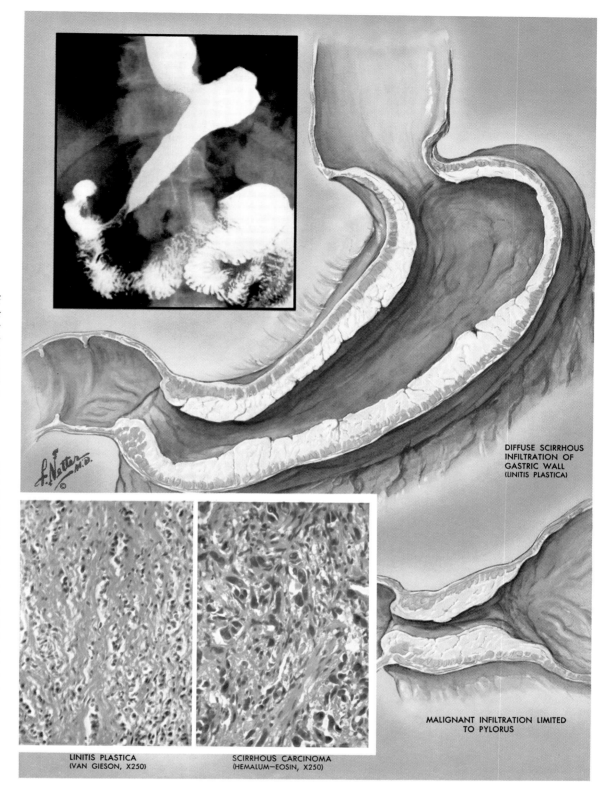

DIFFUSE SCIRRHOUS INFILTRATION OF GASTRIC WALL (LINITIS PLASTICA)

LINITIS PLASTICA (VAN GIESON, X250)

SCIRRHOUS CARCINOMA (HEMALUM—EOSIN, X250)

MALIGNANT INFILTRATION LIMITED TO PYLORUS

impossible. In view of such proliferation of connective tissue, it is not surprising that the primary cause was formerly considered to be a chronic reactive inflammatory process and received, accordingly, the designation "linitis plastica".

The roentgenographic appearance of scirrhous carcinoma varies, of course, depending upon the extent to which the gastric wall has become involved. If limited to the pyloric region, a localized area of narrowing, distinct irregularities of the contour and the disappearance of the normal mucosal markings leave no doubt as to the diagnosis. With the *fibrotic process* sufficiently *advanced at the pyloric canal* to cause a more or less complete obstruction and the more proximal parts of the wall still maintaining their normal structure and extensibility, the stomach is markedly dilated and can retain food ingested during the previous 24 hours or even over a longer period of time. If,

however, the neoplasm has spread over a larger segment or, as happens not infrequently, over the entire inner aspect of the stomach, the cavity of the stomach presents itself as a narrow tube with no mucous membrane pattern visible. The *contour* in such cases may be *erratically distorted,* and the barium meal rushes through the organ because of the rigidity of the pylorus, which, under these circumstances, is permanently opened. Gastric peristalsis in these patients is conspicuously absent. As the obstruction in advanced "linitis plastica" is located at the cardia, it is the esophagus which eventually becomes dilated.

With X-ray findings as clear as those described above, the diagnosis of scirrhous carcinoma presents no difficulties, and laboratory data, such as achlorhydria, hypo- or hyperchromic macrocytic anemia or occult blood resulting from the destruction of the glands or

(Continued on page 184)

CARCINOMA OF STOMACH

(Continued from page 183)

from erosions, respectively, provide little more than mere additional supporting or confirming information. Gastroscopy, at times difficult to perform because of the rigidity and lack of air in the stomach, may help establish the diagnosis, although the gastroscopic picture of an infiltrating carcinoma may now and then resemble that of a lymphoma or hypertrophic gastritis, necessitating a biopsy for differentiation. The unfortunate feature of the situation, however, is that these characteristic X-ray pictures are seen only in a late stage of the disease when the presence of lymph node metastases can be expected with fair certainty. Symptoms develop rather insidiously, and the patients come for medical care at a time when total gastrectomy — the only sensible treatment for this condition — can scarcely be more than palliative. The prognosis may become more favorable for the infiltrating type of carcinoma, as for other types of cancer of the stomach, when the methods for early recognition improve and when institutions, such as cancer prevention clinics, are more widely used.

Ulcerating Carcinoma of Stomach

Many pathologists, following Borrmann's classification, separate ulcerative cancer as a special type and consider it the most common form of early detectable gastric carcinoma. Though all forms of cancer of the stomach may become necrotic in parts and undergo ulcerative degeneration, it is particularly the adenocarcinoma and its papillary and polypoid varieties that tend to ulcerate while still relatively small. Necroses and loss of substance on the surface of a diffuse, infiltrating, scirrhous carcinoma are relatively rare and only superficial, whereas the funguslike, proliferating and more circumscribed — but still broadly infiltrating — neoplasms (see page 181) tend often to become deeply ulcerated by the sloughing of substantial parts of their central segments, probably because their blood supply cannot keep pace with their rapid growth. In such cases, especially with the early superficially spreading type, it may be extremely difficult, if not

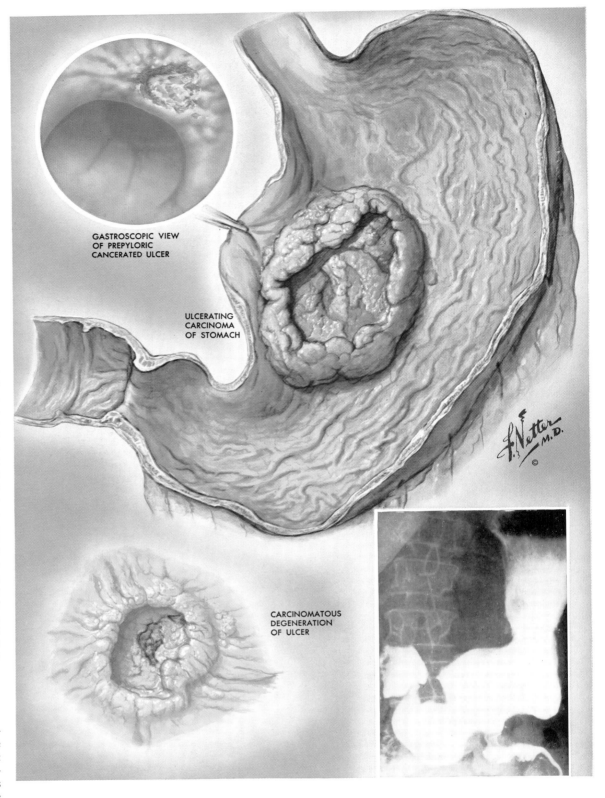

GASTROSCOPIC VIEW OF PREPYLORIC CANCERATED ULCER

ULCERATING CARCINOMA OF STOMACH

CARCINOMATOUS DEGENERATION OF ULCER

impossible, to separate the ulcerating carcinoma diagnostically from a benign chronic, callous and penetrating peptic ulcer. Neither age nor the duration of the patient's complaints can contribute to the final decision, in spite of the fact that, statistically, patients with cancer more frequently come under the older age group and have a comparatively short history of functional disturbances. Likewise, all other criteria, be they radiologic, gastroscopic or cytologic, are unreliable, which is not surprising if one bears in mind that even the histopathologic examination of biopsy or autopsy material not infrequently fails to arrive at a clear-cut diagnosis. That, as discussed above (see page 180), a not negligible percentage of ulcers originally benign may undergo *malignant alteration* complicates the issue further. The practical consequence of this situation is that patients with clinical or other signs of ulcer should receive the

benefit of a surgical exploration and appropriate intervention whenever the faintest doubts persist as to the presence of a malignancy.

The functional disturbances brought about by cancer of the stomach depend essentially on the location and on the size the tumor has attained at the time. The great majority of patients feel no discomfort or pain in the early stages and report to their physician only when the neoplasm has reached dimensions which cause obstruction of the pylorus or cardiac orifice, or reduction of the entire gastric lumen or secreting surface. At this time a gamut of manifestations, from vague epigastric discomfort, nausea, anorexia, etc., to weight loss and cachexia, may be present, pointing to a serious digestive dysfunction. If the tumor happens to invade the nerves, pain may become one of the early or actually the earliest

(Continued on page 185)

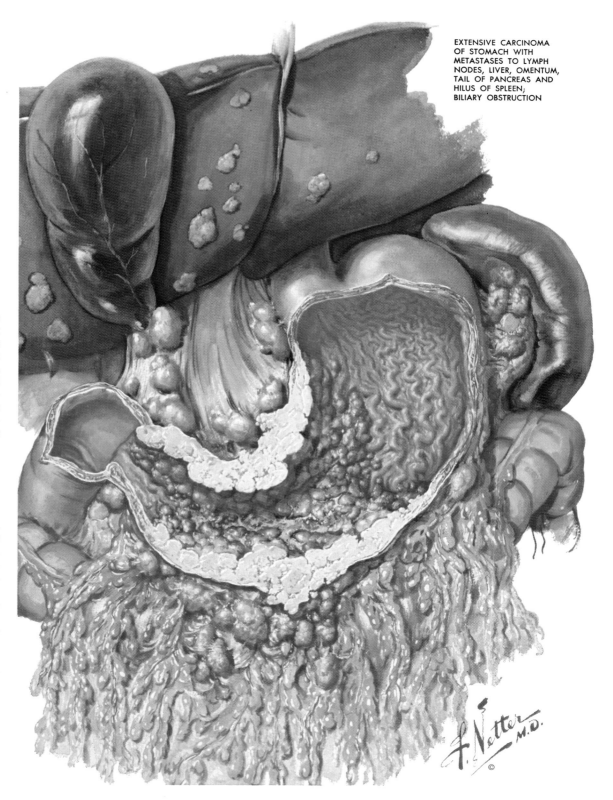

EXTENSIVE CARCINOMA
OF STOMACH WITH
METASTASES TO LYMPH
NODES, LIVER, OMENTUM,
TAIL OF PANCREAS AND
HILUS OF SPLEEN;
BILIARY OBSTRUCTION

CARCINOMA OF STOMACH

(Continued from page 184)

symptom. In such cases, as well as with manifestations of an ulcerating tumor (see above), the physician faces the most difficult problem of differentiation between a cancer and a benign ulcer. In any event, whatever the symptoms and whenever they appear, it has been estimated that at least half of the patients with gastric carcinoma do not seek medical attention until the tumor has extended beyond the stomach.

Spread of Carcinoma of Stomach

All types of carcinoma of the stomach either spread by direct extension to neighboring organs or metastasize by means of the lymphatics or blood stream. Some types have a greater, some (like the scirrhus) a lesser tendency to produce metastases. The regional lymph nodes become involved, sometimes very early and usually, though by no means always, in a definite sequence. With the lesser curvature being, to a certain degree, the preferred site, the lymph nodes of the upper left, anterior and posterior walls of the stomach (Region I of diagram on page 63) and their drainage system along the left gastric artery and the coronary vein are those first and most frequently affected. A rather serious prognostic significance must be attached to an early *involvement of the nodes in the pyloric area* (Region IV of the diagram on page 63), including the suprapancreatic nodes and those near the hilus of the liver (see CIBA COLLECTION, Vol. 3/III, pages 30 and 20, respectively), which excludes any possibility of radical removal of the malignancy. Secondary growth of malignant tumor cells in the *lymph nodes of the prepyloric, pyloric and pancreatic regions* and in the *hepatoduodenal ligament* may be accompanied clinically by icterus, as a result of an obstruction of the common bile duct, subsequent biliary stasis and dilatation of the gallbladder (Courvoisier's law or sign, see CIBA COLLECTION, Vol. 3/III, page 82). The *liver* is held as a site of predilection for *metastases* of gastric cancer (see CIBA COLLECTION, Vol. 3/III, page 115), either by direct spread or through the lymphatic routes just mentioned. (It is

possible, but probably not common, that cancer cells enter the liver by way of the portal circulation.) Similarly, though less frequently, metastases develop in the lower part of the esophagus, colon, pancreas and gallbladder.

Metastatic involvement of the lymph nodes along the greater curvature, in the gastrocolic ligament and in the *omentum majus* occurs less regularly than in those structures along the lesser curvature. Occasionally, the cancer cells are carried via celiac lymph nodes to the thoracic duct and the mediastinal and supraclavicular lymph nodes (Virchow's node).

Hematogenic metastases in lung, bone and brain (in that order of frequency) are relatively rare and are encountered, of course, only in far-advanced cases.

The direct transplantation of aberrant *cancer cells* upon the *peritoneum* represents a special type of spread. It requires complete penetration of the stom-

ach wall and, thus, is again a phenomenon of an advanced stage of gastric cancer. Once the serosa has become involved, cancer cells may be set free and may settle on the surface of any organ within the peritoneal cavity. The ovaries seem to be the most frequent site, sometimes the only location of such implanted metastases, which, in this organ, develop into a histologically rather characteristic secondary neoplasm, known as Krukenberg tumor (see CIBA COLLECTION, Vol. 2, page 210). If conditions permit, the simultaneous resection of the primary tumor and the ovarian metastases seems justified and worth serious consideration.

Another, certainly not infrequent, site of metastases is the pelvic peritoneum, where they may project into the rectum as a shelflike structure, the so-called "rectal shelf" of Blumer, and can be felt on rectal examination.

PRINCIPLES OF OPERATIVE PROCEDURES

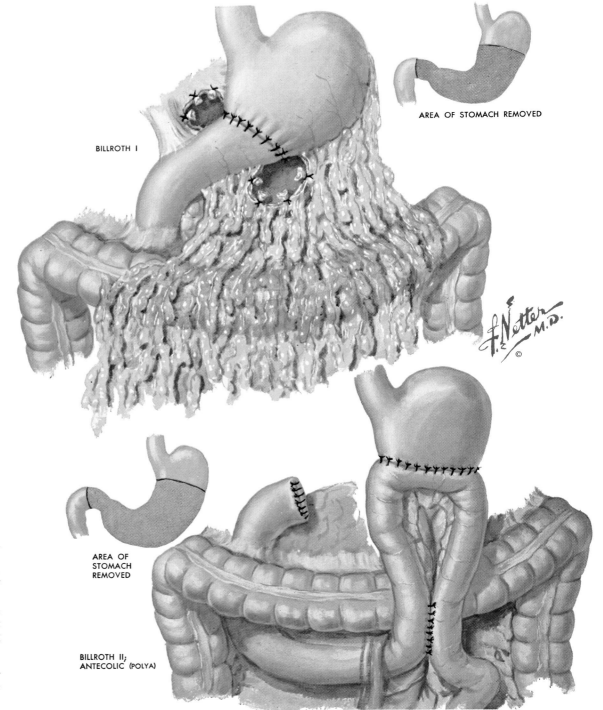

BILLROTH I

AREA OF STOMACH REMOVED

AREA OF STOMACH REMOVED

BILLROTH II; ANTECOLIC (POLYA)

With even a suspicion that a patient's complaints are not definitely and exclusively explained by a benign gastric lesion, an immediate surgical exploration is imperative. The precise operative procedure in the presence of an established, or even suspected, malignancy depends largely upon the size, site and extent of the lesion, but the situation will require, in the majority of cases, if an extensive procedure is at all feasible, nothing short of a subtotal or total gastrectomy, leaving the fundus, if the tumor occupies the antrum or the distal part of the corpus, and leaving the antrum when the tumor is confined to the most proximal gastric regions (see below and page 180).

Treatment of a peptic, gastric or duodenal ulcer begins with medical management (diet, antacid therapy, antisecretory drugs) and caring for the patient's psychologic and emotional problems. No rule of thumb can be given or used to fix the period of time during which medical treatment should be continued in the hope of improvement in subjective or objective symptoms. A great variety of individual factors must be considered before concluding that further medical efforts to regulate diet, habits and gastric secretion will be useless. In general, however, physician and patient should avail themselves of the benefit of an early consultation with the surgeon if the symptoms do not abate after a few weeks of adhering strictly to sound medical therapy. Failure of response after 2 weeks of hospitalization with a well-planned regimen, repeated recurrences of severe symptoms, intractable ulcer pain, lack of roentgenologic (or gastroscopic) evidence that the ulcer has not

completely healed after a few months (even though marked subjective improvement is noted), persistence of blood in the stool and any other signs of a threatening complication are fairly universally accepted as indications for surgical intervention. The patient's inability to co-operate with the physician's attempts to bring an ulcer under control, his unwillingness to accept the necessary restrictions imposed on him or his difficulties in assuming the financial burden accompanying more or less regular recurrences are further circumstances favoring the decision to operate.

The procedure of choice for the surgical treatment of a gastric or duodenal ulcer is a subtotal gastrectomy, by which from two thirds to three quarters of the distal portion of the stomach is removed, aiming to reduce the acid-secreting mucosa to such a degree that the gastric juice becomes anacid or at least hypoacid. Since only complete extirpation of the entire antrum can guarantee a permanent ablation of acid production, the distal line of the resection must lie beyond the pylorus.

Several types of operations and modifications

thereof have been developed, some of which have stood the test of time. Others were abandoned when their results did not live up to expectations, or when comparative studies regarding the frequency of post-operative complications (see pages 188 and 189) demonstrated their inferiority as opposed to other procedures.

The Viennese surgeon Billroth was the first to perform a partial gastrectomy, which included the pylorus and connected the distal end of the remaining stomach with the open end of the duodenum. The mobilization of the duodenum, necessary for such an end-to-end gastroduodenostomy, can, as a rule, be obtained tension-free without technical difficulties, even in the case of an extremely extensive resection of the stomach. This type of operation, known as "Billroth I", deserves preference over all other operative procedures, because with it the physiologic pathway for food transport is preserved, and the sequence of the digestive processes is less disturbed than with any other procedure. Execution of

(Continued on page 187)

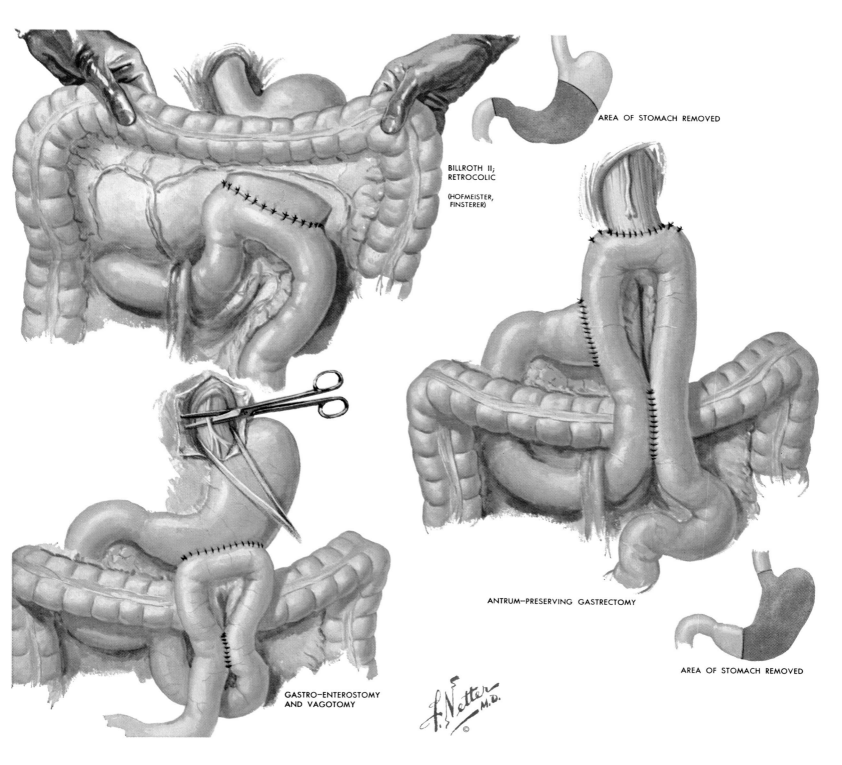

BILLROTH II;
RETROCOLIC

(HOFMEISTER,
FINSTERER)

AREA OF STOMACH REMOVED

ANTRUM–PRESERVING GASTRECTOMY

AREA OF STOMACH REMOVED

GASTRO–ENTEROSTOMY
AND VAGOTOMY

(*Continued from page 186*)

"Billroth I", however, is restricted by the prime necessity of a healthy and wide enough duodenal cuff for the end-to-end anastomosis. Consequently, this type of operation is technically precluded, in many cases, by fibrotic or cicatricial alterations of the duodenal wall.

Faced with cases where the first type of procedure was unfeasible, Billroth developed another type of gastrectomy, known as *"Billroth II"*, in which, after closing the duodenal opening, he connected the stump of the stomach to a loop of jejunum. Such a gastrojejunostomy can be constructed either in front of the transverse colon or in retrocolic fashion, by pulling the needed length of the jejunum upward through a slit made in the transverse mesocolon. In the antecolic procedure it has proved imperative to provide a side-to-side anastomosis of the afferent to the efferent limb of the jejunum at some distance from the stomach. This (Braun's) anastomosis prevents stasis in the afferent limb of the

loop and, thereby, the danger of a blowout of the by-passed duodenal stump.

Bilateral *vagotomy*, i.e., the severing of both vagus nerves at the level of the juxtacardial portion of the esophagus, aims at an elimination or reduction of the cephalic phase of the gastric secretion (see page 82). The hopes entertained that this simple procedure would permanently cure an ulcer have not been fulfilled. As experience has shown, the effect of vagotomy on acid production is often inadequate and, in most cases, only transient. Furthermore, this severance of the nervous pathway tends to induce a persistent pylorospasm and dyskinesia of the small and large intestine, resulting in a severe spastic constipation. If vagotomy is performed as the sole procedure to relieve the patient from his ulcer symptoms, because for one reason or another the surgeon cannot carry out a subtotal gastrectomy, it is always imperative to perform at least a gastrojejunostomy or pyloromyotomy to prevent a holdup of the gastric evacuation.

With a less radical gastrectomy, the proximal stomach is removed, but the antrum is preserved. The continuity of the digestive tract is maintained by an esophagojejunostomy, and the remaining antrum is implanted in the loop of the jejunum, which serves as a connection with the esophagus. Here again, the use of a Braun's anastomosis (see above) is advisable to prevent the reflux of duodenal secretions into the esophagus. The chief indication for this operation is carcinoma of the upper parts of the stomach (see page 180). The advantages of this procedure, as against a total gastrectomy, have been demonstrated clinically and experimentally. The preservation of the antrum not only assists in a better assimilation of proteins, fats and iron, but the threat of inanition, possible after all total gastric resections, will be removed. The intercalation of antrum and duodenum into the digestive pathway probably provides a more physiologic regulation of the duodenal secretory activity by the direct contact of food and mucosa.

POSTGASTRECTOMY COMPLICATIONS I

A small number of patients who have been subjected to gastrojejunostomy, with removal of a more or less large part of the stomach, suffer from distressing manifestations which have become known as postprandial or *"dumping" syndrome.* Its incidence seems to fluctuate, some authors having encountered it in about 6 per cent, others in 8 to 10 per cent, of the population who have undergone gastric resection. It has been observed after any of the various operative procedures presently accepted for the treatment of peptic ulcer (see pages 186 and 187) but seemingly is seen slightly more often after a Billroth II anastomosis than after the Billroth I type of operation. The chief features cover a wide range, from epigastric discomfort and a vague feeling of oppression to sudden episodes of profuse sweating, tachycardia, tremor and a tendency to faint. Painful sensations or vomiting are less regular manifestations. In the majority of cases, these symptoms occur while the patients are eating their meals or immediately thereafter and may be prevented or promptly improved if a supine position is assumed while eating or at the moment any discomfort is felt. The "dumping" syndrome appears a few weeks after operation and may disappear gradually within another few weeks or months. In some cases it may persist for years and will then have a deleterious effect on the general condition of the patient, so that attempts must be made to correct the situation by means of a second operation, which, however, is unfortunately not always successful. Some cases have been reported in which a cure was obtained by transforming the Billroth II type into a Billroth I. But, in general, further operations can be avoided and improvement may be expected in time if the patient can be trained to lie flat while eating, to take

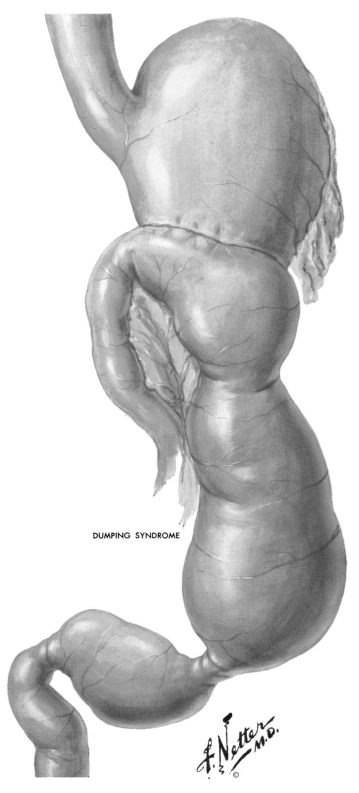

DUMPING SYNDROME

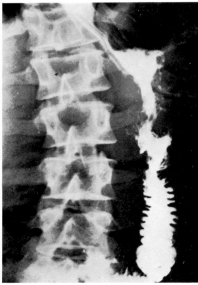

DUMPING SYNDROME

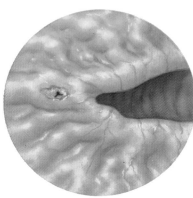

STOMAL GASTRITIS
(INFLAMMATION OF ANASTOMOTIC REGION)
(ANASTOMOSITIS)

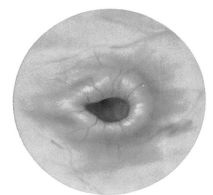

STENOSIS OF ANASTOMOTIC ORIFICE
(GASTROSCOPIC VIEW)

only small meals, to masticate thoroughly every single bite and to avoid drinking with his meals.

The true cause of the "dumping" syndrome has not yet been found, though many efforts have been made to explain it. The sudden filling of the efferent jejunal loop, hypoglycemia, traction on the mesentery, disturbances of the balance of the autonomic innervation and irritative effects of gastric juice on the jejunal mucosa have been considered as triggering mechanisms for this syndrome.

On X-ray studies one may observe a rapid emptying, with complete evacuation of the opaque meal from the esophagus and remaining parts of the stomach into a strongly dilated efferent jejunal loop. This dilatation is probably supported by spasms in the more distal portions of the jejunum.

Anastomositis, a name coined for the inflammation of the anastomotic area between the residual portion ("pouch") of the stomach and the "stoma loop" of the jejunum, is a frequent postoperative complication. The high incidence of this inflammatory reaction should not be surprising in view of the fact that this region is destined to be the meeting point of what is left of the gastric secretion and of the intestinal juice, the latter being anything but physiologic for the gastric mucosa, and the former being irritating to the intestinal tissue structures. Broadened, hyperemic, edematous mucosal folds can be readily seen on gastroscopy, as well as on X-ray films, after all anastomosing operations, indicating the presence of a stomal gastritis. But the degree of the visible inflammation does not always correspond to the clinical picture. A chronic condition with local signs of irritation and inflammation may take a completely symptom-free course. The sensation of pain, as a rule, indicates the presence of an anastomotic ulcer (see page 189).

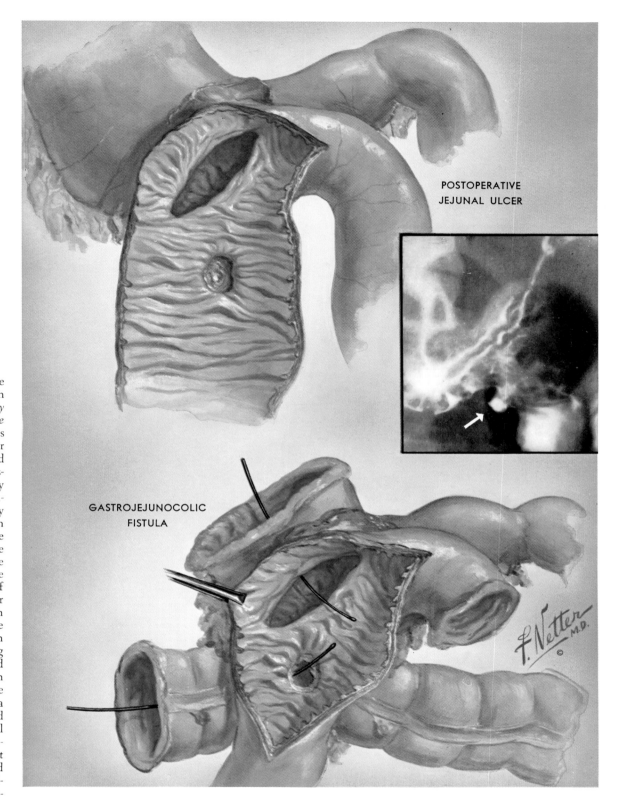

POSTOPERATIVE
JEJUNAL ULCER

GASTROJEJUNOCOLIC
FISTULA

P. Netter M.D.

POSTGASTRECTOMY COMPLICATIONS II

While a primary peptic ulcer of the jejunum is and always has been an extremely rare condition, a *secondary ulcer,* situated *on the jejunal side of the stoma* of gastrojejunal anastomoses, has been a well-known complication ever since gastro-enterostomy was introduced as a rational treatment for an ulcer disease that proved to be unmanageable by other means. The frequency of this complication has, however, markedly decreased with the steady progress in the techniques of gastric surgery, the improvement of suture material and the judicious choice of the various operative procedures now available. With a simple gastro-enterostomy or with those types of operations that preserve the pylorus or part of the antrum, the incidence with which a new ulcer may develop at the stoma itself or somewhat distal to it in the jejunal wall is still quite disturbing (up to 16 per cent), a fact explained undoubtedly by the high concentration of hydrochloric acid deriving from the preserved antrum. On the other hand, a secondary jejunal ulcer is encountered in not more than 0.2 per cent of all patients submitted to a typical gastro-duodenal resection, quite independent of the mode by which the passage of food has been restored. Pain, almost invariably most severe, is the dominating symptom of this type of ulcer, which, in addition, exhibits a pronounced tendency to perforate and bleed. The diagnosis of peptic, postoperative jejunal ulcer may be conjectured, based on the intensity and persistence of the pain, and can, as a rule but by no means in all cases, be confirmed by X-ray examination or gastroscopy.

When the gastrojejunostomy has been performed in the retrocolic fashion, a perforation may lead to a *gastrojejunocolic fistula,* a very serious condition, particularly if the digestive activity of the gastric juice starts to act upon the colonic wall. Chronic diarrhea, with undigested food in the stool, fecal odor of the breath and stercoraceous vomiting point to the presence of a gastrojejuno-colic fistula. The latter may be ascertained roentgenologically if the contrast medium, given orally, enters the colon immediately or, vice versa, when given rectally, enters the remaining stomach.

A trial to treat the uncomplicated stomal ulcer by diet and medicaments (anticholinergics) seems justified, although these efforts are seldom successful. If the ulcer symptoms continue unabated or if signs of hemorrhage appear, further surgery becomes inevitable. With any sign of a perforation or an established gastrojejunocolic fistula, the operative indications are clear-cut.

What can or must be done operatively in such cases depends largely upon the type of surgery performed previously. Should the ulcer follow a simple gastro-enterostomy, a gastroduodenal resection, including the old ulcer-bearing portion of the anastomosis, will have to be carried out. In patients whose duodenal ulcer has been circumvented by the so-called "exclusion operation", by which the pylorus and parts of the antrum are preserved, an additional excision of antral parts may prove sufficient for a cure of an anastomotic ulcer, without touching the anastomosis itself. Reduction of the size of the stomach stump and/or resection of the anastomosis in toto with construction of a new channel is often necessary after a primary gastroduodenal resection. Every one of these procedures should be combined with a bilateral vagotomy to decrease further the acid-secreting potential. The gastrojejunocolic fistula presents a serious preoperative nutritional problem and requires removal of the jejunal loop, shortening of the residual part of the stomach and the closure of the fistula into the colon. Excision of the ulcerated portion of the colon is, in the majority of instances, avoidable, but preliminary proximal colostomy is sometimes advisable.

REFERENCES

Section I

	PLATE NUMBER
ANSON, B. J., AND MADDOCK: *Callander's Surgical Anatomy*, W. B. Saunders Company, Philadelphia, 1953.	3, 15, 17-23
BASSETT, D. L.: *Stereoscopic Atlas of Human Anatomy*, Sec. 2, Head and Neck, Williams & Wilkins Company, Baltimore, 1954.	1-13, 14-21
BRASH, J. C., AND JAMIESON: *Cunningham's Textbook of Anatomy*, Oxford University Press, London, 1951.	1-29
DIAMOND, M.: *Dental Anatomy*, Macmillan Company, New York, 1952.	10, 11
GOSS, C. M.: *Gray's Anatomy of the Human Body*, Lea & Febiger, Philadelphia, 1954.	1-29
HAMILTON, W. J.: *Textbook of Human Anatomy*, Macmillan & Company, Ltd., London, 1957.	1-29
HOLLINSHEAD, W. H.: *Anatomy for Surgeons, Vol. I, The Head and Neck*, Paul B. Hoeber, Inc., New York, 1954.	1-29
JAMIESON, E. B.: *Illustrations of Regional Anatomy, Vol. II, Head and Neck*, Williams & Wilkins Company, Baltimore, 1947.	4-7, 14-23
KRONFELD, R.: *Histopathology of the Teeth and Their Surrounding Structures*, Lea & Febiger, Philadelphia, 1955.	4, 5, 10, 11, 15
LAST, R. J.: *Anatomy, Regional and Applied*, Little, Brown and Company, Boston, 1954.	1-29
LERCHE, W.: *The Esophagus and Pharynx in Action*, Charles C Thomas, Publisher, Springfield, Ill., 1950.	16, 17, 19-21
MAINLAND, D.: *Anatomy as a Basis for Medical and Dental Practice*, Paul B. Hoeber, Inc., New York, 1945.	3-7, 10-12
MESCHAN, I.: *An Atlas of Normal Radiographic Anatomy*, W. B. Saunders Company, Philadelphia, 1957.	3
MORRIS, H.: *Morris' Human Anatomy*, Blakiston Company, New York, 1953.	5-11, 14-26
SARNAT, B. G., EDITOR: *The Temporomandibular Joint*, Charles C Thomas, Publisher, Springfield, Ill., 1951.	2, 3
SCHAEFFER, J. P.: *Morris' Human Anatomy*, Blakiston Company, New York, 1953.	1-29
SOBOTTA, J.: *Atlas of Descriptive Human Anatomy*, Hafner Publishing Company, New York, 1954.	3-15, 17-23
SPALTEHOLTZ, W.: *Hand Atlas of Human Anatomy*, J. B. Lippincott Company, Philadelphia, 1955.	3-15, 18-29
TAYLOR, G. W., AND NATHANSON: *Lymph Node Metastases; Incidence and Surgical Treatment in Neoplastic Disease*, Oxford University Press, New York, 1945.	25, 26
TOBIAS, M. J.: *Anatomy of the Lymphatic System (A Compendium Translated from Anatomie des Lymphatiques de l'Homme, by H. Rouvière)*, Edward Brothers, Ann Arbor, 1938.	25, 26
WOODBURNE, R. T.: *Essentials of Human Anatomy*, Oxford University Press, New York, 1957.	1-29

Section II

	PLATE NUMBER
ABEL, W.: *The arrangement of the longitudinal and circular musculature of the upper end of the esophagus*, J. Anat. Physiol., 47:381, 1913.	3, 4
ADACHI, B.: *Das Venensystem der Japaner*, Kenyusha Druckanstalt, 1940.	9
ALLISON, P. R.: *Reflux esophagitis, sliding hernia and the anatomy of repair*, Surg. Gynec. Obstet., 92:419, 1951.	6
AUERBACH, L.: *Fernere vorläufige Mittheilung über den Nervenapparat des Darmes*, Virchow's Arch., 30:457, 1864.	13
BENEDICT, E. B.: *Endoscopy*, Williams & Wilkins Company, Baltimore, 1951.	2
BODIAN, M., CARTER AND WARD: *Hirschsprung's disease*, Lancet, 1:302, 1951.	13
BUTLER, H.: *The veins of the esophagus*, Thorax, 6:276, 1951.	9
CHAMBERLIN, J. A., AND WINSHIP: *Anatomic variations of the vagus nerves; their significance in vagus neurectomy*, Surgery, 22:1, 1947.	11-13
CICERI, C.: *Morfolgia e struttura della membrana diaframmatico esofageo*, Monit. zool. ital., 40:501, 1929.	5, 6
COLLIS, J. L., KELLY AND WILEY: *Anatomy of crura of diaphragm and surgery of hiatus hernia*, Thorax, 9:175, 1954.	6
——, SATCHWELL AND ABRAMS: *Nerve supply to crura of diaphragm*, Thorax, 9:22, 1954.	6
COWDRY, E. V.: *Special Cytology, The Forms and Functions of the Cell in Health and Disease*, Paul B. Hoeber, Inc., New York, 1928.	7
DEMEL, R.: *Die Gefässversorgung der Speiseröhre; ein Beitrag zur Oesophaguschirurgie*, Arch. klin. Chir., 128:453, 1924.	8
DOGIEL, A. S.: *Ueber den Bau der Ganglien in den Geflechten des Darmes und der Gallenblase des Menschen und der Säugethiere*, Arch. Anat. Physiol. (LPZ), Anat. Abtg., 130, 1899.	13
FLEISCHNER, F. G.: *Hiatal hernia complex: Hiatal hernia, peptic esophagitis, Mallory-Weiss syndrome, hemorrhage and anemia and marginal esophagogastric ulcer*, J. Amer. med. Ass., 162:183, 1956.	5
HAECKERMANN, K.: *Beitrag zur Lehre von der Entstehung der Divertikel des Oesophagus*, Dissertation, Göttingen, 1891.	3, 4
HILL, C. J.: *A contribution to our knowledge of the enteric plexuses*, Philos. Trans., Ser. B, 215:355, 1927.	13
HOVELACQUE, A.: *Anatomie des nerfs craniens et rachidiens et du système grand sympathique chez l'homme*, Paris, G. Doin et Cie, 1927.	13
INGELFINGER, F. J., AND KRAMER: *Dysphagia produced by a contractile ring in the lower esophagus*, Gastroenterology, 23:419, 1953.	5
IRVIN, D. A.: *The anatomy of Auerbach's plexus*, Amer. J. Anat., 49:141, 1931.	13
JACKSON, C.: *Diaphragmatic pinchcock in so-called "cardiospasm"*, Laryngoscope (St. Louis), 32:139, 1922.	3, 4
—— AND JACKSON: *Bronchoscopy, Esophagoscopy and Gastroscopy*, W. B. Saunders Company, Philadelphia, 1934.	2
JACKSON, R. G.: *Anatomy of the vagus nerves in the region of the lower esophagus and stomach*, Anat. Rec., 103:1, 1949.	11
KEGARIES, D. L.: *Venous plexus of oesophagus*, Surg. Gynec. Obstet., 58:46, 1934.	9
KELLY, A. B.: *Ascending fibrosis of esophagus and its relation to presence of gastric islets of gastric mucosa*, J. Laryng. Otol., 54:621, 1939.	5
KNIGHT, G. C.: *Relation of intrinsic nerves to functional activity of esophagus*, Brit. J. Surg., 22:155, 1934.	8
KUNTZ, A.: *On the occurrence of reflex arcs in the myenteric and submucous plexuses*, Anat. Rec., 24:193, 1922.	13
——: *The autonomic nervous system*, Lea & Febiger, Philadelphia, 1953.	13
LAIMER, E.: *Beiträge zur Anatomie des Oesophagus*, Med. Jahrbücher (Wien), 333, 1883 (quoted from Lerche).	3-5
LENDRUM, F. C.: *Anatomic features of the cardiac orifice of the stomach*, Arch. intern. Med., 58:474, 1937.	5
LERCHE, W.: *The muscular coat of the esophagus and its defects*, J. thorac. Surg., 6:1, 1936.	3-5
——: *The Esophagus and Pharynx in Action*, Charles C Thomas, Publisher, Springfield, Ill., 1950.	2-5, 7
LOW, A.: *A note on the crura of the diaphragm and the muscle of Treitz*, J. Anat. Physiol., 42:93, 1907.	6
MAXIMOW, A. A., AND BLOOM: *Textbook of Histology*, W. B. Saunders Company, Philadelphia, 1931.	7
MEISSNER, G.: *Ueber die Nerven der Darmwand*, Zschr. rat. Med., 364, 1857.	13
MITCHELL, G. A. G.: *Anatomy of the autonomic nervous system*, E. & S. Livingstone, Edinburgh, 1953.	11-13
——: *Cardiovascular innervation*, E. & S. Livingstone, Edinburgh, 1956.	11-13
—— AND WARWICK: *The dorsal vagal nucleus*, Acta Anat. (Basel), 25:371, 1955.	13
MOSHER, H. P., AND McGREGOR: *Study of lower end of esophagus*, Ann. Otol. (St. Louis), 37:12, 1928.	5
——: *Lower end of oesophagus at birth and in adult*, J. Laryng., 45:161, 1930.	5
PALMER, E. D.: *The Esophagus and Its Diseases*, Paul B. Hoeber, Inc., New York, 1952.	2
——: *Attempt to localize normal esophagogastric junction*, Radiology, 60:825, 1953.	5
PETERS, P. M.: *Closure mechanism at the cardia with special reference to diaphragmatico-oesophageal elastic ligament*, Thorax, 10:27, 1955.	5, 6
REICH, L.: *Ueber die Lokalisation der Kardia*, Mitt. Grenzgeb. Med. Chir., 40:481, 1927.	5
ROUVIÈRE, H.: *Anatomy of the Human Lymphatic System* (Translation), J. W. Edwards Publisher, Inc., Ann Arbor, 1938.	10
SHAPIRO, A. L., AND ROBILLARD: *The esophageal arteries*, Ann. Surg., 131:171, 1950.	8

STÖHR, P., JR.: *Mikroskopische Studien zur Innervation des Magen-Darmkanales*, Zschr. Zellforsch., 34:1, 1948.   13

SWIGART, A. L., SIEKERT, HAMBLEY AND ANSON: *The esophageal arteries*, Surg. Gynec. Obstet., 90:234, 1950.   8

TAFURI, W. L.: *Auerbach's plexus in the guinea pig. I. A quantitative study of the ganglia and nerve cells in the ileum, caecum and colon*, Acta Anat. (Basel), 31: 522, 1957.   13

TOREK, F.: *First successful resection of thoracic portion of esophagus*, J. Amer. med. Ass., 60:1533, 1913.   8

WHITE, J. C., SMITHWICK AND SIMEONE: *The autonomic nervous system*, H. Kimpton, London, 1952.   13

Section III

ADACHI, B.: *Das Venensystem der Japaner*, Kenyusha Druckanstalt, 1940.   14

BALL, C. F.: *Left paraduodenal hernia; two cases, one with rupture through wall of hernial sac*, Amer. J. Surg., 29:481, 1935.   3

BARGMANN, W.: *Histologic und Mikroskopische Anatomie*, Georg Thieme, Stuttgart, 1956.   4, 7

BELLOCQ, P.: *Anatomie Médico-Chirurgicale, Fasc. IX-X*, Masson et Cie, Paris, 1947-52.   1-7

BODIAN, M., CARTER AND WARD: *Hirschsprung's disease*, Lancet, 1:302, 1951.   13

BRYAN, R. C.: *Right paraduodenal hernia*, Amer. J. Surg., 28:703, 1935.   3

CHAMBERLIN, J. A., AND WINSHIP: *Anatomic variations of the vagus nerves; their significance in vagus neurectomy*, Surgery, 22:1, 1947.   13

COLE, L. G.: *Living stomach and its motor phenomenon*, Acta radiol. interamer., 9: 533, 1928.   1

COLLIS, J. L., KELLY AND WILEY: *Anatomy of crura of diaphragm and surgery of hiatus hernia*, Thorax, 9:175, 1954.   3

CORNING, H. K.: *Lehrbuch der Topographischen Anatomie*, J. F. Bergmann, München, 1949.   1-3, 6, 15

DOUGLASS, B., BAGGENSTOSS AND HOLLINSHEAD: *The anatomy of the portal vein and its tributaries*, Surg. Gynec. Obstet., 91: 562, 1950.   9-11, 14

GOSS, C. M.: *Gray's Anatomy of the Human Body*, Lea & Febiger, Philadelphia, 1954.   1-7

HAFFERL, A.: *Lehrbuch der Topographischen Anatomie*, Springer-Verlag, Berlin-Göttingen-Heidelberg, 1957.   1-3

HALEY, J. C., AND PEDEN: *Suspensory muscle of duodenum*, Amer. J. Surg., 59:546, 1943.   3

—— AND PERRY: *Further study of suspensory muscle of duodenum*, Amer. J. Surg., 77: 590, 1949.   3

HEALEY, J. E., JR., AND SCHROY: *Anatomy of the biliary ducts within the human liver; analysis of the prevailing pattern of branchings and the major variations of the biliary ducts*, Arch. Surg. (Chicago), 66: 599, 1953.   8-12

——, —— AND SÖRENSEN: *The intrahepatic distribution of the hepatic artery in man*, J. int. Coll. Surg., 20:133, 1953.   8-12

HORTON, B. T.: *Pyloric musculature, with special reference to pyloric block*, Amer. J. Anat., 41:197, 1928.   5

IVY, A. C., GROSSMAN AND BACHRACH: *Peptic Ulcer*, Blakiston Company, Philadelphia, 1950.   1, 6

JACKSON, R. G.: *Anatomy of the vagus nerves in the region of the lower esophagus and stomach*, Anat. Rec., 103:1, 1949.   13

KUNTZ, A.: *The Autonomic Nervous System*, Lea & Febiger, Philadelphia, 1953.   16, 17

LOW, A.: *A note on the crura of the diaphragm and the muscle of Treitz*, J. Anat. Phys., 42:93, 1907.   3

MICHELS, N. A.: *The hepatic, cystic and retroduodenal arteries and their relations to the biliary ducts; with samples of the entire celiacal blood supply*, Ann. Surg., 133:503, 1951.   8-12

——: *Collateral arterial pathways to the liver after ligation of the hepatic artery and removal of the celiac axis*, Cancer, 6:708, 1953.   8-12

——: *Blood Supply and Anatomy of the Upper Abdominal Organs; With a Descriptive Atlas (172 illustrations)*, J. B. Lippincott Company, Philadelphia, 1954.   8-12

MILLS, R. W.: *Relation of body habitus to viscera*, Amer. J. Roentgenol., 4:155, 1917.   1

MITCHELL, G. A. G.: *Anatomy of the autonomic nervous system*, E. & S. Livingstone, Edinburgh, 1953.   16, 17

MOODY, R. O., VAN NUYS AND KIDDER: *Form and position of empty stomach in healthy young adults as shown in roentgenograms*, Anat. Rec., 43:359, 1929.   1

MOYNIHAN, B. G. A.: *On Retroperitoneal Hernia*, Bailliere, Tindall and Cox, London, 1906.   3

PERNKOFF, E.: *Topographische Anatomie des Menschen, Bd. II, Bauch, Becken und Beckengliedmasse, 1. Teil*, Urban & Schwargenberg, Berlin-Wien, 1941.   1-3, 6, 15

ROUVIÈRE, H.: *Anatomie des Lymphatiques de l'Homme*, Masson et Cie, Paris, 1932.   15

SCHABADASCH, A.: *Die Nerven des Magens der Katze. Intramurale Nervengeflechte des Darmrohrs*, Zschr. Zellforsch., 10:254, 320, 1930.   16, 17

SHAPIRO, A. L., AND ROBILLARD: *Morphology and variations of the duodenal vasculature. Relationship to the problems of leakage from a postgastrectomy duodenal stump, bleeding peptic ulcer and injury to the common duct*, Arch. Surg., 52:571, 1946.   10, 12

SHORT, A. R.: *Retroperitoneal hernia*, Brit. J. Surg., 12:456, 1925.   3

TAFURI, W. L.: *Auerbach's plexus in the guinea pig. I. A quantitative study of the ganglia and nerve cells in the ileum, caecum and colon*, Acta Anat., 31:522, 1957.   13

THOREK, P.: *Six subphrenic spaces; applied anatomy and surgical considerations*, Surgery, 21:739, 1947.   3

TORGERSEN, T.: *The muscular build and movements of the stomach and duodenal bulb*, Acta radiol. (Stockh.), Suppl. 45, 1942.   1

TREVES, F.: *The anatomy of the intestinal canal and peritoneum in man*, Brit. med. J., 1:415, 470, 527 and 580, 1885.   1-7

WILKIE, D. P. D.: *The blood supply of the duodenum, with special reference to the supraduodenal artery*, Surg. Gynec. Obstet., 13:399, 1911.   8-12

WOODBURNE, R., AND OLSEN: *The arteries of the pancreas*, Anat. Rec., 111:255, 1951.   8-12

Section IV

ALVAREZ, W. C.: *An Introduction to Gastro-Enterology*, Paul B. Hoeber, Inc., New York, 1940.   1-5, 9-22

ANDRESEN, A. F. R.: *Office Gastroenterology*, W. B. Saunders Company, Philadelphia, 1958.   25, 27, 28

ARDRAN, G. M., AND KEMP: *Some aspects of mechanism of swallowing*, Gastroenterologia, 78:347, 1952.   6, 7

—— AND ——: *Protection of laryngeal airway during swallowing*, Brit. J. Radiol., 25: 406, 1952.   7

AYRE, J. E.: *A rotating gastric brush for rapid cancer detection*, Ciba Clin. Symposia, 8: 179, 1956.   29

—— AND OREN: *New rapid method for stomach cancer diagnosis: gastric brush*, Cancer, 6:1177, 1953.   29

BABKIN, B. P.: *Secretory Mechanism of the Digestive Glands*, Paul B. Hoeber, Inc., New York, 1944.   11-15

——: *Die sekretorische Tätigkeit der Verdauungsdrüsen*, Hdbch. der norm. und pathol. Physiol., Bd. 3, B/III, p. 689, J. Springer, Berlin, 1927.   11-15

—— AND KITE: *Central and reflex regulation of motility of pyloric antrum*, J. Neurophysiol., 13:321, 1950.   9, 10

—— AND ——: *Gastric motor effects of acute removal of cingulate gyrus and section brain stem*, J. Neurol., 13:335, 1950.   13

BARCLAY, A. E.: *Mechanics of digestive tract*, Lancet, 1:11, 1934.   4-15

BEATTIE, J., AND SHEEHAN: *Effects of hypothalamic stimulation on gastric motility*, J. Physiol., 81:218, 1934.   13

BERK, J. E., THOMAS AND REHFUSS: *Acid factor in duodenal ulcer as evaluated by acidity and neutralizing ability in duodenal bulb*, Amer. J. dig. Dis., 9:371, 1942.   10

BERNSTEIN, L. M., AND BAKER: *A clinical test for esophagitis*, Gastroenterology, 34: 760, 1958.   25

BLUNTSCHLI, H., AND WINKLER: *Kaubewegungen und Bissenbildung*, Hdbch. der norm. und pathol. Physiol., Bd. 3, B/III, p. 295, J. Springer, Berlin, 1927.   4, 5

BORISON, H. L., AND WANG: *Functional localization of central coordinating mechanism for emesis in cat*, J. Neurophysiol., 12:305, 1949.   18

—— AND ——: *Physiology and pharmacology of vomiting*, Pharmacol. Rev., 5:193, 1953.   18

BROBECK, J. R.: *Neural regulation of food intake*, Ann. N. Y. Acad. Sci., 63:44, 1955.   1

——, LARSON AND RAYES: *A study of the electrical activity of the hypothalamic feeding mechanism*, J. Physiol. (Paris), 132:358, 1956.   2

Section IV (continued)

PLATE NUMBER

BRODY, M., AND GOETZ: *Studies on the gastrointestinal effects of Marsilid®*, J. Clin. exp. Psychopath., 19, Suppl. 1:146, 1958. — 19

CARBONE, J. V., AND LIEBOWITZ: *The effect of adrenal corticoids on gastric secretion and the suppression of corticoid-induced hypersecretion by anticholinergics*, Metabolism, 7:70, 1958. — 19

CARLSON, A. J.: *The Control of Hunger in Health and Disease (Psychic Secretion in Man)*, University of Chicago Press, Chicago, 1916. — 1, 9

——: *The secretion of gastric juice in health and disease*, Physiol. Rev., 3:1, 1923. — 11, 12, 14, 15

CHINN, H. L., AND SMITH: *Motion sickness*, Pharmacol. Rev., 7:33, 1955. — 18

CODE, C. F.: *The inhibition of gastric secretion*, Pharmacol. Rev., 3:59, 1951. — 14, 15

CORAZZA, L. J., AND MYERSON: *The influence of various clinical disorders and drugs on excretion of uropepsin*, J. Amer. med. Ass., 165:146, 1957. — 12

CORBIN, B., AND HAMILTON: *Function of mesencephalic root of fifth cranial nerve*, J. Neurophysiol., 3:423, 1940. — 13

COUNCIL ON PHARMACY AND CHEMISTRY: *Present status of cinchophen and neocinchophen*, J. Amer. med. Ass., 117:1182, 1941. — 19

CRIDER, J. O., AND THOMAS: *The influence of certain conditions in the duodenum on the rate of secretion and acidity of the gastric juice*, Amer. J. Physiol., 101:25, 1932. — 11

DAMIANI, R.: *Le alterazioni del plessi nervosi intramurali dell' esofago nel cardiospasmo*, Chir. Pat. sper., 2:101, 1954 (abstract Gastroenterology, 28:679, 1955). — 29

DOLL, R., FRIEDLANDER AND PYGOTT: *Dietetic treatment of peptic ulcer*, Lancet, 1:5, 1956. — 16

DONALDSON, R. M., VOM EIGEN AND DWIGHT: *Gastric hypersecretion, peptic ulceration and islet cell tumor of the pancreas (the Zollinger-Ellison syndrome. Report of a case and review of the literature)*, New Engl. J. Med., 257:965, 1957. — 16

DOUTHWAITE, A. H., AND LINTOTT: *Gastroscopic observation on the effect of aspirin and certain other substances on the stomach*, Lancet, 2:1222, 1938. — 19

DRAGSTEDT, L. R.: *A concept of the etiology of gastric and duodenal ulcer*, Amer. J. Roentgenol., 75:219, 1956. — 16

EINHORN, M.: *Ueber die Wichtigkeit der Fadenimprägnatious probe für die Erkennung von Geschwüren im oberen Verdanungstrakt*, Arch. Verdau.-Kr., 17:150, 1911. — 26

ELLISON, E. H.: *The ulcerogenic tumor of the pancreas*, Surgery, 40:147, 1956. — 16

FLOOD, C. A., JONES, ROTTON AND SCHWARZ: *Tubeless gastric analysis; a study of 100 cases*, Gastroenterology, 23:607, 1953. — 19

FRIEDMAN, M.: *Peptic ulcer and functional dyspepsia in armed forces*, Gastroenterology, 10:586, 1948. — 25

FULTON, J. F.: *Physiology of the Nervous System*, Oxford University Press, New York, 1949. — 3, 13

FYKE, F. E., AND CODE: *Resting and deglutition pressures in the pharyngo-esophageal region*, Gastroenterology, 29:24, 1955. — 6, 7

Section IV (continued)

PLATE NUMBER

——, —— AND SCHLEGEL: *Gastroesophageal sphincter in healthy human beings*, Gastroenterologia, 86:135, 1956. — 6, 7

GIANTURCO, C.: *Some mechanical factors of gastric physiology; pyloric mechanism; effect of various foods on emptying of stomach*, Amer. J. Roentgenol., 31:745, 1934. — 10

——: *Some mechanical factors of gastric physiology; empty stomach and its various ways of filling. Pressure exerted by gastric walls on gastric content. Physical changes occurring to foodstuff during digestion*, Amer. J. Roentgenol., 31:735, 1934. — 10

GOODMAN, L. S., AND GILMAN: *The Pharmacological Basis of Therapeutics*, Macmillan Company, New York, 1955. — 19

GRAY, S. J., RAMSEY, REIFENSTEIN AND BENSON: *The significance of hormonal factors in the pathogenesis of peptic ulcer*, Gastroenterology, 25:156, 1953. — 13, 14

GREGORY, R. A., AND IVY: *Humoral stimulation of gastric secretion*, Quart. J. exp. Physiol., 31:111, 1941. — 11

GROSSMAN, M. I.: *Gastrointestinal hormones*, Physiol. Rev., 30:33, 1950. — 11

——: *The caffeine gastric analysis as an aid in diagnosis of duodenal ulcer*, Gastroenterology, 28:1047, 1955. — 28

——: *Integration of current views on the regulation of hunger and appetite*, Ann. N. Y. Acad. Sci., 63:76, 1955. — 1, 2

——, ROBERTSON AND IVY: *Proof of hormonal mechanism for gastric secretion; humoral transmission of distention stimulus*, Amer. J. Physiol., 153:1, 1948. — 11

——, ROTH AND IVY: *Pepsin secretion in response to caffeine*, Gastroenterology, 4:251, 1945. — 19

HATCHER, R. A.: *Mechanism of vomiting*, Physiol. Rev., 4:479, 1924. — 18

HAVERBACK, B. J., STEVENSON, SJOERDSMA AND JERRY: *The effects of reserpine and chlorpromazine on gastric secretion*, Amer. J. med. Sci., 230:601, 1955. — 19

HELLEBRANDT, F. A., AND TEPPER: *Studies on influence of exercise on digestive work of stomach; its effect on emptying time*, Amer. J. Physiol., 107:355, 1934. — 15

HIGHTOWER, N., OLSEN AND MOERSCH: *A comparison of the effects of acetyl-beta-methylcholine chloride (mecholyl) on esophageal intraluminal pressure in normal persons and patients with cardiospasms*, Gastroenterology, 26:592, 1954. — 25

HOLLANDER, F.: *Current views on the physiology of gastric secretion*, Amer. J. Med., 13:453, 1951. — 11-15

HUNT, J. N., AND MACDONALD: *The relation between volume of a test-meal and the gastric secretory response*, J. Physiol., 117:289, 1952. — 11

HURST, A., AND LINTOTT: *Aspirin as cause of hematemesis: clinical and gastroscopic study*, Guy's Hosp. Rep., 89:173, 1939. — 19

HURST, A. F., AND STEWART: *Gastric and Duodenal Ulcer*, Oxford University Press, London, 1929. — 11

HWANG, K.: *Mechanism of transportation of the content of the esophagus*, J. appl. Physiol., 6:781, 1954. — 8

Section IV (continued)

PLATE NUMBER

—— AND GROSSMAN: *A note on the innervation of the cervical portion of the human esophagus*, Gastroenterology, 25:375, 1953. — 8

IMBRIGLIA, J. E., STEIN AND LOPUSNIAK: *Cytological study of the upper gastrointestinal sediment. Its value, as correlated with roentgenologic and clinical findings in the diagnosis of cancer*, J. Amer. med. Ass., 147:120, 1951. — 27

IVY, A. C.: *Physiology of the Gastro-intestinal Tract*. Unpublished manuscript. — 9-22

——, GROSSMAN AND BACHRACH: *Peptic Ulcer*, Blakiston Company, Philadelphia, 1950. — 11, 12, 14-16

JANOWITZ, H. D.: *Hunger and appetite. Physiologic regulation of food intake*, Amer. J. Med., 25:327, 1958. — 1

——: *Quantitative tests for gastrointestinal function*, Amer. J. Med., 13:465, 1952. — 27, 28

KAHLSON, G.: *Nervous and humoral control of gastric secretion*, Brit. med. J., 2:1091, 1948. — 11

KAY, A. W.: *Effect of large doses of histamine on gastric secretion of HCl; augmented histamine test*, Brit. med. J., 2:77, 1953. — 28

KRAMER, P.: *What is cardiospasm?*, Amer. J. dig. Dis., N.S., 2:1, 1957. — 25

—— AND INGELFINGER: *I. Motility of the human esophagus in control subjects and in patients with esophageal disorders*, Amer. J. Med., 7:168, 1949. — 7

——, —— AND ATKINSON: *The motility and pharmacology of the esophagus in cardiospasm*, Gastroenterologia, 86:174, 1956. — 25

—— AND ——: *Esophageal sensitivity to mecholyl in cardiospasm*, Gastroenterology, 19:242, 1951. — 25

KUNTZ, A.: *The autonomic nervous system*, Lea & Febiger, Philadelphia, 1953. — 8, 13

LERCHE, W.: *The Esophagus and Pharynx in Action*, Charles C Thomas, Publisher, Springfield, Ill., 1950. — 6, 7

LITTMAN, A., FOX, KAMMERLING AND FOX: *A single aspiration caffeine test in duodenal ulcer and control patients*, Gastroenterology, 28:953, 1955. — 28

MACDONALD, I., AND SPURRELL: *Sham feeding with pectin meal*, J. Physiol., 119:259, 1953. — 11

MAGOUN, H. W., RANSON AND FISHER: *Corticifugal pathways for mastication, lapping and other motor functions in cat*, Arch. Neurol. Psychiat., 30:292, 1933. — 8, 13

MALACH, M., AND BANKS: *Experience with a tubeless method of gastric analysis*, New Engl. J. Med., 247:880, 1952. — 19

MARGOLIN, S. G., ORRINGER, KAUFMANN, WINKELSTEIN, HOLLANDER, JANOWITZ, STEIN AND LEVY: *Variations of gastric functions during conscious and unconscious conflict states*, Ass. Res. nerv. Dis. Proc., 29:656, 1950. — 14

MILLER, H. R.: *Central Autonomic Regulations in Health and Disease, with Special Reference to the Hypothalamus*, Grune & Stratton, Inc., New York, 1942. — 1, 8, 13

MITCHELL, G. A. G.: *Anatomy of the Autonomic Nervous System*, E. & S. Livingstone, Edinburgh, 1953. — 13

MUSICK, V. H., AVEY, HOPPS AND HELLBAUM: *Gastric secretion in duodenal ulcer*

Section IV (continued)

PLATE NUMBER

in remission; response to the caffeine test meal, Gastroenterology, 7:332, 1946. — 19

NASIO, J.: *A new test for gastric function,* Amer. J. dig. Dis., 11:227, 1944. — 27

NECHELES, H.: *The physiology of the stomach; in Portis, Diseases of the Digestive System,* page 110, Lea & Febiger, Philadelphia, 1944. — 9-12

NEGUS, V. E.: *The second stage of swallowing,* Acta oto-laryng., Suppl. 78, 1948. — 6, 7

——: *The Comparative Anatomy and Physiology of the Larynx,* Grune & Stratton, Inc., New York, 1949. — 6, 7

NIELSEN, N. A., AND CHRISTIANSEN: *Passage of food through human stomach,* Acta radiol., 13:678, 1932. — 9, 10

NORTHROP, J. H., AND HERRIOTT: *Chemistry of crystalline enzymes,* Ann. Rev. Biochem., 7:37, 1938. — 12

PALMER, E. D.: *Clinical Gastroenterology,* Paul B. Hoeber, Inc., New York, 1957. — 25-28

PALMER, W. L.: *The mechanism of pain in gastric and duodenal ulcer. II. The production of pain by means of chemical irritants,* Arch. intern. Med., 38:694, 1926. — 25

——: *The "acid test" in gastric and duodenal ulcer. Clinical value of experimental production of the typical distress,* J. Amer. med. Ass., 88:1778, 1927. — 25

PANICO, F. G.: *Improved abrasive balloon for diagnosis of cancer,* J. Amer. med. Ass., 149:1447, 1952. — 29

——, PAPANICOLAOU AND COOPER: *Abrasive balloon for examination of gastric cancer cells,* J. Amer. med. Ass., 143:1308, 1950. — 29

PAVLOV, I.: *The Work of the Digestive Glands,* Griffin, London, 1910. — 11

RAFSKY, H. A., LOEWENBERG AND PETERSON: *Evaluation of the Einhorn string test,* Rev. Gastroenterology, 19:390, 1952. — 26

RAKE, G. W.: *On the pathology of achalasia of the cardia,* Guy's Hosp. Rep., 77:141, 1927. — 25

RAMSAY, G. H., WATSON, GRAMIAK AND WEINBERG: *Unifluorographic analysis of the mechanism of swallowing,* Radiology, 64:498, 1955. — 6, 7

RIDER, J. A., VON DER REIS AND LEE: *Special gastroenterological diagnostic procedures,* Amer. J. Gastroent., 25:137, 1956. — 23-28

RIOCH, J. M.: *Neural mechanism of mastication,* Amer. J. Physiol., 108:168, 1934. — 4, 5

ROSENTHAL, H. L., AND BUSCAGLIA: *Tubeless gastric analysis,* J. Amer. med. His., 168:409, 1958. — 28

ROSENTHAL, M., AND TRAUT: *The mucolytic action of papain for cell concentration in the diagnosis of cancer,* Cancer, 1:147, 1951. — 29

ROSS, J. R., MCGRATH, CROZIER, ROHART AND MIDDLETON: *Exfoliative cytology: its practical application in the diagnosis of gastric neoplasms,* Gastroenterology, 34:24, 1958. — 29

ROTH, J. A., AND IVY: *The effect of caffeine upon gastric secretion in the dog, cat and man,* Amer. J. Physiol., 141:454, 1944. — 19

——, —— AND ATKINSON: *Caffeine and peptic ulcer,* J. Amer. med. Ass., 126:814, 1944. — 19

RUBIN, C. E., MASSEY, KIRSNER, PALMER AND STONECYPHER: *The clinical value of*

Section IV (continued)

PLATE NUMBER

gastrointestinal cytologic diagnosis, Gastroenterology, 25:119, 1953. — 29

SANCHEZ, G. C., KRAMER AND INGELFINGER: *Motor mechanism of the esophagus, particularly of its distal portion,* Gastroenterology, 25:321, 1953. — 7

SEGAL, H. L., AND MILLER: *Present status and possibilities of ion-exchange compounds as tubeless agents for determining gastric acidity,* Gastroenterology, 29:633, 1955. — 19

SEYBOLT, J. F., PAPANICOLAOU AND COOPER: *Cytology in the diagnosis of gastric cancer,* Cancer, 4:286, 1951. — 29

SLEISENGER, M. H., LEWIS, LIPKIN AND WIERUM: *Uropepsin and 17-hydroxycorticoid excretion in normal subjects and patients with peptic ulcer during both states of activity and quiescence,* Amer. J. Med., 25:395, 1958. — 29

——, STEINBERG AND ALMY: *The disturbance of esophageal motility in cardiospasm: studies on autonomic stimulation and autonomic blockade of the human esophagus, including the cardia,* Gastroenterology, 25:333, 1953. — 25

TEMPLETON, F. E.: *X-ray Examination of the Stomach,* University of Chicago Press, Chicago, 1944. — 9

THOMAS, J. E.: *A further study of the nervous control of the pyloric sphincter,* Amer. J. Physiol., 88:498, 1929. — 10

——: *The mechanism of gastric evacuation,* J. Amer. med. Ass., 97:1663, 1931. — 10

——: *Mechanics and regulation of gastric emptying,* Physiol. Rev., 37:453, 1957. — 9, 10

—— AND KUNZ: *A study of gastro-intestinal motility in relation to the enteric nervous system,* Amer. J. Physiol., 76:606, 1926. — 9, 10

——, CRIDER AND MORGAN: *Study on reflexes involving the pyloric sphincter and antrum and rôle of gastric evacuation,* Amer. J. Physiol., 108:683, 1934. — 10

TUTTLE, S. G., AND GROSSMAN: *Detection of gastro-esophageal reflux by simultaneous measurement of intraluminal pressure and pH,* Proc. Soc. exp. Biol., 98:225, 1958. — 26

TYLER, D. B., AND BARD: *Motion sickness,* Physiol. Rev., 29:311, 1949. — 18

ULFELDER, H., GRAHAM AND MEIGS: *Further studies on the cytologic method in the problem of gastric cancer,* Ann. Surg., 128:422, 1948. — 29

UMIKER, W. O., BOLT, HOERZEMA AND POLLARD: *Cytology in the diagnosis of gastric cancer: the significance of location and pathologic type,* Gastroenterology, 34:859, 1958. — 29

WALKER, A. E., AND GREEN: *Electric excitability of motor face area; comparative study in primates,* J. Neurophysiol., 1:152, 1938. — 13

WANG, S. C.: *Localization of salivatory center in medulla of cat,* J. Neurophysiol., 6:195, 1943. — 3

—— AND BORISON: *Vomiting center; critical experimental analysis,* Arch. Neurol. Psychiat., 63:928, 1950. — 18

WEISMAN, A. D., AND COBB: *Neurological aspects of gastrointestinal disease; in Portis, Diseases of the Digestive System,* p. 209, Lea & Febiger, Philadelphia, 1953. — 11, 13

Section IV (continued)

PLATE NUMBER

WHEELON, H., AND THOMAS: *Rhythmicity of the pyloric sphincter,* Amer. J. Physiol., 54:460, 1921. — 10

WILLNER, V., BANDES AND HOLLANDER: *The normal anatomy and physiology of the esophagus,* J. Mt. Sinai Hosp., 23:3, 1956. — 8

WILSON, M. J., DICKSON AND SINGLETON: *Rate of evacuation of various foods from normal stomach (preliminary communication),* Arch. intern. Med., 44:787, 1929. — 10

WOLF, B. S.: *The roentgen diagnosis of minimal hiatal herniation, motor phenomena in the terminal esophageal segment ("vestibule"),* J. Mt. Sinai Hosp., 23:90, 1956. — 7

WOLF, S., AND WOLFF: *Human Gastric Function,* Oxford University Press, New York, 1943. — 14

ZOLLINGER, R. M., AND ELLISON: *Primary peptic ulcerations of jejunum associated with islet cell tumors of pancreas,* Ann. Surg., 142:709, 1955. — 16

Section V

BESAUCON, L. J.: *Les Avitaminoses,* Flammarion, Paris, 1948. — 16

BEUBE, E.: *Periodontology,* Macmillan Company, New York, 1953. — 3-5

BLACK, G. V., AND MCKAY: *Mottled teeth; an endemic developmental imperfection of the enamel of the teeth heretofore unknown in the literature of dentistry,* Dent. Cosmos, 58:129, 1916. — 4

BURKET, L.: *Oral Medicine,* J. B. Lippincott Company, Philadelphia, 1946. — 1-12, 19-26

CAHN, L.: *Pathology of the Oral Cavity,* Williams & Wilkins Company, Baltimore, 1941. — 1-12, 19-26

CHURCHILL, H.: *Occurrence of fluorides in some waters of United States,* J. Ind. Eng. Chem., 23:996, 1931. — 4

FRAZELL, E. L.: *Clinical aspects of tumors of the major salivary glands,* Cancer, 6:637, 1954. — 22

GOLDMAN, H.: *Periodontia,* C. V. Mosby Company, St. Louis, 1949. — 5

GOODMAN, L., AND GILMAN: *The Pharmacological Basis of Therapeutics,* Macmillan Company, New York (Chapter 44, page 1002), 1955. — 13

HARRIS, S.: *Clinical Pellagra,* C. V. Mosby Company, St. Louis, 1941. — 16

LEDLIE, E. M., AND HARMER: *Cancer of the Mouth. A report on 800 cases,* Brit. J. Cancer, 4:6, 1950. — 23-26

MARTIN, H.: *Cancer of the Head and Neck,* Am. Cancer Soc., Inc., New York, 1953. — 23, 24, 26

MCKAY, F. S.: *Mottled enamel; the prevention of its further production through a change of water supply at Oakley, Idaho,* J. Amer. dent. Ass., 20:1137, 1920. — 4

——: *The present status of the investigation of the cause and of the geographical distribution of mottled enamel, including a complete bibliography on mottled enamel,* J. dent. Res., 10:561, 1930. — 4

MORGAN, W. S.: *The probable systemic nature of Mikulicz's disease and its relation to Sjögren's syndrome,* New Engl. J. Med., 251:5, 1954. — 12

Section V (continued)

	PLATE NUMBER
Orban, B.: *Oral Histology and Embryology*, C. V. Mosby Company, St. Louis, 1944.	I
Padgett, E. C.: *Surgical Diseases of the Mouth and Jaws*, W. B. Saunders Company, Philadelphia, 1938.	19-22, 24-26
Pancoast, H. K., Pendergrass and Schaeffer: *The Head and Neck in Roentgen Diagnosis*, Charles C Thomas, Publisher, Springfield, Ill., 1940.	24-26
Prinz, H., and Greenbaum: *Diseases of the Mouth and Their Treatment*, Lea & Febiger, Philadelphia, 1939.	1-26
Sarnat, B. G., Editor: *The Temporomandibular Joint*, Charles C Thomas, Publisher, Springfield, Ill., 1951.	2
Shapiro, H. H., and Truex: *The temporomandibular joint and the auditory function*, J. Amer. dent. Ass., 30:1147, 1943.	2
Sieben, H.: *Temporomandibular articulation in mandibular overclosure*, J. Amer. dent. Ass., 36:13, 1948.	2
Szanto, L., Farkas and Gynlai: *On Sjögren's disease*, Rheumatism, 13:60, 1957.	12
Thoma, K. H.: *Oral Pathology*, C. V. Mosby Company, St. Louis, 4th Ed., 1954.	1-26
——, Howe and Wenig: *Tumors of the mouth and jaws. Multiple pregnancy tumors*, Am. J. Orthodont. (Oral Surg. Sec.), 31:260, 1945.	21, 22
Wardand, H.: *Tumors of the Head and Neck*, Williams & Wilkins Company, Baltimore, 1950.	21-26
Wynder, E. L., Bross and Feldman: *A study of the etiological factors in cancer of the mouth*, Cancer, 10:1300, 1957.	23
Ziskin, D. E.: *Pregnancy Gingivitis*, Am. J. Orthodont. (Oral Surg. Sec.), 32:390, 1946.	8

Section VI

	PLATE NUMBER
Adams, A. D.: *Diverticula of the thoracic esophagus*, J. thorac. Surg., 17:639, 1948.	6
Adlersberg, D., and Som: *Esophagitis and esophageal ulcer*, Med. Clin. N. Amer., 40:317, 1956.	9-11
Allison, P. R., Johnstone and Royce: *Short esophagus with simple peptic ulceration*, J. thorac. Surg., 12:432, 1943.	2, 10
—— and ——: *Esophagus lined with gastric mucous membrane*, Thorax, 8:87, 1953.	2, 10
Barrett, N. R.: *Chronic peptic ulcer of oesophagus and oesophagitis*, Brit. J. Surg., 38:175, 1950.	2, 10
Benedict, E. B.: *Endoscopy*, Williams & Wilkins Company, Baltimore, 1951.	4, 6, 9-11, 13, 15, 17-19
Bigger, I. A.: *Treatment of congenital atresia of esophagus with tracheo-esophageal fistula*, Ann. Surg., 129:572, 1949.	I
Blakemore, A. H.: *Portacaval shunting for portal hypertension*, Surg. Gyn. Obst., 94:443, 1952.	15
Einhorn, N.: *A case of dysphagia with dilatation of the esophagus*, Med. Rec., 34:751, 1888.	8
Ellis, F. H., Olsen, Holman and Code: *Surgical treatment of cardiospasm (achalasia of the esophagus); considerations of aspects of esophagomyotomy*, J. Amer. med. Ass., 166:29, 1958.	8

Section VI (continued)

	PLATE NUMBER
Fincher, F. F., and Swanson: *Esophageal rupture complicating craniotomy*, Ann. Surg., 129:619, 1949.	14
Findlay, L., and Kelly: *Congenital shortening of oesophagus and thoracic stomach resulting therefrom*, J. Laryng. & Otol., 46:797, 1931.	2
Fleischner, F. G.: *Hiatal hernia complex; hiatal hernia peptic esophagitis, Mallory-Weiss syndrome, hemorrhage and anemia and marginal esophagogastric ulcer*, J. Amer. med. Ass., 162:183, 1956.	2, 10
Harvington, S. W.: *Pulsion diverticulum of hypopharynx at the pharyngo-esophageal junction. Surgical treatment in 140 cases*, Surgery, 18:66, 1945.	6
Holinger, P. H., and Johnston: *Benign strictures of the esophagus*, Surg. Clin. N. Amer., 31:135, 1951.	16
Hurst, A. F.: *Treatment of achalasia of the cardia*, Lancet, 1:618, 1927.	8
——: *Some disorders of the esophagus*, J. Amer. med. Ass., 102:582, 1934.	8
—— and Rake: *Achalasia of the cardia*, Quart. J. Med., 23:491, 1930.	8
Ingelfinger, F. J., and Kramer: *Dysphagia produced by contractile ring in lower esophagus*, Gastroenterology, 23:419, 1953.	7
Kirschner, P.: *Benign tumors of the esophagus*, J. Mt. Sinai Hosp., 23:14, 1956.	16
Kramer, P., and Ingelfinger: *Motility of the human esophagus in control subjects and in patients with esophageal disorders*, Amer. J. Med., 7:168, 1949.	8
—— and ——: *Cardiospasm, a generalized disorder of esophageal motility*, Amer. J. Med., 7:174, 1949.	8
Lahey, F. H.: *Pharyngo-esophageal diverticulum: Its management and complications*, Ann. Surg., 124:617, 1946.	6
Leven, N. L.: *Surgical management of congenital atresia of esophagus with tracheo-esophageal fistula; report of 2 cases*, J. thorac. Surg., 6:30, 1936.	I
Lindskog, G. E., and Kline: *The problem of hiatus hernia complicated by peptic esophagitis*, New Engl. J. Med., 257:110, 1957.	9
MacMahon, H. E., Schatzki and Gary: *Pathology of a lower esophageal ring. Report of a case with autopsy observed for nine years*, New Engl. J. Med., 259:1, 1958.	7
Marshak, R. H.: *The Roentgen findings of benign and malignant tumors of the esophagus*, J. Mt. Sinai Hosp., 23:75, 1956.	16-19
Ochsner, A., and De Bakey: *Surgical aspects of carcinoma of the esophagus; review of the literature and report of four cases*, J. thorac. Surg., 10:401, 1941.	17-19
Palmer, E. D.: *The Esophagus and Its Diseases*, Paul B. Hoeber, Inc., New York, 1952.	1-19
Peters, P. M.: *Pathology of severe digestion oesophagitis*, Thorax, 10:269, 1955.	9, 13
Plass, E. D.: *Congenital atresia of the esophagus with tracheo-esophageal fistula, associated with fused kidney. A case report and a survey of the literature on congenital anomalies of the esophagus*, Johns Hopk. Hosp. Rep., 18:259, 1919.	I

Section VI (continued)

	PLATE NUMBER
Potts, W. J.: *Congenital deformities of the esophagus*, Surg. Clin. N. Amer., 31:100, 1951.	I
Rake, G. W.: *On the pathology of achalasia of the cardia*, Guy's Hosp. Rep., 77:141, 1927.	8
Richman, A.: *Achalasia of the esophagus*, J. Mt. Sinai Hosp., 23:34, 1956.	8
Schatzki, R., and Gary: *Dysphagia due to diaphragm-like, localized narrowing in the lower esophagus (lower esophageal ring)*, Amer. J. Roentgenol., 70:911, 1953.	7
—— and Gary: *The lower esophageal ring*, Amer. J. Roentgenol., 75:246, 1956.	7
Sifers, E. C., and Crile: *Cardiospasm. A review of 100 cases*, Gastroenterology, 16:466, 1950.	8
Som, M. L.: *Endoscopy in diagnosis and treatment of diseases of the esophagus*, J. Mt. Sinai Hosp., 23:56, 1956.	8, 13, 15, 16
——: *Laryngo-esophagectomy; primary closure by laryngotracheal autograft*, Arch. Otolaryng., 63:474, 1956.	17
—— and Arnold: *Esophagoscopy in the diagnosis and treatment of esophageal diseases*, Amer. J. Surg., 93:183, 1957.	6, 15
—— and Wolf: *Peptic ulcer of the esophagus and esophagitis in gastric-lined esophagus*, J. Amer. med. Ass., 162:641, 1956.	11
Sweet, R. H.: *Esophageal hiatus hernia of the diaphragm. The anatomical characteristics, technic of repair and results of treatment in 111 consecutive cases*, Ann. Surg., 135:1, 1952.	8
——: *Surgical treatment of achalasia of the esophagus*, New Engl. J. Med., 254:87, 1956.	8
Templeton, F. E.: *Movements of the esophagus in the presence of cardiospasm and other esophageal diseases; a roentgenologic study of muscular action*, Gastroenterology, 10:96, 1948.	8
Terracol, J., and Sweet: *Diseases of the Esophagus*, W. B. Saunders Company, Philadelphia, 1958.	1-19
Vogt, E. C.: *Congenital esophageal atresia*, Amer. J. Roentgenol., 22:463, 1929.	I
Winkelstein, A., Wolf, Som and Marshak: *Peptic esophagitis with duodenal or gastric ulcer*, J. Amer. med. Ass., 154:885, 1954.	9-11
——: *Peptic esophagitis and peptic ulcer of the esophagus*, J. Mt. Sinai Hosp., 23:18, 1956.	9-11
Wolf, B. S., Som and Marshak: *Short esophagus with esophagogastric or marginal ulceration*, Radiology, 61:473, 1953.	2

Section VII

	PLATE NUMBER
Akerlund, A.: *Roentgenologische Studien über den Bulbus Duodeni, mit besonderer Berücksichtigung der Diagnostik des Ulcus duodeni*, Acta radiol. Supp., 1921.	13, 14
Allison, P. R.: *Reflux esophagitis, sliding hiatal hernia and the anatomy of repair*, Surg. Gynec. Obstet., 92:419, 1951.	I
Andresen, A. R. R.: *Office Gastroenterology*, W. B. Saunders Company, Philadelphia, 1958.	7-9, 19, 23-28

BEAUMONT, W.: *Experiments and Observations on the Gastric Juice and Physiology of Digestion*, F. P. Allen, Plattsburg, N.Y., 1833.   7

BOCKUS, H. L.: *Gastroenterology*, W. B. Saunders Company, Philadelphia, 1944.   4, 7-11, 15-19, 23-28

BOLLER, R.: *Der Magen und seine Krankheiten*, Urban und Schwarzenberg, Wien, 1954.   7-10, 16-19, 20, 21, 23-28

BORRMANN, R.: *In Henke-Lubarsch: Handbuch der Speziellen Pathologischen Anatomie und Histologie*, Vol. 4, pt. 1, p. 865, J. Springer, Berlin, 1926.   7-11, 19, 23-28

BOYD, W.: *A Textbook of Pathology*, Lea & Febiger, Philadelphia, 1949.   2, 3-10, 20-28

BRENNER, R. L., AND BROWN: *Primary carcinoma of the duodenum; report of 15 cases*, Gastroenterology, 29:189, 1955.   22

BUCKSTEIN, J.: *Clinical Roentgenology of the Alimentary Tract*, W. B. Saunders Company, Philadelphia, 1940.   13, 14, 22, 25-28

CARBONE, J. V., AND LIEBOWITZ: *The effect of adrenal corticoids on gastric secretion and the suppression of corticoid-induced hypersecretion by anticholinergics*, Metabolism, 7:70, 1958.   8

CORNER, B. D.: *Hypertrophic pyloric stenosis in infancy treated with methylscopolamine nitrate*, Arch. Dis. Childh., 30:377, 1955.   3

DONOVAN, E. J.: *Congenital hypertrophic pyloric stenosis*, Ann. Surg., 124:708, 1946.   3

DRAGSTEDT, L. R., RAGINS, DRAGSTEDT AND EVANS: *Stress and duodenal ulcer*, Ann. Surg., 144:450, 1956.   10

EUSTERMAN, G. B.: *Benign Tumors; in Portis, Diseases of the Digestive System*, p. 277, Lea & Febiger, Philadelphia, 1944.   20, 21

FABER, K.: *Gastritis and Its Consequences*, Oxford University Press, London, 1935.   7, 15-19

GUTMANN, R. A.: *Les Syndromes Douloureux de la Région Epigastrique*, C. Doin et Cie, Paris, 1952.   12

HARRINGTON, S. W.: *Diaphragmatic Hernia; in Monographs on Surgery, 1951*, Thomas Nelson & Sons, New York, 1950.   1

——: *Various types of diaphragmatic hernia treated surgically*, Surg. Gynec. Obstet., 86:735, 1948.   1

HASTINGS, N., HALSTED, WOODWARD, GASSTER AND HISCOCK: *Subtotal gastric resection for benign ulcer; a follow-up study of three hundred fifty-three patients*, Arch. Surg., 76:74, 1958.   16

HEFKE, H. W.: *Reliability of roentgen examination in hypertrophic stenosis in infants*, Radiology, 53:789, 1949.   3

HENDERSON, J. L., BROWN AND TAYLOR: *Clinical observations on pyloric stenosis in premature infants*, Arch. Dis. Childh., 27:173, 1952.   3

IVY, A. C., GROSSMAN AND BACHRACH: *Peptic Ulcer*, Blakiston Company, Philadelphia, 1950.   8-19

JENNINGS, D., AND RICHARDSON: *Giant lesser-curve gastric ulcers*, Lancet, 2:343, 1954.   12

JUDD, E. S., AND NAGEL: *Duodenitis*, Ann. Surg., 85:380, 1927.   13

KIRSNER, J. B.: *Current status of therapy in peptic ulcer*, J. Amer. med. Ass., 166:1727, 1958.   8-10

——: *(On frequency of ulcers in corticoid-treated patients)* quoted in Allen, Harkins, Moyer and Rhoads: *Surgery, Principles and Practice*, p. 602, J. B. Lippincott Company, Philadelphia, 1957.   8

—— AND PALMER: *The problem of peptic ulcer*, Amer. J. Med., 13:615, 1952.   8-10

KOLLER, P. C.: *The Genetic Component of Cancer; in R. W. Raven: Cancer*, Butterworth & Co., Ltd., London, 1957.   23

KORYETZNY, G. E.: *Der Magenkrebs*, F. Enke, Stuttgart, 1931.   23-30

LAHEY, F. H.: *Experiences with Gastrectomy, Total and Subtotal, in Surgical Practice of the Lahey Clinic*, W. B. Saunders Company, Philadelphia, 1949.   29-30

MacCALLUM, W. S.: *Textbook of Pathology*, W. B. Saunders Company, Philadelphia, 1942.   8-10

MARSHAK, R. H., YARNIS AND FRIEDMAN: *Giant benign gastric ulcer*, Gastroenterology, 24:339, 1953.   12

MAYO, H. W., JR.: *The Physiological Basis of Operations for Duodenal, Gastric and Gastrojejunal Ulcer*, C. V. Mosby Company, St. Louis, 1941.   29, 30

MEISSNER, W. A.: *Leiomyoma of the stomach*, Arch. Path., 38:207, 1944.   20, 21

MOYNIHAN, B. G. A.: *Addresses on Surgical Subjects*, W. B. Saunders Company, Philadelphia, 1928.   16

——: *On the recognition of some acute abdominal diseases*, Practitioner, 126:5, 1931.   16-18

——: *Duodenal Ulcer*, W. B. Saunders Company, Philadelphia, 1912.   13-18

MYERS, H. C.: *Early diagnosis of carcinoma of the stomach*, J. Amer. med. Ass., 163:159, 1957.   23

NISSEN, R.: *Magen und Duodenum; in Hellinger, Nissen und Vossschulte, Lehrbuch du Chirurgie*, p. 587, Georg Thieme Verlag, Stuttgart, 1958.   1, 2, 7-32

OCHSNER, S., AND KLECKNER: *Primary malignant neoplasms of the duodenum. Discussion based on seventeen cases, with emphasis on radiologic diagnosis*, J. Amer. med. Ass., 163:413, 1957.   22

PALMER, E. D.: *Gastritis; a revaluation*, Medicine, 33:199, 1954.   7

PALMER, W. L.: *Peptic Ulcer; in Portis, Diseases of the Digestive System*, p. 184,

Lea & Febiger, Philadelphia, 1944.   8-11, 14-18

PERMAN, E.: *The so-called dumping syndrome after gastrectomy*, Act. Med. Scand., "Hilding Berglund" Suppl. (No. 196) 361, to Vol. 28, 1947.   31

PORTIS, S. A., AND JAFFE: *A study of peptic ulcer based on necropsy records*, J. Amer. med. Ass., 110:6, 1938.   11

RANSOM, H. K., AND KAY: *Abdominal neoplasms of neurogenic origin*, Ann. Surg., 112:700, 1940.   21

RICHARDSON, J. E.: *Papilloedema with recovery following severe gastro-intestinal bleeding*, Brit. J. Surg., 42:108, 1954.   12

RIVERS, A. B., STEVENS AND KIRKLIN: *Diverticula of the stomach*, Surg. Gynec. Obstet., 60:106, 1935.   4

ROMINGER, E.: *Ueber Wandlungen im Erscheinungsbild typischer Sanglingskrankheiten unter einer zeitgemässen Behandlung*, Ann. Paediat. Fenn., 3:645, 1957.   3

ROTH, L. A., BECKER, VINE AND BOCKUS: *Results of subtotal gastric resection (Billroth 2 type) for duodenal ulcer; influence of preoperative acidity on postoperative acidity and relation to extent of resection and relation to postoperative sequelae to extent of resection*, J. Amer. med. Ass., 161:794, 1956.   30

SANDWEISS, D. J.: *Effects of adrenocorticotropic hormone (ACTH) and of cortisone on peptic ulcer. Clinical review*, Gastroenterology, 27:604, 1954.   10

SCHINDLER, R.: *Gastritis*, Grune & Stratton, Inc., New York, 1947.   7

SCHROEDER, F.: *Beitrag zur Klinik des Magenmyoms*, Arch. klin. Chir., 184:738, 1936.   20, 21

SMITH, G. K., AND FARRIS: *Rationale of vagotomy and pyloroplasty in management of bleeding duodenal ulcer*, J. Amer. med. Ass., 166:878, 1958.   29, 30

SMITH, L. A., AND RIVERS: *Peptic Ulcer, Pain Patterns, Diagnosis and Medical Treatment*, Appleton-Century-Crofts, Inc., New York, 1953.   8-11, 15-19

STEWART, M. J.: *General relation of carcinoma to ulcer*, Brit. Med. J., 2:882, 1925.   23

WALLENSTEIN, S., AND GÖTHMAN: *An evaluation of the Billroth I operation for peptic ulcer*, Surgery, 33:1, 1953.   31

WALLGREN, A.: *Preclinical stage of infantile hypertrophic pyloric stenosis*, Amer. J. Dis. Child., 72:371, 1946.   3

WANGENSTEEN, O. H., AND LANNIN: *Criteria of an acceptable operation for ulcer. The importance of the acid factor*, Arch. Surg., 44:489, 1948.   29, 30

WINTERS, W. L., AND EGAN: *Incidence of hemorrhage occurring with perforation in peptic ulcer*, J. Amer. med. Ass., 113:2199, 1939.   16, 18

mouth — *continued*
  roof, 3, 7
  skin disease, 121
  syphilis, 106, 113, 114, 120, 121, 126, 127
  tobacco misuse, 70, 111, 126, 127
  tumor, benign, 95, 122, 124, 125
    malignant, 95, 126, 127, 128, 129
  ulcer, 111, 114, 116, 118, 120
  venous drainage, 26
  vestibule, 3, 6, 109
mucocele, 123
mucoperiosteum, 7, 13
mucosa
  buccal, 3, 6, 15, 107, 114, 117, 126
    tumor and ulcer, 124, 131
  duodenal, 55
  esophageal, 38, 39, 40, 139
  gastric, diseased, *see* **gastritis**; **stomach, ulcer**
    heterotopic, 38, 39, 139, 147, 148, 158
    normal, 40, 52, 161
  jejunal, 188
  labial, 3, 16, 17, 107, 114, 117
  lingual, 10, 11
  oral, *see* **gingiva; mucosa**, buccal, etc.
  palatine, 7, 114
  pharyngeal, 17
mucus, gastric, 52, 84
mumps, 115
muscle
  abdominal, 90, 91, 94
  accessory (from temporal bone), 23
  arytenoid, oblique, 37
    transverse, 18, 23, 37
  buccinator, 3, 7, 8, 9, 14, 15, 17, 21, 22, 24, 29, 72, 109
  caninus, 8
  capitis longus, 15, 18
  chondroglossus, 11
  constrictor of pharynx, inferior, 20, 21, 22, 23, 35, 36, 37, 143
    middle, 21, 22, 23, 26, 37, 78
    superior, 7, 9, 11, 15, 16, 21, 22, 23, 24, 25, 26, 37, 74, 75, 78, 132
  crico-arytenoid (posterior), 23, 37
  cricopharyngeus, 21, 22, 23, 34, 35, 36, 37, 74, 75, 76, 90, 91, 96, 132, 143
  cricothyroid, 22
  depressor labii, 8
  diaphragmatic, *see* **diaphragm**
  digastric, 4, 6, 9, 11, 14, 15, 20, 22, 23, 24, 25, 26, 27, 28, 29, 30, 72, 78, 109
  esophageal, circular, 21, 23, 36, 37, 38, 40, 45
    longitudinal, 18, 21, 23, 36, 37, 38, 40, 45
  facial expression (for), 15, 109
  gastric, 38
  genioglossus, 4, 6, 11, 15, 18, 30, 74
  geniohyoid, 4, 6, 9, 11, 18, 21, 30, 72, 78, 109, 123
  glossopharyngeus, 11, 21, 22
  hyoglossus, 6, 11, 15, 16, 21, 22, 24, 26, 29, 30, 109
  incisivus labii, 8
  infrahyoid, 9, 72, 78
  intercostal, 78, 90, 91, 94

muscle — *continued*
  levator anguli oris and labis, 8
  levator veli palatini, 7, 16, 19, 21, 22, 23, 78
  lingual, intrinsic, longitudinal, transverse and vertical, 10, 11, 15, 72, 74, 78
  longitudinal pharyngeus, 21, 23
  longus colli, 18, 34, 35
  (of) Low, 39
  masticatory, 8, 9, 14, 15, 25, 26, 29, 72, 73, 109
  mentalis, 8
  mylohyoid, 4, 6, 11, 14, 15, 18, 21, 22, 24, 30, 72, 78, 109, 123
  omohyoid, 6, 24, 27
  orbicularis oris, 3, 8, 9, 15, 17, 18, 24, 72
  palatoglossus, 7, 11, 15, 16
  palatopharyngeus, 7, 10, 11, 15, 16, 21, 22, 23, 37, 74
  platysma, 9, 15, 109
  psoas major, 50
  pterygoid, external, 5, 8, 9, 24, 25, 26, 72, 105
    internal, 7, 8, 9, 14, 15, 23, 25, 29, 72, 109
  quadratus labii (inferior and superior), 8
  salpingopharyngeus, 16, 19, 21, 23
  scalenus (anterior and medius), 24, 26, 34
  sternocleidomastoideus, 14, 15, 24, 26, 27, 28, 143
  sternohyoid, 6, 24
  styloglossus, 11, 15, 21, 22, 24, 30, 109
  stylohyoid, 6, 11, 14, 15, 22, 23, 24, 25, 26, 29
  stylopharyngeus, 11, 15, 16, 20, 21, 22, 23, 24, 30, 37, 75, 78, 109
  suprahyoid, 9
  suspensory duodeni, *see* **ligament**, Treitz's
  temporal, 8, 9, 72
  tensor veli palatini, 7, 16, 17, 20, 21, 22, 29, 30, 78
  thyrohyoid, 6, 22, 29
  tongue, *see* **m.**, lingual
  triangular, 8
  uvular, 7, 23
  zygomatic (major and minor), 8
myasthenia gravis, 73
myeloma, 129
myoblastoma, 133, 134
myxedema, *see* **hypothyroidism**
myxoma, 125

N

nails, brittle, 142
nares, posterior, *see* **choanae**
nasal cavity (relation to mouth), 7, 18, 109
nasopharynx, *see* **pharynx**, naso-
nausea, *see* **vomiting**
nerve (*see also* **plexus**, nervous)
  accessory, 7, 11, 27; 29, 30
  acoustic, 90, 91, 114
  alveolar, inferior, 4, 5, 6, 9, 15, 25, 29, 30, 72
    superior, 29, 30
  auriculotemporal, 5, 9, 14, 25, 29, 31

nerve — *continued*
  autonomic, *see* **sympathetic** *and* **parasympathetic innervation**
  buccinator, 25, 29, 30
  carotid, internal, 31
  cervical, 6, 29, 30
  chorda tympani, 11, 29, 31, 69, 71, 90
  cranial, I, *see* **n.**, olfactory
    II, *see* **n.**, optic
    V, *see* **n.**, trigeminal
    VII, *see* **n.**, facial
    VIII, *see* **n.**, acoustic
    IX, *see* **n.**, glossopharyngeal
    X, *see* **n.**, vagal
    XI, *see* **n.**, accessory
    XII, *see* **n.**, hypoglossal
  dorsal root, 31, 64
  facial, anatomic relation, 15, 25, 29
    compression, 128
    course, 29, 31
    inflammation, 115
    masticatory muscle branches, 6, 9
    oral cavity innervation, 30, 69, 71, 90
    paralysis, central, 73
    salivary gland branches, 14, 71, 90
    temporal branches, 14
  gastric, anterior and posterior, greater, 44, 64, 65
  glossopharyngeus, anatomic relation and course, 11, 15, 16, 21, 23, 29, 30, 31
    function and mouth innervation, 29, 30, 69, 71, 78, 90, 91, 132
  hypoglossal, 6, 11, 15, 24, 26, 29, 30, 72, 78, 95, 132
  infra-orbital, 29
  intercarotid, 29
  intercostal, 44
  intermedius, 30, 31
  laryngeal, recurrent, 22, 29, 30, 34, 37, 43, 44, 78, 132, 154
    superior, 19, 22, 23, 29, 30, 37, 44, 78
  lingual, 3, 5, 6, 9, 11, 14, 15, 25, 29, 30, 31, 72, 78
  mandibular, 5, 8, 29, 30, 31
  masseteric, 8, 25, 29
  maxillary, 29, 30, 31
  mental, 29
  mylohyoid, 5, 6, 9, 15, 25, 29, 78
  nasal, superior, posterior, 31
  olfactory, 69, 71, 73
  ophthalmic, 29, 31
  optic, 69, 71
  palatine, descending, 31
    greater, 7, 29, 30, 31
    lesser, 7, 16, 29, 30, 31
  petrosal, deep and superficial, 30, 31
  pharyngeal, 30, 31
  phrenic, 29, 34, 39, 65, 90
  pterygoid, external, 8, 29
    internal, 9, 29
  pterygopalatine, 30
  ramus, communicans, 31, 44, 45, 64
  root, *see* **n.**, dorsal root and ventral root
  splanchnic (thoracic), 44, 45, 64, 65, 78, 85, 90, 91

nerve — *continued*
  sympathetic, *see also* **trunk**, sympathetic *and* **sympathetic**, innervation
    pulmonic branches, 44
  temporal, 25, 29
  tonsillar, 16, 30
  trigeminal, course, 29, 31
    deglutition (function in), 78, 79
    divisions, 29, 30, 72
    inflammation, 115
    masticatory muscle branches, 5, 6, 8, 72, 78
    mouth innervation, 30, 69, 71, 72, 78
    nucleus, motoric, 72, 78, 79
      sensory, 71, 72, 78, 79
    root, 29, 72
    tensor veli palatini (for), 7
  tympanic, 30, 31
  vagal, anatomic relation, 15, 24, 29, 34
    cardia branch, 44, 65
    cardiac branch, 29
    celiac branch, 64, 65
    course, 30, 44, 64, 65
    deglutition (function in), 78, 79
    esophageal trunk, anterior and posterior, 44, 45, 65
    fundic branch, 44
    gastric branch, 64, 65
    gastric innervation, 46, 64, 65, 69, 73, 84, 85
    hepatic branch, 44, 64, 65
    palatine branch, 7
    paralysis, 132
    pharyngeal branch, 44, 78, 132
    prepyloric branch, 44
    pulmonic branch, 44
    pyloric branch, 64, 65
    reflex spasm, 143
    root, 31, 64
    section, *see* **vagotomy**
    vomiting (function in), 90, 91
  ventral root, 31
  Vidian, 31
  zygomatic, 29
neuritis, 115
neurofibroma, 133, 177, 178, 179
neurofibromatosis, *see* **Recklinghausen's disease**
neuroma, 134, 140
nicotinic acid, 119
nose, *see* **nasal; harelip**
nucleus
  ambiguus, 44, 79, 91
  glossopharyngeal nerve, 78
  hypoglossal nerve, 72, 79
  mesencephalic of trigeminal nerve, 72, 73
  salivatory, 31, 71, 91
  solitary tract, 69, 71, 72, 73, 79, 85, 91
  trigeminal nerve, motoric, 72, 78, 79
    sensory, 71, 72, 73, 79
  vagal, dorsal, 44, 65, 69, 71, 73, 78, 79, 85, 91
  vestibularis, 91
Nuhn, glands of, 11, 123
nutritional deficiency (*see also* **pellagra; rickets; scurvy**), 70, 104, 106, 107, 111, 112, 113, 118, 119, 126, 127, 145

INFORMATION ON NETTER COLLECTION VOLUMES

The Netter Collection of Medical Illustrations has enjoyed an enthusiastic reception from members of the medical community since the publication of its first volume. The remarkable illustrations by Frank H. Netter, M.D., and text by leading specialists make these books unprecedented in their educational, clinical, and scientific value.

Volume 1: I   **NERVOUS SYSTEM: Anatomy and Physiology**
"…this volume must remain a part of the library of all practitioners, scientists and educators dealing with the nervous system." *Journal of Neurosurgery*

Volume 1: II   **NERVOUS SYSTEM: Neurologic and Neuromuscular Disorders**
"…Part I is a 'work of art.' Part II is even more grand and more clinical!…This is a unique and wonderful text…rush to order this fine book." *Journal of Neurological and Orthopaedic Medicine and Surgery*

Volume 2   **REPRODUCTIVE SYSTEM**
"…a desirable addition to any nursing or medical library." *American Journal of Nursing*

Volume 3: I   **DIGESTIVE SYSTEM: Upper Digestive Tract**
"…a fine example of the high quality of this series." *Pediatrics*

Volume 3: II   **DIGESTIVE SYSTEM: Lower Digestive Tract**
"…a unique and beautiful work, worth much more than its cost." *Journal of the South Carolina Medical Association*

Volume 3: III   **DIGESTIVE SYSTEM: Liver, Biliary Tract and Pancreas**
"…a versatile, multipurpose aid to clinicians, teachers, researchers, and students…" *Florida Medical Journal*

Volume 4   **ENDOCRINE SYSTEM and Selected Metabolic Diseases**
"…another in the series of superb contributions made by CIBA…" *International Journal of Fertility*

Volume 5   **HEART**
"The excellence of the volume…is clearly deserving of highest praise." *Circulation*

Volume 6   **KIDNEYS, URETERS, AND URINARY BLADDER**
"…a model of clarity of language and visual presentation…" *Circulation*

Volume 7   **RESPIRATORY SYSTEM**
"…far more than an atlas on anatomy and physiology. Frank Netter uses his skills to present clear and often beautiful illustrations of all aspects of the system…" *British Medical Journal*

Volume 8: I   **MUSCULOSKELETAL SYSTEM: Anatomy, Physiology, and Metabolic Disorders**
"This is another outstanding volume…" *Journal of Bone and Joint Surgery*